QUADALAJARA

www.QuadMexico.com

Best Wishes 2008!

Jack Tumidajski

Quadalajara

The Utopia That Once Was

Jack Tumidajski

BRUNDAGE PUBLISHING

Quadalajara

The Utopia That Once Was

Jack Tumidajski

BRUNDAGE PUBLISHING
Room 203 Executive Office Building
33 West State Street
Binghamton, NY 13901
www.BrundagePublishing.com

Edited by Patricia Bourdon and Rachel A. Edwards
Jacket design by Angela Capria

Library of Congress
Control Number: 2005934079

ISBN Number: 1-892451-34-4

Printed in the United States of America

To the caregivers

Acknowledgments

To Mom and Pop for being the decent, honest, caring, self-sacrificing, and loving parents they were. Diane, Kathy, Debbie, and I were truly blessed. Thanks for being our Mom and Pop—may you rest in peace.

I wish I could personally thank those who left a record of Quadalajara, keeping this special period of history from being forever forgotten. Thanks to Raymond "Doc" Foland for maintaining copies of Mexico Chapter PVA documents, along with his personal records, and thanks to Bill Bailey for painting a history from memories of the early years through countless hours of casual conversation so many years gone by.

Thanks to Keith Zeigler for holding onto files and documents for so long and allowing me to interview and continually ask questions of him.

A special thanks to my comadre, Maria Elena Bailey, for telling her story as one of the first Mexican señoritas to meet and assist many of the early Gringo Explorers and Pioneers.

To Maria Foland for her enthusiastic support and sharing of her precious memories and pictures.

I am blessed to have the friendship and support of people such as JoAnn Kirch, Teresa Beilsmith, Sofia Lietz, Imelda Myrick, Josefina Ziegler, and my Godchild, Lucia Bailey. Their interviews and photos were valuable contributions.

Thanks to Charlie Newbold, Joe Cicero, Bill Kahler, Jerry Fesenmyer, Pete Mirche, Bob Flowers, Bill Christensen, and Gabriel Chavez for allowing me to interview them and for the information they provided.

To the little brother I never had, Charlie "CT" Tempinski, for encouraging me to look into a small publishing house in Binghamton, New York. Thanks to Frank, Rachel, Patricia, Barrie, Amanda, Angela and the folks at Brundage Publishing for their encouragement and tolerance of my never-ending search for information and photos.

I would like to express my gratitude to Mona Oge, Annelise Hopkins, and Charlottle Naufahu for their priceless motivation and feedback; to my caregivers, Jose Miguel Lopez and Azucena Gonzalez, for all of their help and support; and to Catalina Lopez for helping correct my Spanish.

Thanks to the folks at the Paralyzed Veterans of America's *Paraplegia News*, one for being located so close to home, and especially for allowing me access to their archives.

I would be remiss if I did not thank everyone else who I may have forgotten to mention.

Finally, I am most grateful to those who cleared this path in history, which enabled me and so many others to have a second chance at life, as well as the opportunity and adventure to travel through this special place and moment in time.

Every effort has been made to ensure that all information provided, including photos and captions, is as accurate as possible. Sources included old documents and articles, interviews with Quadalajara survivors and widows, and the author's own recollections from this life-changing journey through time.

It has been a challenging and rewarding experience to help preserve this special place in time and memorialize those who shared it and contributed so much in helping one another and others less fortunate.

I apologize for any errors and to anyone who might feel slighted by anything included or omitted within these pages.

Quadalajara: The Utopia That Once Was

Appendix

Part One

War and Relaxation

Chapter 1

The Tet Blowback: Vietnam

The flight from Seattle-Tacoma International Airport to South Vietnam was the most surreal event of my young life. Leaving behind a rainy Seattle, after a couple of days of record processing at Fort Lewis, Washington, I was on my way into a future filled with uncertainty, apprehension, and downright fear. I was part of another planeload of military cargo—U.S. replacement soldiers—winding its way to Southeast Asia.

I remember thinking the obvious, what every other young man and a few grizzled old vets were also contemplating. Will I someday be returning home on a flight filled with relieved and happy conquering heroes, or will I die in a foreign land that I had never heard of until a few years before?

Eighteen hours of flying time equaled eighteen hours of thinking time. I don't believe anyone could have slept on this flight into the unknown. I had lost my grandmother a few weeks before my enlistment date of October 31, 1967—Halloween. Now I was wearing my new costume to a special party that was being thrown for us in the name of fighting communism, compliments of good old LBJ.

I thought about my grandmother. I wondered how she felt and what she thought about when she made a trip into the unknown as a teenaged girl, leaving her family behind in Poland in hopes of a better life; a better life for herself and her future children and grandchildren. I wondered now how my decision to enlist in the Army during this time of war might have added to her stress. She was a strong woman who, along with my late grandfather, raised ten children; five of whom would see action in World War II defending her adopted homeland, the United States of America. Two of her sons would be seriously wounded, but her prayers would be answered as all five survived America's war with Hitler and his allies. Could the thought of a grandson possibly going off into harm's way be too much for her eighty-three-year-old heart?

I thought about Mom and how much she worried about everything all the time. Would I ever see her again? Would I see the rest of my family? I remembered when I was a small boy and I asked my father if he had ever killed anyone when he was in the war. He didn't answer; he never talked about it.

I thought about my sisters. My baby sister Debbie was only eleven years old. Debbie was very sickly as a child and we were all very protective of her. Would she ever see her big brother again? Then there were Kathy and Diane. Kathy was still in high school. Diane was married and had a son. My nephew David would soon be one year old; his birthday was only days away. Would he ever get to know me? Thoughts of what lay ahead and what was left behind danced in and out of my head like some form of mental torture.

My mind drifted to the night that I left my friends behind; the night that Mike, Charlie, Paul, and I boarded the bus that would take us to Boston. It was a macabre Halloween night; an endless night that singer Gladys Knight would later immortalize in our minds with her song *Midnight Train to Georgia.* It was another bizarre journey, by train, that would take us to Fort Gordon in Augusta, Georgia. (The last ninety miles were actually by bus from Fort Jackson, South Carolina to Fort Gordon after initial processing at Fort Jackson.)

I remembered the ride from Boston to Fort Gordon, the train stopping along the way to pick up other young men—boys, really. Nineteen-year-old draftees and enlisted "men" as young as seventeen and eighteen were all on their way to uncertainty on that "Midnight Train To Georgia." For someone who lived a sheltered life (the farthest I had been away from home was the forty-five miles from Pawtucket to Boston to see a Red Sox game), this Halloween night was truly eye-opening. I was amazed at how different each group of young men was as the train stopped in cities from New York to South Carolina. The most striking difference was between the various young men of African descent; from the "Soul Brothers" of inner city New York neighborhoods to the more timid and reserved descendants of slaves who grew up in rural areas of the South. Despite our differences, all of us were bound together by the same destination: uncertainty, hopes, and fears.

Arriving the next night, travel weary and frightened of the unknown, we were awakened after three hours of sleep by screaming drill sergeants barking at us to "Get up! Fall out!" It was five o'clock in the morning and we were already beginning our indoctrination. It was still dark outside and a steady November rain was welcoming us to military life in this strange baptismal ceremony. We were a new company of America's future defenders beginning to take shape.

After jogging in the early morning rain, we had our first official U.S. Army breakfast. Following breakfast we were issued our olive drab uniforms and had our heads shaven. I remembered coming out of the Army's discount hair stylist building into the sunshine only too happy to cover my now naked head with the newly issued military cap. The Army had succeeded in something—reducing all of us down to look-a-like, would-be soldiers. Our collective future was very much in doubt.

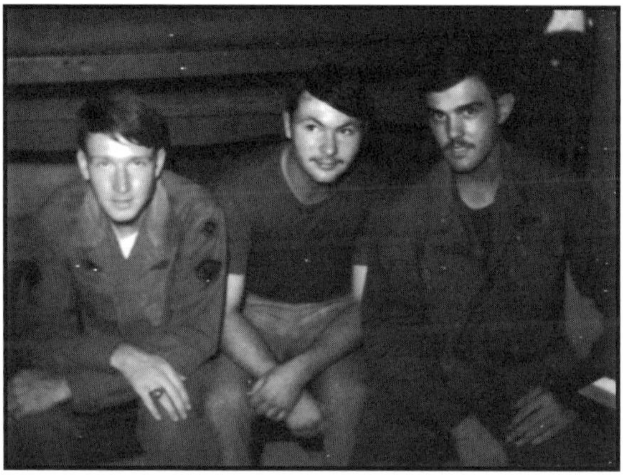

Jack (left) with two unidentified buddies
Qui Nhon, South Vietnam, 1968/1969

My daydream was interrupted by the captain's announcement that we would soon be arriving at Yokohama Air Force Base in Japan. After fourteen hours on the plane, it would be good to stretch and walk around a bit. As we debarked from the plane, I was surprised to find it snowing in Japan—in April. My education was continuing.

It was the middle of the night, or so it seemed, as we made our way to the Air Force eatery. I bumped into Ruffin, one of the rural black kids from down South who I had gone through basic training with. We had been in the same platoon, but we had never gotten much of an opportunity to get to know one another, and he only knew me by the drill sergeant's moniker that had been given to me on day one, "Alphabet Number Two." (If your last name was difficult to pronounce, as mine was, you could expect to be called just about anything. But my nickname was preferable to "Dickhead" or "Fat SOB," as others had been renamed.)

Ruffin and I had also run into one another upon arriving in

Seattle, but I had no idea he was on the same flight. It was somewhat reassuring to meet someone I knew. We went through the chow line together to receive our square hamburger patty on a bun, compliments of the U.S. Air Force.

After the Yokohama stop, I sat with Ruffin for the remaining four hours of the trip. Conversation became non-existent once we boarded. Thoughts of what lay ahead now dominated all others. The apprehension and fear again took grip.

As the plane finally touched down on the airfield at Cam Ranh Bay, the sense of an end to a journey came over me. As we climbed down the steps of the aircraft and walked up onto a waiting military bus—complete with rifle toting escorts—the sense of an even longer and more important journey took its place.

* * *

I had been stationed in and around Qui Nhon, South Vietnam since having arrived in April 1968 as a Tet replacement. The Tet Offensive was one of the major turning points in the Vietnam War and took everyone by surprise. The Viet Cong offensive touched areas of South Vietnam that had been hitherto considered "safe." Our unit had suffered a number of casualties, mostly on "the Hill," where our troops were responsible for guarding Qui Nhon's northern front from the invisible enemy. On January 31, 1968, all that changed as the Viet Cong, or VC (Victor Charlie in military jargon), captured parts of Qui Nhon, as well as many other cities and areas that had yet to experience the hell those out in the boonies lived with on a daily basis.

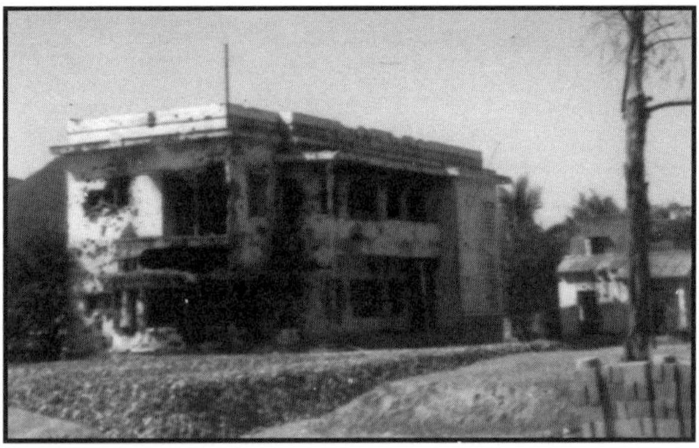

Aftermath of a January 31, 1968 Tet Offensive
Qui Nhon, South Vietnam, June 1968

It was now three and a half months after Tet and we were still re-fortifying our positions around the city of Qui Nhon, with its telltale signs of conflict and damage to the terrain, buildings, and state-of-mind. My first week in South Vietnam had been a marathon sandbag filling session. Considering the alternative, being stationed to some remote part of the country or one of the combat units, I could not and would not ever complain.

Eventually, I got out of sandbag duty and was assigned to the Director of Transportation (DOT), United States Army Support Command Qui Nhon, as a clerk. It appeared that eight weeks of basic training at Fort Gordon followed by eight weeks of clerical training at Fort Jackson had paid off after all. The personnel officer in Qui Nhon had been impressed by my still-thin military file and decided to keep me, along with a few other GIs, for duty with the 1st Logistical Command (1st Log). The other half-dozen guys would be sent farther into South Vietnam to the cities of AnKhe and Pleku. From what I was told by those who came before me, I had lucked out for duty assignment.

* * *

Although our first compound was located within the city itself, a secure location with air-conditioned buildings and high-ranking military officers everywhere, the reality of war soon became apparent. I developed a severe pain in my lower back. It was so excruciating that I was literally doubled over for the slightest relief. I was ordered to walk to the infirmary about a quarter mile away. Once there and doing my best to stand in line, I gradually inched forward closer to the desk clerk.

When I finally reached the desk, I began, “I have this tremendous pain.” Before I could finish my sentence, the clerk checked the column titled VD, as most before me had been quickly diagnosed. “No, it can’t be,” I explained. I was soon escorted to a private room and told to lie still on my back. I was finally diagnosed with having a kidney stone.

The next five days were spent in the military hospital at the Qui Nhon Airport. My orders were to stay in bed and force fluids. There was a pitcher of Kool-Aid constantly by my bedside. Whenever the pain subsided, I was to assist hospital personnel as a sort of roving untrained hospital orderly. In the bed next to mine was a GI with testicular cancer. He and many others weren’t as fortunate as I was to have such a curable problem.

It wasn't long before the first helicopter of injured servicemen touched down, bringing with it my first close look at the horrors of war. It carried young men with blood-drenched uniforms, grotesque open wounds, missing limbs, and worse. The wounded came with sounds of screams of pain mixed with moans from those who already had their shot of Morphine. An Army doctor was attending to one young man with his guts hanging out. Some memories have been blocked out by my mind over time, while others linger vividly as if they just happened.

The GI with testicular cancer was shipped back to the States. He was one of the "lucky" ones. Every day I would witness doctors and nurses treating the young man with his guts torn apart, watching what looked like alcohol being poured into his open abdomen as his screams sent chills down my spine. Daily trips taking gurneys and supplies down to the bottom floor where the amputee ward was located were interrupted by other helicopters landing on the helipad.

I was given one week to pass my kidney stone; surgery would be the next option. Straining urine through white gauze pads was how they would know if the Kool-Aid treatment worked. On my fifth day of this nearly hourly ritual, I was surprised to see what looked like a chunk of brown sugar in the gauze pad. My days of playing hospital orderly were over, and I was sent back to my unit the next morning.

When back on duty, one of the jobs I acquired was that of Air Force liaison. Daily contact with my Air Force counterpart at Phu Cat Air Base north of Qui Nhon was maintained to alert those further up the logistical line of what supplies were needed and what supplies were being sent from our port city up north. I remembered my first phone conversation with my Air Force contact at Phu Cat. I was still a naïve newcomer. After informing him of what cargo was headed his way, I was told that three cadavers would be on the return flight. I remember being taken aback by his routine manner of speech. I wasn't sure if I heard him correctly or understood the magnitude of what I'd just been told. After sheepishly asking him to repeat what he had told me, I froze for a moment. This was anything but routine for me. I was assured that I understood correctly. Thus began one of my daily duties: learning the always-unpleasant news that another mother's son was returning home to a heartbroken family.

After ten months of duty in South Vietnam, I was finally being rewarded with R&R (Rest and Relaxation). My destination: Bangkok, Thailand.

Chapter 2

Bangkok Belle

After ten months in Vietnam I was ready for my Rest and Relaxation in Bangkok. Hearing some of the stories from the guys who had been there had only made my hormones kick into overdrive. "Rest and Relaxation" was the furthest thing from my mind; girls—beautiful exotic Thai girls—were driving my thoughts. The California Bar, the Rhapsody Bar, Happy Happy Turkish Steam Bath, and the other places the guys had told me about had me reeling with anticipation for my R&R in Bangkok.

I arrived at the hotel, home base for my stay, and saw that it was more than adequate; it even had a swimming pool on the rooftop. I began unpacking my things for my six-day/five-night Bangkok visit. It felt so good to be out of Vietnam and out of harm's way for a few days. I had saved $250 for this trip and I planned to "let it all hang out" and have a great time. The sunshine was pouring into my fourth floor room as I delighted in pulling civilian clothing from my duffel bag; clothes that I hadn't worn since leaving the States for Vietnam ten months before. I couldn't stop thinking about the attractive girl at the reception desk. Her dark complexion and big round eyes were such a contrast to the Vietnamese girls I hadn't developed much of an interest in—not to mention her pretty smile. Were all the girls in Thailand so beautiful? They had certainly gained quite a reputation from GIs for their exotic looks. I couldn't wait to get out and investigate on my own.

A knock on the door "woke" me from my daydream.

"Hello, my name is Kam," the man said. "I am a taxi driver, and if you would like I can take you wherever you want to go in Bangkok. I am also available on a weekly basis. For $30 I can be your driver and tour guide."

I wasn't sure whether I wanted to part with $30 for a taxi service, but the idea of having my own guide to the city was intriguing. I kind of wished that some of the guys from Qui Nhon were here with me, but I was going to make the best of this trip no matter what.

I asked Kam how this arrangement would work. He had no trouble explaining how he would be on-call twenty-four hours a day. He would be waiting in the hotel coffee shop whenever I needed him, and his sleep time and time off would work around my schedule. He assured me that he could take me to the California Bar, Happy Happy Turkish Steam Bath, or any other place I wanted to go. He had obviously done this before. Most of his customers were probably guys just like me who were experiencing this needed break away from the war; looking for a good time in this mysterious, exotic, Thai city with the funny name: Bangkok.

* * *

I don't know why I had decided to check out the Happy Happy Turkish Steam Bath first, but I found myself looking through a glass window at a number of young women sitting on a long bench. Each was wearing a short, sexy dress. Each girl also wore a button with a number on it—the number to give if you wanted to spend some time with them. At this point, it was late afternoon. Kam had disappeared into the background of the near empty place after pointing me in the direction of this interesting window of Thai beauties on display. Welcome to Bangkok's world of sex.

At first I had been anxious to explore these places, but now I felt uncomfortable here. Something didn't seem right. I looked through the invisible partition that separated me from these supposed objects of desire. Different sizes and shapes of the female form were right in front of me in their red dresses, white dresses, black outfits—all with the common denominator of their buttons. The girls weren't sitting in any particular order; number thirty-seven was sitting next to number four who was sitting next to number fifteen and so on. It was so impersonal—that's what felt so wrong about it. There sat a dozen or so young Thai women waiting to be "chosen" by some total stranger for who knows what. I couldn't relax. Had I done the right thing by coming to Thailand for my R&R and what exactly would I be paying for?

Whether it was the little voice in my head that said "you're here now, just pick one," or a sudden surge of hormones, I can't say—it was probably a combination of the two. I told the "housemother," who had appeared out of nowhere just as Kam had disappeared, that I'd take number four. She then disappeared to go get my chosen girl. With my mind made up, I followed my new "friend" up a set of stairs to a narrow hallway with rooms on each side. She escorted me into one of the rooms and opened the door to reveal a fancy bathtub in the center.

My companion spoke some English, which helped to set me at ease a bit. I kept thinking to myself, *How does this work?* I had already given some money to the "housemother," but was still apprehensive since I didn't know what to expect next. How could I do anything with someone I didn't know? What exactly was going to happen? She told me her name was Patricia (at least for the purposes of this afternoon). Sensing my anxiety, she immediately tried to help me relax.

"Just get into the water, and I will give you a nice bath. Relax and enjoy yourself," she told me.

With that, I took the plunge into this erotic adventure soothed by Patricia's comforting words and the calming effect of the hot water. I had never had a girl give me a bath before—much less done anything sexual—having grown up before the "sexual revolution." I was literally in uncharted waters.

As I became even more relaxed, I asked Patricia about the Happy Happy Turkish Steam Bath and if she could explain to me the ground rules. Jerry from Indiana, one of the guys in my unit in Nam who had been here a few months earlier, had bragged about this place. I could see what he meant as I became even more relaxed. Yet, he was married, or claimed to be. He even showed us a picture of a beautiful blonde who he said was his wife. But why come here, to Bangkok, if he was married? Why not go to Hawaii like most of the married guys and reunite with his wife?

Patricia began to explain things as she soaped me up and massaged me with her experienced hands and fingers.

"We used to be able to massage you guys all over your body, even down there, but the authorities changed the rules. We cannot do that anymore. Only if you take me out of here am I able to get undressed and do things with you," she said, dropping an obvious hint.

Finally, the picture was coming into focus for me, but I didn't feel comfortable with Patricia. Though she had told me many things about herself in the short time we had been together, who knew if any of it was true? She told me she was a widow and that her husband had been a police officer recently killed in Bangkok. She had two children, and they were the reason she was working here. She didn't look as attractive or sexy up close as she had from behind the window. Maybe the uncomfortableness of the moment was coming into play. Maybe I suddenly came to the realization that this woman would sleep with me for my money to support her children. The mood wasn't right and my hormones had amazingly settled down. There I was, a twenty-year-old, healthy man with very limited sexual experience in the company of a young Thai woman who was willing to have sex with me. I thought to myself, *What's the problem, Jack?*

Patricia must have had a clock in her head signaling that my time was up; it was time that I paid the "house" for this service. There was no way I was going to pay another "housemother" or other honcho of the Happy Happy Turkish Steam Bath for the privilege of going back to my hotel room to have sex with this girl. The uncomfortable sense that I didn't belong here had returned with a vengeance. Patricia had long sensed there would be no further opportunity for her to make more money. What had she gotten from this experience with me? Probably next to nothing. The house probably got the lion's share. It was apparent in Patricia's manner what she was thinking; she didn't have to say anything—I knew: "Why did you waste my time? I hate doing this anyway. I didn't really want to go with you either. I just need the money."

I soon left and decided to go back to the hotel for dinner. My enthusiasm was somewhat dampened, but my driver assured me that I would be more comfortable at the California Bar if I wanted him to take me there later that evening. After dinner and a brief nap (the jetlag had hit me), I was ready to take Kam up on his suggestion. Bangkok at night looked quite intriguing from my fourth floor vantage point overlooking the city. I felt good about checking a few places out. I decided to check out the California Bar.

On my way out to meet Kam, I bumped into a guy in the hallway. We started talking and were surprised to find out that we were both New Englanders; my new friend, Bob, was from Boston. He was headed out on the town. He had met a really cute girl in one of the bars the night before and was anxious to see if she would be there again. If he couldn't find her, however, he said he would probably stop by the California Bar and try to find me.

"It was nice meeting you, Jack, good luck tonight. I'll give you a call tomorrow at lunchtime if I don't catch you later," he said while walking back down the hall.

I headed down to the lobby where Kam would be waiting for me. It was reassuring to have met someone here in Bangkok in my same situation, and it also helped that Bob was from my neck of the woods.

I arrived at the California Bar after a short trip through downtown. I was impressed by the sights and sounds of Bangkok at night; it was like some exotic light show designed to get my adrenaline pumping for what lay ahead. The club was extremely dark inside with brightly colored lights placed strategically throughout that made for the ambiance of this popular night spot. My companion led me to a table at the right side of the club. It was my first time in a nightclub, and I was truly impressed with the feeling. I was finally glad to be in Bangkok. With all the anticipation behind me, I was ready to kick back, relax, and observe. Whatever I would do here, I was not in any hurry.

As I sipped my beer, my eyes were scanning the rest of the California Bar. There were young American servicemen and attractive Thai women mingling everywhere; on the dance floor, seated at tables, standing, and moving around in a constant sea of raging hormones and sexual tension. Rock and Roll music filled the air and added to the atmosphere. This was why I came here, to Bangkok, on R&R: to put Vietnam as far from my mind as possible. This would be a five-day adventure and escape from the reality of what was behind me—and what lay ahead of me.

* * *

After a while, the combination of the music, the lighting, the hormones, and the alcohol took affect. I wanted to meet one of these beauties. I wanted to talk to someone. I was ready.

I had been watching some of the girls; waiting for the opportunity when one would be free. I walked around the California Bar to familiarize myself with this adult playground. As I was returning to the table my driver had secured for us, I spotted one of the more attractive young ladies sitting alone.

"Kam, do you think she is with anyone?" I asked him. I had been away from the table for only five or ten minutes.

"I know this girl," he replied "She is a good girl. I will ask her for you."

My trusty guide walked over to her table. She came back with him.

"She was talking to another GI, but he is very drunk. She can speak English," he informed me. Since I was still new to this scene, I didn't want any problems.

"Can I buy you a drink?" I asked her. "We can move to another table back there." I pointed to an area on the far side of the club from where I had just returned. I was sure we could get lost in the crowd of GI hunters and their pretty game in this corner table.

"I'll be over there," reassured Kam, signaling an area by the entrance. With that, we moved to an out of the way spot across the room.

This young lady was definitely a looker. I was surprised that no one else had approached her in the short time she had been sitting alone.

"My name is Jack," I said. "What's yours?"

"My name is Belle," she replied. "Thank you for inviting me to have a drink with you. I was afraid of that other GI."

She seemed genuinely relieved to get away from her other admirer. We both were able to relax back in the corner, and the conversation flowed freely and easily; Belle's English was more than adequate. She was a bit taller than most of the petite young women I had observed. She was probably 5'3" or 5'4"; not tall by Western standards, but definitely taller than most of the competition. Belle was slender but shapely, with very stunning features; long black hair, and dark eyes that reminded me of the girl at the reception desk.

We had a second drink. I don't know what it was I ordered for her. It was blue and came in a rounded glass that looked like a mini goldfish bowl. At least it wasn't "Saigon Tea." (Saigon Tea was what the bar hustlers in Vietnam would order at $2 a pop. It was tea in a shot glass. Many a GI had gone through a pocket full of money in hopes that doing so might lead to a romantic liaison…it usually didn't.)

Belle asked if I wanted to taste her odd, blue drink. "No thanks, I'll stick to beer," I told her as I counted the number of beers I had consumed so far that night. I was probably on my fifth beer (definitely a record for me), but I didn't feel drunk. This girl was so friendly and likable. Could it be the alcohol? Maybe the hormones. Who was I kidding—it was both.

"Would you like to leave with me?" I asked her.

"You will have to give me $12 for the house," she explained. "That way I won't have to come back until tomorrow. But Jack, there is something that I have to do in the afternoon, is that okay?"

"Whatever you have to do is fine with me," I said without hesitation.

She gave me a kiss on the cheek and said, "Please wait for me near the entrance."

I couldn't believe my luck as I made my way through the club and met Kam by the door. "I'm waiting for Belle," I informed him. Somehow, I don't think he was surprised.

I had met a few "bar girls" in Qui Nhon. Mostly innocent flirting occurred, but this seemed different. Belle didn't seem like a bar girl. This was more like a date; a date between two consenting adults—one with five beers in his system and raging hormones.

We left the club, and by the time my confidante and driver dropped us off at the hotel it must have been around midnight. The ride back had been nothing but one big flirting session. If Belle had intended on getting any sleep that night she was going about it entirely the wrong way. If she disliked me or was indifferent toward me, she didn't show it—in fact, it was just the opposite. We were like two teenagers returning from the prom. We were two young people who had known each other and been dating for a long time, only I wasn't dropping her off to beat her curfew. We were going back to the hotel—back to my room. There was no curfew and no feeling that we shouldn't be doing this.

The next few hours were like something out of a dream. There was no guilt and no feeling that I was with a "bar girl." I was with Belle and she was with me. There was no clock on the wall and no time concerns, only the physical pleasures that a man and woman can enjoy together.

* * *

In the morning, we managed to get a breakfast call in to room service around 11:00. It was like Vietnam didn't exist. Belle's flirtatious ways didn't disappear with the morning sun. It was as if sleep was merely an interval, like breaks between rounds of a boxing match. We managed to get in quite a bit of morning conversation. I was so comfortable and relaxed with her; something that I would not have believed possible only a day before.

The phone rang just after breakfast. It was Bob.

"Sorry I didn't make it to the club last night," he said. "Remember that girl I told you about? I found her at the other place, the Rhapsody Bar, and I'm gonna be with her today."

I understood…completely.

"We're going to go to that dinner show with the traditional dance and theater tonight. Did you hear about it?"

While he was talking I thought, *Hey, that let's me off the hook for the forgotten lunch date*. "I'll talk to you later, Bob," I told him and then hung up.

"What time is your appointment, Belle?" I asked.

She had momentarily forgotten. "I'm supposed to be there at 2:00," she replied, "if it's okay with you. I'm sorry, but I'll have to leave soon."

"Do you want me to give you a ride?" I asked Belle, not

wanting to see her leave. "I can call the coffee shop. I'm certain that Kam will be there by now."

She seemed surprised by my offer, which surprised me. Within the hour we were walking down the hall holding hands. She continued to talk and make me laugh. This girl had a dynamite personality. I wouldn't allow myself to think of Belle as anything but a very attractive, personable new friend, regardless of how we came to be together.

Belle's errand turned out to be some family commitment with an aunt. I waited with my driver in the car around the corner. I told Belle I would drop her off at her home so she wouldn't have to pay for transportation. She seemed very appreciative. I thought this was how a gentleman was supposed to act, especially a gentleman who had just spent the night with her. Then I had an idea.

"Can you go with me to the dinner show tonight?" I asked as she got into Kam's taxi.

Her face beamed a bright smile as she said, "Yes, if you want me to go with you. But there is one problem, Jack. The bar will want another $12. I'm sorry."

"What time do you have to be there?" I inquired.

"Nine o'clock, but if we can go by the bar now I can give them the money. If that is okay with you, Jack."

After stopping by the now lifeless California Bar, I dropped Belle off a few doors from her home.

"I'll meet you in the hotel lobby at six o'clock," Belle said as she disappeared into a maze of look-alike houses.

Belle was right on time. She was wearing a long black dress that only made her all that more attractive. Kam dropped us off at the restaurant where we met Bob and his date. We joined a few other people at a large table for ten. The restaurant itself was very ornate and colorful with a stage at the far end.

Belle joined the conversation of the ladies as I got to know my new guy friends a little better. After a short while, Belle gave me a slight elbow in the ribs as if to say, "Did you come here to talk to your friends or to be with me?" It was almost time to eat as I put my arm around Belle and pulled her playfully to me.

"What's the food like here? Is it like the American food back at the hotel?"

She gave me a little giggle and a roll of her beautiful dark eyes signaling me that I was in for a surprise. Just looking at her pretty face and those beautiful eyes, I had forgotten dinner for the moment and thought back to our flirting sessions and how wonderful it felt to hold her in my arms. We ordered another round of drinks just as our meal was arriving.

"Meat and potatoes" Jack now knew what Belle's giggle was about.

Dinner was traditional Thai food: fish with rice and noodles. The only problem was that the fish didn't look cooked. As I tried to decide what, if anything, I was brave enough to eat, I felt a soft, seductive, playful foot brushing against my leg. Bob's girl had gotten my attention. She smiled slyly, not wanting to attract anyone else's attention. What was this all about? As everyone began to eat and I continued to stare at the food on my plate, the petite temptress was at it again. She seemed to enjoy my reaction, and the more she got away with it the more she kept doing it.

"Aren't you going to try it?" Belle interrupted as I struggled to concentrate with Bob's cutie playing footsies with me. What's the protocol here? I'm with a beautiful young Thai woman who I'm growing fonder of by the minute, while being distracted by another pretty vixen who seems to delight in teasing me. Somehow I didn't think my new buddy would be too thrilled if he knew. I could hardly avoid making eye contact since she was seated directly in front of me. Without fail she would flash a coy smile at me every time I looked ahead, and the foot was never far behind, rubbing against my calf. I'd have to say I did enjoy it, but I was afraid her bold flirting would catch someone's attention.

I managed to survive dinner. The show was anti-climactic and paled in comparison to what took place under the dinner table between my leg and the playful foot of my seductress. I couldn't imagine that anyone else in Bangkok could have a sexier pair of bookends this evening than I did between Belle and my new temptress. Nor could I imagine anyone possibly distracting me from my date. But then again, this was Bangkok

"Let's go back to the hotel," Belle turned and whispered.

As we parted company from our friends to meet outside with Kam, she asked, "Do you like Mai?"

Apparently the marathon game of footsies hadn't gone unnoticed.

"Which one was Mai?" I sheepishly replied.

"You know," was the answer. I sure did, but that was the extent of my grilling. As Belle took my hand, I instantly felt the sense of our being a couple again, and Mai faded quickly from my thoughts.

At the hotel, I told Kam I wouldn't need his services until around one o'clock the next afternoon; better give the poor guy some time with his family, since I had no idea what day three would bring.

I sensed that Belle was becoming as fond of me as I was of her, but there seemed to be a little feeling of vulnerability coming from her. Was it because of Mai? Maybe not knowing the future from day to day was troubling her. She was obviously comfortable with me. I'd probably treated her better than most GIs she had known. As we walked along the corridor to my room still holding hands, I didn't think of her as someone I had just met in a bar.

"Jack, do you like me?" Belle asked as we embraced once inside the room. She felt so right in my arms. I held her tightly.

"You know I do," I replied. "You're so beautiful. I'm so happy I met you."

Night would soon become morning with Belle in my arms; a night of passionate lovemaking with my Thai "girlfriend." My second night in Bangkok was just like my first; I hadn't yet realized that there were now only three nights left on my R&R. Three more nights and I would be heading back to Nam; heading back to another two months of uncertainty. I couldn't allow myself to think of going home after those two months—not yet, and not until I got back to Qui Nhon and marked off another six days from my "short-timers" calendar. (It was customary for GIs to start marking off a day on the calendar whenever they reached approximately one hundred days left on their scheduled tour of duty. The fewer days left to serve in Vietnam, the "shorter" the calendar and GI were.)

* * *

I awoke to the rays of sunlight straining to get through the small crack that separated the curtains. As my eyes focused on the surroundings telling me where I was and that a new day was beginning, I found myself amused by the lack of bed covers protecting Belle and me. I didn't know if she had cast them aside during the night, or if they had been merely a casualty of last night's activities. We were now attired as we were when we originally entered this world. I watched Belle for a moment as her breathing moved her abdomen up and down rhythmically. Her long black hair teasingly covered one shoulder reaching down to her breasts. As I debated waking her, I noticed for the first time that my Thai princess seemed a bit larger around the waist than the slender image she presented in her black dress. Why hadn't I noticed before? Had her clothing fit just enough to hide Belle's small gut? Maybe the excitement of the Bangkok nightlife was the reason I hadn't noticed. Maybe it was the beer. Or maybe the last thing I wanted to think about was the possibility of Belle being pregnant.

I emerged from the shower to find my companion yawning and stretching the sleep out of her body; a body now modestly covered by the bedspread.

"Good morning, sleepy," I said. "That must have been some dream."

"Aren't you coming back to bed?" she inquired coquettishly. "It's too early to go anywhere."

If only Belle knew that the stakes had just been raised in this game of flirting and frolicking in bed. If my suspicion was correct, the game was over. I knew I could never sleep with her again. The thought of making love to someone carrying a child was as foreign to me as any thought I had had since arriving in Bangkok. It didn't matter that she was just starting to show; if she was pregnant, I would not be able to look at her in the same way. If Belle was pregnant, she would no longer be the beautiful exotic Thai girl whose looks and personality had first attracted me—she would be totally off limits.

I laid down on the bed next to Belle. Before she had a chance to do or say anything, I placed my hand on her stomach. I didn't have to ask. She now knew why I had acted differently towards her.

"I'm going to have a baby," she said as she looked at me with the innocence of a schoolgirl. She again seemed so vulnerable. I held her in my arms for what would be the last time.

Before I had spoken a word, Belle asked, "Can I show you something? I don't read English very well," she said. With that she reached for her purse and took out a letter. "Can you read this to me?" She snuggled up next to me.

The letter was postmarked from the Midwest. As I opened it, I felt like I was invading someone's privacy. Belle was anxiously waiting for me to tell her what it said and to find out what the writer was telling her in this language that she spoke but couldn't read very well.

"It's from Joe, he's an American GI like you," she explained. "I think he wants to marry me. He told me that when he was here in Thailand. It is his baby."

> *Dear Belle,* I read to her, *I got back to the States last week. I never thought that I would come back alive. We lost*

so many guys in our unit. I can't possibly explain how great it feels to be home. It's like a dream. Maybe it's like waking up from a nightmare, but it wasn't a nightmare. I told my mother about you, that I want to marry you. She doesn't understand. She doesn't believe that I love you. I think about you all the time. I wonder if you are all right. I get discharged in a couple of months. I am going to go to Bangkok to bring you to the United States. We can get married when we get here. It is so different from Thailand here. I know that you will like it when you get used to it. Please answer my letter soon, and if there is some way that you can call me, I'll pay for the call. I love you very much and can't wait until I see you again. Joe.

Belle was all smiles. That look of vulnerability seemed to vanish with the letter from her GI boyfriend. I felt sorry for this guy. I didn't know how long they had been together and didn't ask. Belle was indeed a beautiful young woman who was fun to be with, but if Joe had only known Belle from a short week's R&R away from the hell that was Vietnam, how could he be in love with her? In a way, I understood. Was I now beginning to see Belle in a different light? Was I seeing her in a way that I had convinced myself I never would just a couple of nights before? I thought about Joe and how surprised he was going to be when he found out Belle was pregnant. Then again, was it even his kid? I decided not to speculate about it—it was none of my business. It was nice to see Belle so happy, if only for the moment. Belle knew that our "dating" had come to an end and that we would be parting ways. I never expected this would be how it would end. I felt somehow empty, like something had sucked the feelings from me, while at the same time realizing that I would again be free to explore Bangkok at night.

* * *

After lunch, Belle and I met Kam in the lobby. He had already been at the coffee shop for a while. I guess he wouldn't want to lose his "gig" to another driver if his boss had suddenly changed plans and wanted to get an earlier start on the day. The ride to Belle's house was different this time; there was no more playful flirting and holding hands. I wondered what would happen to her; would Joe come to Bangkok and take his now pregnant bride-to-be back to the U.S., or would Belle's dreams of marriage and a better life in America become a casualty like so many other dreams that had died in Southeast Asia?

As I dropped her off at the familiar spot by her house, Belle gave me one last kiss on the cheek and disappeared once again into the maze of look-alike houses—this time for good.

While my thoughts momentarily wandered, my trusty guide asked me, “Where would you like to go, Mr. Jack?”

“Take me to where you live. I would like to see your home and meet your family. Is that okay with you?” I requested.

“Sure,” he replied. With that, my thoughts turned from Bangkok’s nightlife and beautiful young women to getting to know the people and understand the city by day. There would be time to resume my nocturnal activities later if I wished. I guess the shock of what transpired that morning had taken me aback. I needed a fresh perspective.

When we arrived in Kam’s part of the city, I was shocked into the reality of the poverty in this Southeast Asian country. The glitter and mystique of exotic Bangkok gave way to unpaved streets with old, broken down cars here and there, and children—oblivious to their plight—playing amongst discarded old tires and pools of stagnant water. Kam had barely turned off the ignition of his taxi when two of these little girls came running up to the vehicle to greet their daddy. The smiling children with the dirty faces and dresses had no sooner done this than, noticing the stranger seated in the family car, suddenly transformed themselves into shy angelic little beings on their best behavior.

Kam disappeared into his humble dwelling with his two daughters, while I remained in the taxi looking about the neighborhood and comparing it to the image of Bangkok I had fostered in my mind from my first two days of R&R. It really wasn’t that different from the poverty I had seen in and around Qui Nhon. This whole military experience was an eye-opener for me and millions of other young men who were sent to far away lands in this geopolitical chess game that was the Cold War.

Kam emerged from his home to inform me that his wife had gone to the market to shop for the family needs. He seemed almost embarrassed; not wanting to invite me into the family home.

“Would you like to take the girls for a ride? We can go somewhere with them,” I suggested.

Kam re-entered his home and soon reappeared with his two little angels, complete with new dresses and freshly washed faces. In a few minutes we found ourselves at a park featuring acts as bizarre as elephants performing with huge telephone pole-type logs, to Bangkok's finest and most brightly colored gamecocks trying to slash one another to death with razor blade styled attachments to their claws.

As I roamed the afternoon away at the park with many other Bangkok visitors, my shy little guests, or rather, my shy little hostesses (since I was in their land) began to warm up to me somewhat. Although Kam's girls spoke only a few words of English, the curious eight- and four-year-olds had what most every child in the world possessed: a universal like of candy and soft drinks. This went nicely with the popcorn we consumed on this sunny afternoon in Thailand.

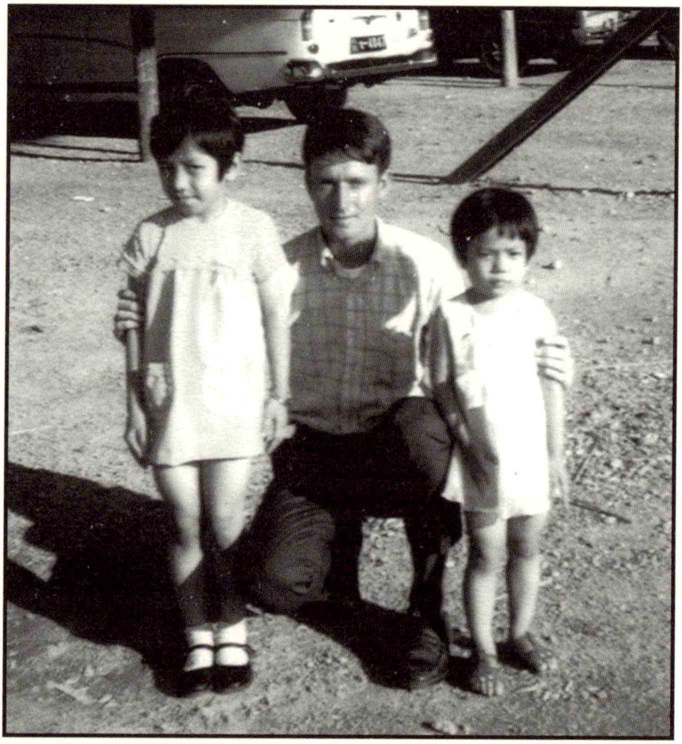

Jack with two little angels
Bangkok, Thailand, February 1969

After a few hours of casually strolling through this scenic park, it was time to return home where Mrs. Kam would be waiting for her little princesses. It was quite a diversion from the other Bangkok I had come to know. The afternoon had taken my mind off Belle and served to enhance my awareness of what life was really all about. Life was neither all about war, nor all about prowling the nightlife of Bangkok in search of a young man's cure for raging hormones; yet, I knew I would go out again that night.

Chapter 3

Sex, Drugs, and R&R

Nighttime had begun to settle on Bangkok as Kam and I returned to the hotel. I decided to take a nap before making any further plans, and told my guide I would meet him in a couple of hours. I had enjoyed my afternoon with Kam and his daughters, but wondered if Mrs. Kam would have approved of the junk food and soft drinks her two daughters had so easily consumed. I drifted off to sleep. By the time my eyes focused on my surroundings, I realized three hours had passed; Kam was probably wondering what happened to me.

I wondered where Bob might be this night. Again, I felt alone in this strange city—good thing I had Kam. I called the coffee shop where my trusty driver answered. He must have known it was me; either that or all the other drivers had already left to go back out on the town with their GIs.

After a quick shower and dinner, I found myself consulting my guide about Bangkok's nightlife. I decided to go to the Rhapsody Bar. I wanted to check out some place different, and besides, I knew I wouldn't bump into Belle there. It was almost like starting my R&R all over again, except now I knew the ground rules.

The Rhapsody Bar was quite a bit smaller than the California Bar. I ordered a beer and decided to just relax and watch the boy-meets-girl action taking place in front of me. Being a "veteran" on my third night in Bangkok, I could tell which guys were "rookies." These newbies were either the reserved onlookers, or the more drunken "let-me-at-'em" guys who hadn't yet found a woman.

I tried not to think about Belle; if she was at the bar, if she was with some other GI, or what would happen to her. I wasn't comfortable being by myself. Kam was a pro at disappearing when he wasn't needed and reappearing when he was. It was close to midnight and I decided to have him take me to a place I would feel more comfortable in; to where Bob might be and hopefully Belle would not: the bigger and better California Bar.

"I think you like this club the best," Kam commented. "Most GIs do."

As we made our way through the crowd, the smoke, and the music toward a table in the back, he asked, "Do you want me to find a nice girl for you? I know you don't want to see Belle. I know many good girls here, Mr. Jack."

"See if you can find my friend from last night, Bob," I replied.

As I sipped my beer, I thought about Belle, and again about the fact that I had only three nights left on my Bangkok R&R—and about Vietnam. I felt as if I was wasting a precious night on the town. I was in a place that had hundreds of pretty young exotic women just waiting for some GI to pay $12 to take them away from the club for a night.

The excitement of my night in Bangkok mingled with the sad reality of the perspective of my hosts and hostesses. Maybe it was because of Belle; I couldn't help but feel sorry for her. Maybe it was the afternoon and getting to know the other side of Bangkok. Whatever the reason, I didn't feel like meeting anyone this night. I tried not to look at the ladies of Thailand as bar girls. I didn't see Belle that way, but there was no one else. I decided to call it a night. I would have time to reflect tomorrow.

* * *

Closing the door to my hotel room intensified the cold, empty feeling of being alone in a foreign land. Although I had enjoyed Bangkok by day, it was quite a different feeling that night. As I stretched out on my bed, the thought of bringing someone new to it felt wrong. Maybe I could bring Belle back here. I didn't have to do any more than hold her in my arms. I wished, at that very moment, that I could have done so. I drifted off to sleep thinking of her, while knowing I would probably never see her again or know what would become of my Thai princess.

The telephone woke me, ushering in day four. It was Bob.

"Did I wake you, Jack?" he inquired.

"No problem," I assured him. "What's up?"

"Can you make it to lunch in half an hour?" he asked.

Lunch? Already? I glanced at the wall clock. 11:45 was too late for breakfast anyway.

"Give me one hour and it's on me," I responded.

As I hung up the phone, I glanced at the clock again and thought of how late I had slept. I thought about the guys back in Nam and getting up at 5:30 every morning for ten months when we weren't staying up all night. Then there were the times we would sleep four hours and then have two hours on guard duty. I deserved sleeping in, especially here in Thailand. After all, wasn't that the purpose of *rest* and *relaxation*?

After lunch, Bob and I took in a little sightseeing before hitting the bars in the late afternoon. Bangkok was still asleep as we downed a few beers and chatted about home and how we ended up here—two Red Sox fans on the other side of the world—and planned the final days of our R&R.

"I'm meeting Mai later on at the club," Bob informed me, "She has a few errands to run today. I dropped her off this morning. Isn't she cute?"

If there were someone in Bangkok who could take my mind off Belle, it would be Mai. But it was useless to even think about her, Bob would never let her go.

Nighttime found us again at the California Bar. As Kam conveniently disappeared into the shadows of the now-throbbing nightclub, Bob and Mai were seated with me at a long table with other GIs and girls meeting and talking. Mai was too far from me to even attempt playing footsies, but every now and then we would make eye contact. Mai had to be the prettiest girl in there. Too bad she was off limits.

As we drank, talked, and listened to the rock and roll music of a local Thai group, I found myself sitting next to a rather attractive young lady with dark round eyes and a pretty smile.

"My name is Jack," I began. "What's yours?"

"I'm Lee," she replied. "I saw you here a few nights ago."

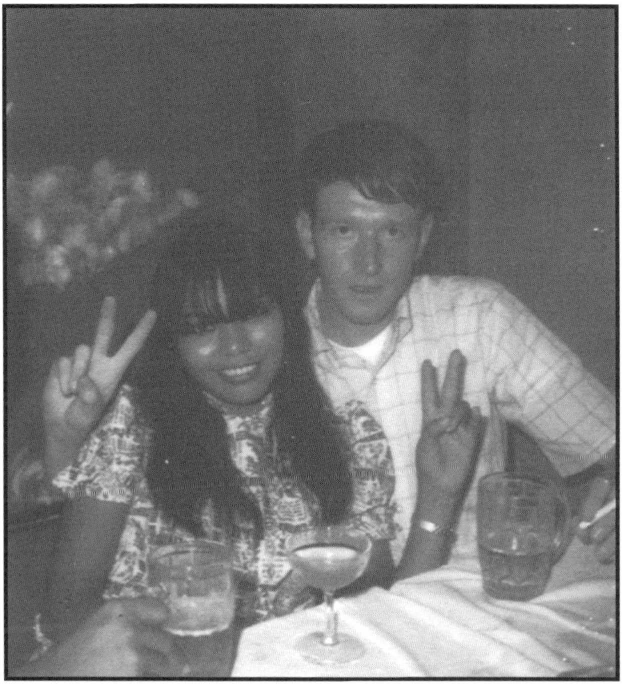

Lee and Jack unwinding at the California Bar
Bangkok, Thailand, February 1969

Lee was short and curvy, not as petite as Mai, but definitely worth getting to know better. I didn't notice her come to our table during the hustle and bustle of the evening, but I was glad that she did.

"Do you want to dance?" I asked.

"Yes," she quickly responded.

Bob had left with his companion, and I had a feeling that I would soon be doing the same.

"Would you like to go with me" I invited Lee.

"Sure," she replied. I would have been shocked by any other answer. "Let me get my things and tip out," she instructed. "I'll meet you by the front of the club."

Lee no sooner left to get her stuff than Kam appeared.

"I'll see you in a few minutes by the doorway," I told Mr. Dependable. "I'm gonna stop by the men's room first."

As the door closed behind me, I realized I was being followed. I turned to find myself face to face with an irate fellow GI in the process of pulling a knife from his pocket.

"She's with me," he said sternly. As my adrenaline began to pump quickly, one of his friends blurted out, "Forget about her. There are plenty of girls here. We're all on the same side."

After cooler heads prevailed and the group of soldiers went back into the nightlife of the California Bar, I couldn't help but think of a couple other such rushes of fear I had experienced back in Nam. I never expected to come so close to becoming a Vietnam War statistic while on R&R. What type of asterisk would have been placed by my name, anyway?

I quickly took care of business and hurried off to meet Kam and Lee. I had a question or two for her before this went any further, like if I was causing trouble by taking her with me?

I asked Lee on the way back to the hotel. She assured me that there would be no surprises like the one I encountered in the men's room.

The ride back to the hotel also lacked the flirting that took place between Belle and me on my first night in the city, but the effects of hours of drinking beer mixed with my crazy hormones and Lee's looks made the anticipation build within me. If I had not met Belle or seen Mai, Lee would have been a prize well worth going after.

Once in my room, Lee turned on the bath water and informed me that we would be taking a bath together. I offered little resistance as my curvy new "girlfriend" took charge of the situation.

"Do you want to know why I chose you in the club?" Lee asked seductively. "Big nose big ____," she giggled. I followed her into the bathroom hoping that she wouldn't be too disappointed.

The warm water was very relaxing to an already tired, alcohol-filled body as Lee splashed water at me whenever I attempted to get closer to her. Extracurricular activities would have to wait until after our bath.

"Let's go to bed now," Lee told me as she stood up in the bathtub. I wasn't going to argue with her as I followed her lead into night number four in Bangkok.

* * *

I awoke with the sunlight. Lee was still asleep next to me. As I focused on the clock that said 11:00 a.m., I couldn't help but think that in a little over twenty-four hours I would be packing for my return flight to Vietnam. These carefree nights in Thailand were nothing but a pleasant distraction from what awaited all of us GIs. How could the time have passed so quickly? Why couldn't Bangkok be reality and the war just some sick fantasy? I wondered for the first time how many guys had lost their lives in the war while I was here having a good time. At least I knew I would be returning to an area in Vietnam where there normally wasn't much action. What about those guys who put their lives on the line every day and night out in the boonies—guys like the crazy GI who was about to pull a knife on me because of Lee?

"Are you awake, Jack?" rose a sexy voice within a sleepy body. "What time is it?"

As I informed Lee that it was just past 11:00, she responded as she cuddled up against me, "We have time before lunch." I already knew that Lee liked to call the shots, so to speak, and I wasn't about to complain.

We had no sooner gotten out of our morning bath than a knock on the door connecting my room to the next interrupted our playtime. We soon found ourselves standing around in my room talking to Bob and Mai, each one of us dressed in the exact same uniform: a white hotel towel wrapped around a naked body. I had no idea that Bob and I had adjoining rooms. Mai had been in the very next room probably the entire time I had been in Bangkok. I guess it just never came up in conversation during our party time in Thailand.

As Lee and Mai spoke in their native tongue, Bob said, "Looks like you found yourself a real beauty." I jumped on his opening line like a tiger on its prey.

"Would you be interested in changing partners?" I asked, hoping that Bob might want to sample some of Bangkok's other forbidden fruit. "Have you been with the same girl since you got here?"

"I'm satisfied," he insisted, "I like this one."

Who could blame him? Bob was with undoubtedly one of the most attractive young ladies in a city famous for its beautiful women. I wondered what the girls were talking about. Mai gave me another flirtatious look as if to say, "I tried." As the door closed behind my two neighbors, a mischievous Mai popped into my room for one last word with Lee. After saying something in Thai to my new "girlfriend," Mai looked at me and said, "Sorry." If she only knew how much I wanted to be with her. Maybe she did.

I had mentioned previously to Kam that I might like to take a drive out of Bangkok, possibly to see the famous "Bridge over the River Kwai," which we were informed was off limits as far as R&R was concerned.

When I mentioned this to Lee after lunch, she said, "I have

better idea." She showed me a plastic bag full of grass that was in her purse. "Do you want to smoke some this afternoon?" she asked.

"I've never tried it before," I replied, remembering the lectures back in Nam from Sergeant Gomez about the evils of "mari-juwwana," as he pronounced it. I thought about it for a moment. I rationalized to myself; *it's probably legal here anyway*, knowing well that it wasn't. I decided to give it a try. What could they do—send me to Vietnam?

Lee and I spent the afternoon "floating in the clouds" as she massaged a few of my Salem's to extract the tobacco and repack them with this funny weed. My last afternoon in Bangkok was spent on a marijuana cloud making love to Lee without a care in the world. Vietnam did not exist; neither did Belle nor Mai. I don't even think Bangkok existed on this cloud; just Lee and I making out in slow motion.

Morning brought with it the finality of my Bangkok R&R. Lee was up before me. "I have something for you," Lee said as she placed a ring in my hand. "I want you to remember me. I will always remember you. I hope you are okay in Vietnam. You are very nice GI. I like you very much."

I was touched by Lee's gesture, even if some other American GI had bought her the gift she left with me. The black star sapphire stone in the ring was easily worth more than what I had spent and paid the California Bar to be with this sexy cutie.

After a quick shower, I laid on my bed for the last time. The phone rang and I could hear Lee speaking in Thai with someone as she softly stroked my face. "It's for you," Lee told me as she handed me the receiver.

"Hello, Jack." It was Belle. "I wanted to come by your room to say goodbye, but you have someone there. I just want to say that I will be praying for you and hoping that you make it home okay."

"Where are you?" I asked Belle, still surprised to be talking to her again.

"I'm here at the hotel, but I don't think it is a good idea that I see you. Be careful in Vietnam."

I got off the phone with Belle and then Lee watched me pack the few things I brought along that weren't Government Issue—a few shirts and pairs of slacks. I thanked her again for her gift as the ever-punctual Kam showed up, camera in hand, for a final photo or two. There would be a bus arriving shortly to transport those going back to their units in Vietnam and, just as assuredly, there would be another arriving here at the hotel full of eager GIs awaiting their turn in

Bangkok—their turn to forget about war and focus on the cure for raging hormones.

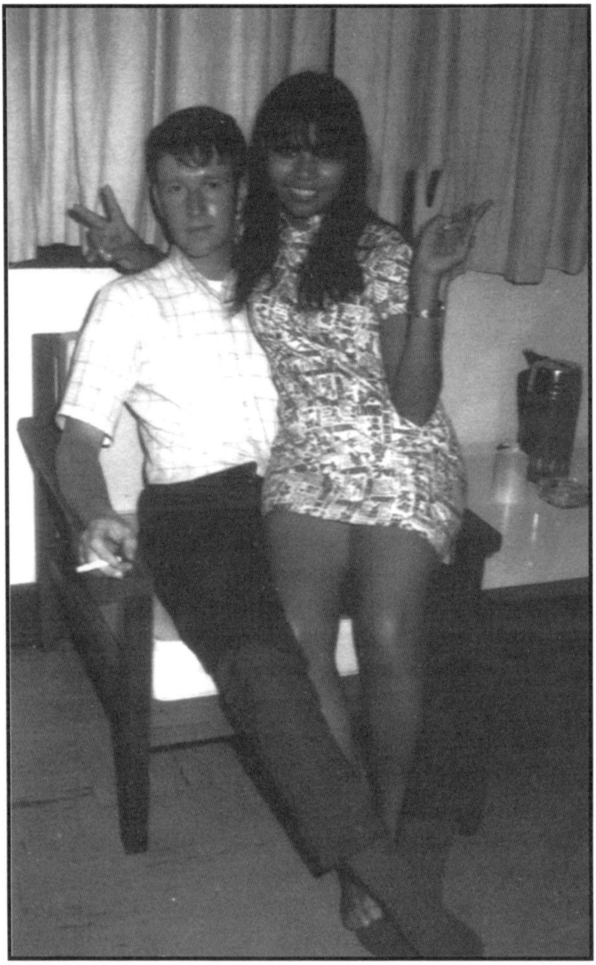

Jack and Lee, one last picture before boarding the bus back to reality
Bangkok, Thailand, February 1969

Chapter 4

A Taste of Reality

On my third night back in Qui Nhon after my exotic R&R in Thailand, I drew perimeter guard duty. We were currently stationed in a compound atop a mountain overlooking “Sand Bag Valley.” That was what I liked to refer to it as, since I felt as though I had personally filled half the sand bags used to build and rebuild bunkers down there. We were also directly across from the infamous “Hill” where the Tet Offensive claimed so many lives. The months we spent up there overlooking the city of Qui Nhon, while providing a first line of defense, had been the eeriest of my tour of duty. The thought of what had happened to those who had made the ultimate sacrifice on the hilltop a half mile away—a bunch of cooks, clerks, and drivers—was never far from my thoughts. I couldn’t imagine the living hell that those who faced combat and a daily fear of dying went through. If it were up to me, I never would.

I had pulled guard duty on many occasions, but this was the first time I drew guard duty on this side of our mountain compound.

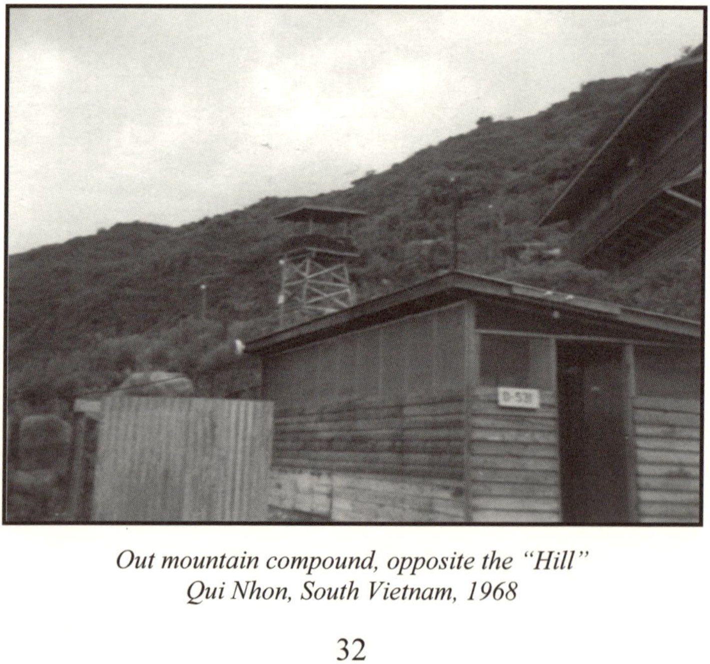

Out mountain compound, opposite the “Hill”
Qui Nhon, South Vietnam, 1968

There was nothing between me and whoever or whatever might be out in the darkness. The strange feeling of living atop this mountain compound never quite left, but climbing up the fifteen-foot guard tower reminded me that I was, in fact, back in Vietnam; this definitely wasn't Bangkok, and my R&R was quickly becoming just a memory.

Looking out from the guard tower, one could get a better appreciation of our position. The steep incline to my left led straight down to the ocean. Over my left shoulder was the tiny fishing village we drove through every day on our way to the port of Qui Nhon and our logistical duties with DOT. To my right was the Hill, easily twice the size of ours, and the only thing separating us from that hill was a radio transmitter in the middle of Sand Bag Valley. I could hear the waves crashing against the base of the mountain as high tide brought with it its own natural sound effects. As I settled into my position peering over the sand bag barrier which lined the guard tower, my buddies were settling in for another uncomfortable night atop this unnamed mountain compound. My relief would come in two hours and after four hours of sleep I would be back up to guard duty. It would be someone else's turn the next night.

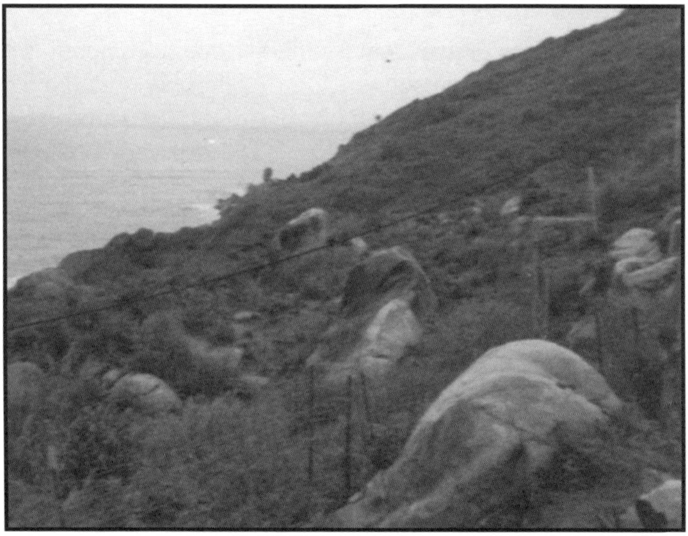

Mountain compound with its steep incline to the South China Sea below Qui Nhon, South Vietnam, 1968

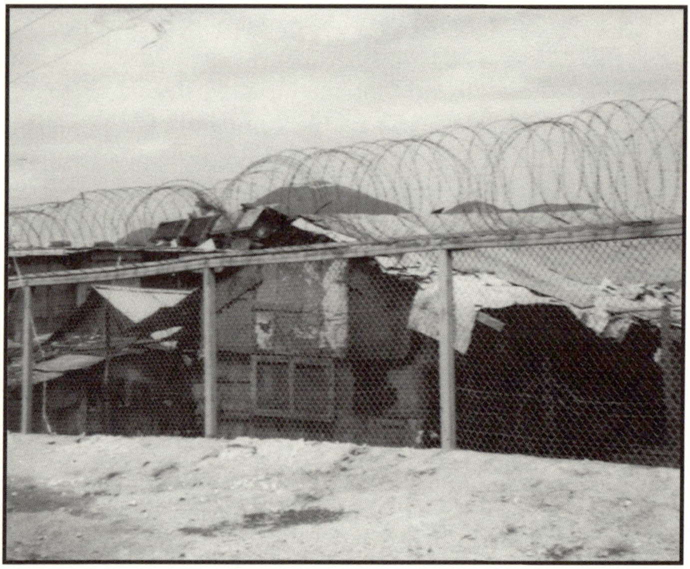

Shanty Town Village adjacent to our Qui Nhon port compound, quite a difference from our mountain side home overlooking Sand Bag Valley Qui Nhon, South Vietnam, 1969

Around midnight, my replacement came accompanied by the sergeant of the guard, the person in charge of those on guard duty. With minimal conversation and use of his flashlight, he stood by as my replacement climbed up into the tower while I descended to get a little sleep before my next turn came up at 4:00 a.m. I went back to the guard shack and stretched out on a bare Army cot—no mattress, just springs—and tried to relax and get some sleep. Two hours later, another set of soldiers were awoken and taken out to their positions, while those they replaced trickled in to claim a bare spring sleeping cot. Half asleep, I knew my turn would be coming up again in another two hours.

* * *

My four hours of "sleep" were up, and as I ascended the steps to the guard tower, I found I would be spelling one of the "provisional guards." One month earlier, someone had decided to beef up our perimeter guard by pulling in some soldiers from one of the infantry companies. I had done a double-duty watch (two guards in the tower) earlier with this soldier, and knew of his inclination to sleep while on watch. As I again settled into my position, I felt uneasy about the darkness in front of me. Did I have reason to be concerned? It had been over a year since the Tet Offensive had taken its toll on our unit on the Hill across Sand Bag Valley.

The night had grown quiet with the low tide taking its music away as it retreated out to sea. I stared into the darkness, ever vigilant for anything out of the ordinary—I couldn't help but think of what happened on the Hill. Twenty-eight young men had been guarding the Hill in four separate bunkers. Twenty-eight sons who probably had reassured their mothers and families of how "lucky" they were to be stationed in Qui Nhon, safely tucked away in this coastal port city so far from the fighting—so far from the war.

Brad was the only survivor of that night on the Hill. The explosion rendered him unconscious. Thinking he was dead, the enemy took his watch, as well as his innocence that horrific night. Brad and I were assigned to DOT. I met him briefly when he returned from his R&R in Australia. He was an emotional wreck, and he came back after less than a week in Australia engaged to a girl he had just met. Was I taking the place of this young man who would, in all likelihood, carry the weight of his nightmare with him for the rest of his life?

Shortly before dawn, the bushes just beyond the little clearing in front of me began to move. Or did they? As my heart began to pound, they moved again. This time it wasn't my imagination. I froze with fear. For the first time since I arrived in Vietnam, I was literally paralyzed with fear—I couldn't move. My mind raced a million miles an hour as I attempted to recall the procedure for placing a round in the chamber of my antiquated M14 rifle. It was useless. My mind and body failed to respond. As we were about to be attacked by the invisible enemy, I summoned all my strength and I managed to raise and point my M14 toward where the enemy would be coming from, unsure if I would be able to pull the trigger or if I had even properly readied my weapon for combat. In an instant it was over. I found myself face to face with my adversary: the cutest little fawn I ever hoped to lay eyes on. A baby deer had done to me what the invisible enemy had yet to do. It scared the living hell out of me.

The last month and a half of my tour was spent at the port of Qui Nhon itself. I was moved into a barracks just inside the main gate. Military police guarded the gate, checking all traffic entering and leaving. It was the same gate we passed through at least twice a day while working at DOT. Sprinkled in between military trucks and jeeps were civilian vehicles, mostly South Korean trucks that hauled cargo from the port to its destination in the Qui Nhon area. There was a stark contrast between the hilltop compound and my new home. The final fifty or so days on my "short-timers" calendar was going to be a breeze to knock off. I would enjoy drawing an "X" across the date every morning, while staring at the picture from an auto magazine of the canary yellow Camaro I would buy once I returned stateside.

I adapted easily to my new surroundings. The duty station was roughly a half mile away. The main difference between my former compound and the new one was that the ocean waves now crashed against the shoreline merely the length of a football field away, as opposed to over a hundred feet below. Resting near the port compound was a dilapidated Vietnamese village. Houses were made from anything the dwellers could piece together, from wood to chicken wire to cardboard. Bare light-bulbs hanging from electrical cords could be seen at night, especially from one of the guard towers. The electricity to power them was tapped into from the compound. While on guard duty, I witnessed the run-down village after-hours from above. Voices in the night, accompanied by modest displays of affection, and money counting occurred every night.

My daily lunchtime routine consisted of a hot dog from the Korean food concession, a bag of chips, and a Dr. Pepper. Whenever I wasn't required to drive for Colonel Kendrick or take the guys to the mess hall, noontime meant snacking, listening to music from the Armed Forces Radio Network on my transistor radio, and slopping on a generous portion of Coppertone suntan lotion. Each passing day I'd mark another "X" on my calendar and continue to bronze my body from the waist up for an hour. The clean white sand above the helicopter pad behind the DOT building served as my own private beach. As I lay there overlooking the inlet cove, I could see fishermen in their sampans and women knee-deep in low tide mud gathering up slippery little shoreline fish that would soon be served as a tasty meal. But mostly, I'd close my eyes and imagine I was back home; back in Pawtucket, Rhode Island driving my yellow Camaro.

The time spent in a now relatively quiet and peaceful Qui Nhon tended to make me forget my first weeks in this country. Memories of filling sandbags and rebuilding bunkers faded. Now that we no longer had the constant reminder of what happened on the Hill one year earlier, it became easy to forget what was going on in other areas of South Vietnam. Soldiers—some still a few years away from being old enough to vote—were dying every day. But for those of us lucky enough to be stationed in the Qui Nhon's and Cam Ranh Bay's of this country, the war was out of sight, and often out of mind as well. Occasionally, guilt or a chance encounter with a fellow soldier just in from the bush would make us appreciate our surroundings that much more.

* * *

On the weekends, the enlisted men were divided into two groups. Since Qui Nhon was once again considered "safe"—no more gray alerts, much less yellow or red—we were given permission to go into the city itself and take a welcome break from our 7:00 a.m. to 7:00 p.m. duty schedules. Half of the guys were allowed to leave after noon on Saturday while the other half got Sunday afternoons off. It was kind of like a mini R&R, but this wasn't exactly Bangkok.

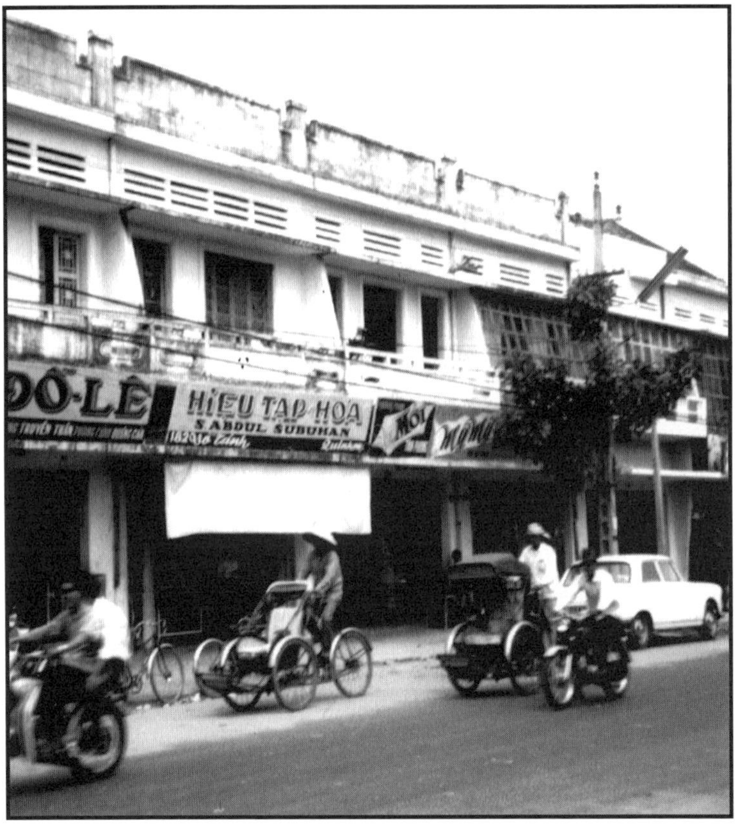

Qui Nhon, South Vietnam, 1968

Sunday afternoons I'd get together with my friend Harget, from advanced training back in Fort Jackson, and two guys from my unit, Garcia and Santiago. Harget was a "soul brother" from Brooklyn, Santiago was a Puerto Rican from Chicago, and Garcia was a Mexican from Los Angeles. It was still the turbulent '60s back in the States, but the military had a way of bringing people of diverse backgrounds together. How else could one account for a Pollack, an inner city Black kid, a Puerto Rican, and a Mexican hanging out together, other than the fact that we were all Americans serving our country.

We quickly established our weekly routine: going from bar to bar searching for the best Vietnamese girls we could find. After a few beers in a few bars, we would top off these special Sunday afternoon downtown adventures with a relaxing steam bath and special massage from one of the local massage places in Qui Nhon—just what a twenty-year-old kid in wartime needed until next Sunday came around. Besides, after playing the "Saigon Tea" game all too often without much luck, a sure thing took the guesswork out of the "will she or won't she" game.

The guys who came before us briefed us on this little game. Although there were a number of bars and places where $5 could produce an instant "love connection," most of these girls and women weren't exactly appealing. In most of the bars an attractive girl would sit down beside you and ask if you would buy her a drink. While you drank beer or whatever, the girl would periodically ask for another drink. Saigon Tea at $2 a pop could add up if the girl was pretty enough, a good hustler, or if GI Joe had had one too many. Occasionally, one of the guys would brag about going to an upstairs or back bedroom with one of these stunningly attractive bar girls, but you never knew if it really happened or if that was the best recollection this GI had of the encounter. One guy in our unit actually bragged of getting a pretty bar girl just by buying her Saigon Tea, except for the fact that he admittedly invested $40. I'm not sure how much Bob should have carried on about his lucky day.

I had my own experience with Saigon Tea. On one of those days when Harget, Santiago, Garcia, and I would go our separate ways for a few hours, I met a petite Vietnamese girl—she had to be only 4'7". I nicknamed her my "Watermelon Girl," because from the first day she came over to my table, she was always eating and feeding me watermelon. Watermelon Girl was a petite cutie and not much of a hustler. She would spend time with me while only hitting me up for one or two teas.

After a few visits to Watermelon Girl's bar, I stopped in one Sunday afternoon to see if she was still working there. My new friend immediately came over to join me, leaving another GI upset by her sudden departure. I didn't know how much this guy had invested in my girl, but I'm sure he'd wasted more than a few dollars on the clear iced tea. After talking for a while, I heard those words that I wasn't sure I'd ever hear from my Watermelon Girl: "Do you want to leave and go to my house?"

We walked quickly along the street directly behind the bar, which was located on the city's main street. I felt apprehensive at first, but there were other GIs and civilian personnel milling around, and by now I was no longer taking orders from my "main" brain anyway. As we entered her house, Watermelon Girl's mother was busy ironing American military uniforms. Her mother was a *mamasan* who must have had a job at one of the Army compounds in the Qui Nhon area. The woman barely glanced at the GI her daughter was escorting to the bedroom. Guess I wasn't the first…

Once inside the bedroom of this exotic Asian cutie, my Watermelon Girl turned toward me. "Ten dollars," she said.

It was too late now. I reached into my pocket for $10 and protection. In a few minutes I was walking alone down the street to meet the guys at the steam bath. I never saw Watermelon Girl again, and I never went back.

* * *

PING! PING! My thoughts of being home in the U.S. were suddenly interrupted, and I quickly scrambled to my feet and took cover behind the latrine. Those weren't bees zipping past me into the sand that interrupted my daydream. My private beach suddenly became a target range and I was the guest target. I ran inside the building, and soon everyone with a weapon was crouched behind whatever they could find to protect themselves from whoever was out there. But where? It was a typical early afternoon with fishermen in sampans and a few people wading. The gunfire had ceased, and after an inspection of the area, two bullet holes were found; one in the wall of the latrine itself and another in the side of our main building. My private beach was permanently deemed off limits, and extra fortification and vigilance was ordered.

As my "short-timer" days dwindled and my twenty-first birthday approached, I got this zany idea to extend my tour of duty another six months so I could spend my birthday at home; back in Rhode Island with family and friends. I decided to leave Vietnam a month early and return for another seven months. I would practically be guaranteed the same duty station with Director of Transportation while celebrating my April Fool's birthday back in the real world. It would also make a five month "early out" option that much more attractive. For the price of spending eighteen rather than twelve months in Vietnam, I'd be able to enjoy my twenty-first birthday at home, as well as get out of the Army in late May/early June 1970. I would have an entire summer to goof off and enjoy civilian life before returning to college in the fall on the GI Bill. It was a brilliant plan.

Fortunately, after doing the required paperwork and submitting it to the orderly on duty, the young sergeant looked up at me as if I'd been out in the sun too long.

"Are you sure?" he questioned. "You want to come back to Vietnam for seven more months just to spend your birthday at home?"

His words hit home. He handed back my papers and I tore them up and threw them in to the trash. Might as well finish out my original tour and get out of this place.

I spent my twenty-first birthday behind the latrine at our seaside compound drinking red wine—Musketell, compliments of Lieutenants Brian and Jerry. Brian Sprague was my immediate supervisor at DOT and we had formed a fairly close friendship. The twenty-four-year-old teacher from Michigan and I were due to depart Vietnam within a couple days of one another. He promised to do whatever he could to get me out of Qui Nhon early on his flight back home.

Soon after, it was my squad's turn to rotate to the front bunkers at the immediate entrance to the compound in the event that an alert alarm sounded. I would be in the first sandbagged bunker facing the compound gate. The only people in front of our position were the two MPs who guarded the main entry to the port of Qui Nhon. Outside of my experience with the sniper at my former private beach, the Qui Nhon area had been "safe" for all of my tour of duty. The Tet Offensive had faded to a distant memory. Besides, I would be out of here in seventeen days or less.

The alarm sounded during the middle of the night. Qui Nhon was on full Red Alert—there was enemy activity in the area.

Our platoon fell out to its designated locals: my squad to the front bunkers, and myself and another soldier to the first bunker. We were startled boys and young men, with our hearts pounding as we joined the confusion of that night. As I took my position in the first bunker, the gate to the compound and the MP post suddenly looked much closer than ever before. The sky was illuminated with flares and there was gunfire at the port's entrance, just fifteen or twenty yards in front of us. The makeshift village of scrap wood and cardboard lean-to's adjacent to the compound was on fire. Distant gunfire sporadically filled the night air. A truck approached the main gate and drew fire from the MPs. It was total chaos. It was as if nobody was in charge or knew what was happening. I could have been back in Rhode Island if I had only extended my tour. Seventeen days from leaving this mixed up war and now this.

It was only the second time in a year I had to chamber a round in my WWII vintage M14. Relief, albeit temporary, was learning that the truck was driven by South Korean civilians just trying to reach the safety of Qui Nhon's port. The MPs waved them by as the gunfire slowed and the confusion lessened.

By morning the fire was out, as villagers inspected what remained. Unofficial word filtered down to us that some GI, in a nearby compound, had opened fire at something suspicious. An errant flare shot into the night sky by another nervous soldier had apparently caused the fire. The events of the past few hours only served to heighten my appreciation of what other scared young men lived and died with on a daily basis.

* * *

The final two weeks passed uneventfully. I learned that my next duty station would be Fort Benning, Georgia. My request to be stationed closer to home or on the West Coast was denied. I had nothing against the South, but after stops in Georgia and South Carolina, the last place I wanted to be stationed—other than South Vietnam—was the South. But I had a plan. I'd do what few other enlisted men had successfully done: go directly to the Pentagon and request a change of duty station.

Leaving Cam Ranh Bay and Vietnam behind, we boarded the plane that would take us back to the States; back to see our families and friends again, back to "the world," and away from this strange land where so many young men had sacrificed their lives.

The excitement of leaving was like no other I had yet

experienced. The anticipation of the aircraft finally taking us from the soil where most of us had set foot twelve months earlier was intense. A year of our youth had been spent in this upside-down country. We all had our memories of what we were called upon to do and what we had seen during our respective tours of duty. We had many unpleasant and unspeakable memories we would carry with us, forever imbedded in our minds.

The excitement soon turned to euphoria as this commercial airliner was finally airborne. Looking out the window I realized that, for most of us, this would be the last time we would see Vietnam. Instead of sitting on our helmets in the belly of some old C-130 cargo plane, we were getting the civilian treatment, complete with attractive young American stewardesses to serve us. It was like a dream; one I had waited so long for. Yet it was not a dream—the war was over for us.

Unlike the endless eighteen-hour flight from Seattle to this strange Southeast Asian country, the thoughts going home were about plans and dreams. I thought about seeing Mom and Pop, my sisters, my nephew David (who would turn two years old in a matter of days), my friends, and my old girlfriends. Would any of them be there to greet me? Why did Lois stop writing? Who might still be single and unattached?

I was returning home not as a confused, depressed, teenaged Army recruit, but as a confident twenty-one-year-old man. I had plans. I was going to be like Nick, the first boy from our isolated Pawtucket neighborhood to return from Vietnam like some sort of hero and buy a new car. Only mine wasn't going to be a dark Mustang convertible, but a canary yellow Camaro—just like the one in the picture I had cut out from the auto magazine and tacked up over my short-timer's calendar.

I thought more about the people I was going home to: about my baby sister Debbie; she would be a teenager in another year. Kathy would be graduating from my old school, Tolman High, in just a couple of months. Diane and everyone would be planning David's birthday party. But most of my thoughts were about Mom; how she worried about everything, and how relieved she would be to have her only son finally home and out of harm's way. I also thought about Pop, recipient of a Bronze Star for valor during World War II, who had never answered my boyhood question, "Did you ever kill anybody during the war?" I had a much greater appreciation now for his silence than when I first posed it so many years before.

For the first time in my young life I knew exactly what I

wanted. I was going to be eligible for an "early out" program offered by the Army. I'd have time to enjoy part of the summer of '70 and go back to college in the fall on the GI Bill. No more confusion, no more uncertainty and depression with my years spent in a fog trying to work my way through school. I would soon be returning to college as a Vietnam veteran, a sophomore at Michigan State or the University of Rhode Island. I would go just about anywhere, but not Providence College. Forget the prestige that PC had to offer as the all-male Catholic university in the state; I wanted to be surrounded by coeds. I was eager to be around girls—American girls. I was especially eager to be around American girls in mini skirts; the fashion trend we'd only heard about. The "sexual revolution" had just started when I went into the military, and I was eager for a social life.

So many dreams...

Part Two

Expect the Unexpected

Chapter 5

Broken Dreams

The plane touching down on U.S. soil only served to magnify the fact that we were truly home, safe and sound. We would be bussed from Seattle-Tacoma Airport to Fort Lewis for processing, and then we'd be left to our own devices from there. Everyone was eager to go home as quickly as their next flight out of Seattle would take them. Everyone, probably—except me. I had something that couldn't wait. I was getting the first flight available to take me from Washington to Washington, as in state to DC. As anxious as I was to get home and see everyone, I had something important to accomplish first. I was going straight to the Pentagon to see if I could have my next duty assignment changed. I'd rather be stationed closer to home, and a day or so delaying my homecoming celebration would be worth it in the long term.

I had enlisted in the Army as a naïve nineteen-year-old boy with no real travel experience, and returned stateside as a well-traveled, but still somewhat naïve, twenty-one-year-old man. I'd traveled up and down the East Coast and flown to the Pacific Northwest and back, with stops in Vietnam, Japan, and Thailand in between. But I was still naïve about many things.

* * *

After arriving in the Nation's Capital and getting a decent night's sleep, I decided to grab a quick bite to eat somewhere within walking distance of the hotel before getting ready for my long planned trip to the Pentagon. As I walked down the block, it soon struck me that I was different, different from everyone who I passed by, met, or spoke with. I was the only person that morning, in this part of Washington, DC, who was of European descent! Man, how naïve was that? And yet, most of the young men called upon to fight for and defend our great country—no matter were it World War II, Korea, Vietnam, or some other unheard of trouble spot—were probably no different than me. We all served our country in time of need before becoming worldly enough to learn about life or take on the responsibility of raising a family, or simply learning life's lessons on our own.

The Pentagon was intimidating at least and confusing at best. I was unfortunately cursed with a lousy sense of direction, but after asking a few staffers how to get to where I needed to report, I found myself saluting an Army officer with more brass on his jacket than I'd seen since driving Colonel Kendrick to an important high level officers' meeting.

"Where are your medals, soldier?" he barked.

"I haven't had time to unpack yet, Sir," I nervously replied. "We were given new uniforms when they processed us through Fort Lewis after returning from Vietnam, Sir."

I was relieved when he told me to sit while he went through my records. I knew I had received a number of glowing endorsements and recommendations since boot camp. I had taken on a number of leadership roles, some thrust upon me and others by volunteering, and my crowning achievement of having graduated at the top of my basic training class was something I worked hard for and was most proud of. The recommendations from Captain Day and Colonel Kendrick were nothing to take lightly either. Somehow, this shy kid who would sit in the back of the classroom and hide throughout his high school years had matured into a confident, young soldier.

"Impressive." was the first word uttered by the officer. "How would you like a position here at the Pentagon? There'll be many administrative responsibilities and long hours involved."

Somehow the U.S. Army had managed to do the impossible. They had transformed a college accounting major into an administrative specialist who was now being considered for a Pentagon assignment as a paper shuffler.

It was an intriguing offer indeed, but after a year of typing, handling TCMDs (Transportation Control and Movement Documents), and handing out and reviewing paperwork for twelve-hour days, the last thing I wanted to do was another year or more of this. I merely wanted some simple typical Army work that would have me stationed as close to home as possible.

"Sir, in all honesty, that's exactly what I've been doing for the past twelve months," I answered. "I'd just like to change my orders from Fort Benning to somewhere closer to home." What's the worst he could say? I knew he wasn't going to send me back to Vietnam.

"Fine," was his answer, "I'm assigning you to Aberdeen Proving Ground—it's near Baltimore. Welcome home, soldier."

I decided to take the train home from DC to Providence, and planned to grab a taxi when I got there. Since I was processed out of Cam Ranh Bay a few days before my original April 19 date, nobody would be expecting me for a couple more days. I loved to surprise Mom. I once obtained a three-day pass from Fort Jackson and flew home from South Carolina to Providence. It was my first flying experience. The arrangements weren't the best, as I had to change planes twice, and I arrived at Green Airport in Providence with a slightly stained uniform from not quite reaching the air sickness bag in time, but the look on Mom's face when I walked through the door was worth every inconvenience.

This was going to be the mother of all surprises. Pop would still be at work, and Kathy and Debbie would still be in school.

I had a few hours to just kick back and think while the train chugged northward to my home. The euphoria was still there and building inside me as I contemplated the past few years of my life. I thought of all that time I spent working full-time while I was still in high school; I even worked the local car wash for some under-the-table money on Saturdays and Sunday mornings. My social life consisted of the weekly high school dance at St. Rafael's Academy on Saturday night, and the rare spontaneous Sunday afternoon date with one of my female friends. Sometimes Bobby Taylor brought his girlfriend Denise and her sister Eileen—and my ex-girlfriend—over for the occasional make-out and argue session. That's probably why we were exes, because our chemistry was almost always out of sync.

Bobby was now doing his infantry training. His brother Mike was still in Nam; the third young man from our Bishop's Bend neighborhood to be sent over. Mike, Charlie, Paul, and I had all enlisted at the same time on the Army's "buddy system" (where they promised to keep friends together, through basic training at least). Mike was in the same financial and educational predicament as I was. We talked for hours between our freshman and sophomore years at Providence College about the financial pressure and the military draft that would surely gobble us up if we ever lost our college deferments.

I would never forget one particular moment in time when a group of us took a break from a marathon basketball game at the playground. We were sitting on the embankment next to the court, just talking about Vietnam, the Army, college, girls, and whatever other thoughts passed through our minds. Mike and I had decided to join the Army. We had each opted out of PC, mainly to "get it over with," rather than apply for student loans. Vietnam would forever be on the horizon; the endless war that was taking so many young men half way around the globe to fight in some place none of us knew much about or understood.

Charlie Hine was a recent graduate of Tolman High with no plans for the future, and Paul was just seventeen and clueless. Paul always seemed to tag along, even when we wished he hadn't. Charlie and Paul decided they wanted to enlist with us on the buddy system. Bobby was enjoying life after high school; an extremely active social life that began when he and Denise temporarily broke up included being the first one of our group of pre-sexual revolution teenage boys to "lose his virginity."

"I'll take my chances with the draft," Bobby proclaimed. His logic: "I'm having too good a time. Two years as a draftee are a lot shorter than a three year enlistment." I'll always remember those words…

Bobby Taylor was the runt of our group, but the toughest. He backed down from no one. He wasn't afraid. He even considered joining the Marines, as his big brother Billy had.

Mike, Charlie, Paul, and myself played a "what if" sort of game that I suggested. Mike grabbed a few sticks. Two were long, one medium in length, and one short straw. The game was simple enough. A Vietnam scenario where two of us would return unharmed, one badly injured, and the person unlucky enough to draw the short straw would be killed in action. I had no idea how prophetically close this stupid game would play out, but I wished to hell that we hadn't done it. Fortunately for the guy who drew the short straw, he was blessed with good luck, rather than bad.

* * *

As the train snaked up into New England and closer to home, I wondered who was still in the neighborhood to hang around with on my thirty day post-Vietnam leave. Each hour that passed only served to put thoughts of Vietnam further and further behind me, and bring to the forefront my current situation. I was finally free to do whatever I wanted. I was now old enough to walk into a bar, stay out as late as I wanted, and do whatever I pleased—as long as it didn't conflict with Mom and Pop's house rules. A good son respected his parent's wishes, as long as he lived under their roof. I wanted to be as good a son as possible.

As I thought about the guys, I realized hardly anyone from my group was still in Bishop's Bend. Charlie had done a stupid thing in Advanced Individual Training (AIT). He decided to go airborne with the 82nd Airborne Division. As things turned out, he pulled a leg muscle, never got into the Airborne, and eventually received the best duty possible—in Germany.

That's where I was supposed to be stationed. I learned that after AIT in a "you didn't hear this from me" conversation with one of the young sergeants who worked in the Orderly Room days before our official orders were handed out. I'd made my parents intensely relieved when I gave them the good news. I actually held my orders in my hands, but sensed by the drill sergeant's sarcastic words and grin that this euphoric high would be short-lived.

Within minutes he explained, in a cheerful way—as though he was happy to burst our bubbles—"Those of you who thought you lucked out and were going to Germany, guess again." The Tet Offensive, which surprised everyone from Vietnam to the Pentagon, changed my entire future. Those of us lucky enough to have received orders for Germany were now officially "on hold," waiting for further orders. One guess was all we needed as to where Uncle Sam most needed us. Calling my parents with the bad news even managed to eclipse having to fess up and tell them I had dropped out of college to join the Army a mere five months before.

My cousin, "Regular Richie," was also in the Army. We called him that after he surprised his mother by asking for permission to stay at Mike and Bobby's house for the extended penny ante poker game during our childhood. My Aunt Steffi had probably never heard her son's voice over the phone before, and when she asked, "Richie who," my cousin replied, "Regular Richie!" Richard Tumidajski would be referred to by his new moniker, "Regular Richie" for years to come.

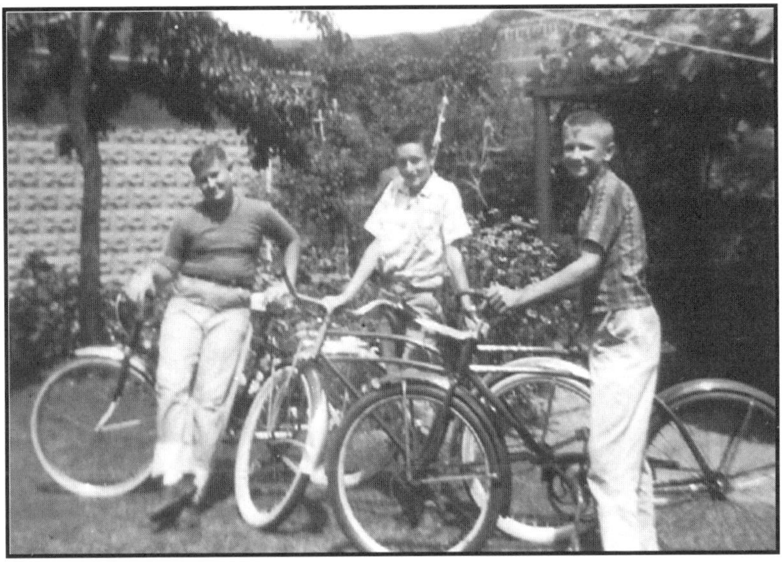

Cousins Charlie, Jack, and Richie (Joe absent from the usual quartet)
"Baby Boomers" enjoying the innocence of being a kid
Early-60s

Cousins Rich, Joe Tumidajski, and Charlie Tempinski functioned as surrogate brothers. Since Rich and Charlie (like myself) had no brothers, and Joe's brother Kenny was six years his junior, the four of us spent significant time together in our formative years. The fact that we all grew up on either Lauder Avenue or neighboring Fortin Avenue, kept us geographically close, as well.

Joe was away at the University of Rhode Island. Charlie, who we affectionately dubbed "CT" when we were kids, was actually a second cousin, but every bit a brother to me. CT was finishing his senior year at Tolman High School while preparing for college. Who was still at home? My good friend and sports rival, Pat McKenna was commuting to Bryant College in Providence, and Jimmy Kaszyk was away at Southeastern Massachusetts University. I heard that Paul, who enlisted with us back in October '67 after getting his parents to sign a waiver so their seventeen-year-old tag-along son could join the Army with us, had eventually cried his way out once we were separated—and he had learned exactly what a Combat Engineer did for Uncle Sam. I was sure to get his exaggerated side of the story when I got home.

And home I'd soon be, as the train pulled into Providence. I couldn't wait to see everyone and how much they'd changed.

Especially Debbie and David. But most of all, I couldn't wait to see the look on Mom's face.

I asked the cab driver to drop me off at the corner. I could carry my duffel bag easily to the house. Rounding the corner, it was impossible not to see our little house, since Pop let me pick the color a few years back when we painted it from standard white (and we did have a white picket fence) to this in-your-face Aztec Gold. It definitely caught the neighbors by surprise, and some of the family, including Mom, had to warm up to the color.

I wouldn't be officially home until I walked through the side door, but each step brought me closer to my objective. When Mom saw me walk in she was practically speechless.

"Jack," was all she said, as she held me tighter than any other time in my life. Mom's year of worrying was over—her son was home.

As the reality began to settle in, she told me all the latest family news. Mom always wrote, so I was pretty much up-to-date with everything, but she refreshed my memory. Then my sisters came home, followed by Pop, and the reunion was on. Finally.

It didn't take as long as I expected to get settled in at home. Seeing all my civilian clothes again brought back forgotten memories of who I was, or had been, up until eighteen months before. That unbelievable feeling made me realize I had never been as high on life as I was now. *I'm on top of the world*, I kept telling myself over and over. I didn't know how long this feeling would last, but after a couple of depressing years leading up to my time served with the Army, and time in a hostile environment, this feeling was beyond belief.

After re-acquainting myself with Mom, Pop, Kathy, Debbie, Diane, and little David, the phone started ringing—and kept ringing—through the weekend and into the beginning of my first full week home. I was Mr. Popular, a neighborhood "hero." Both Jimmy and Paul made the same offer: "My girlfriend has a friend we think you'd like. Are you interested in a double date next Saturday night?" Could it get any better than this?

My first night on the town was with my good friend Pat McKenna. Pat and I were very competitive, anything from chess to selecting the guys we wanted in our pickup basketball games made us rivals. We were two of Bishop's Bend's best athletes. We almost always served as our team's captains. Basketball was the number-one pastime for us before we discovered girls. We had a sort of Wilt Chamberlain/Bill Russell rivalry. I was the better shooter and scorer, and Pat was the better rebounder and defender. We had some epic battles sometimes, just playing one-on-one.

My parents weren't too thrilled about my driving the family car since I was no longer covered under their insurance policy. Since Mom worried about everything, she wasn't all that supportive of my plan to buy my dream car, the '69 canary yellow Camaro, either. She worried I might overdo weekend trips driving home from my new duty assignment near Baltimore. But that was the whole point of my Pentagon trip—to be stationed closer to home.

That night Pat and I decided to have a beer at a local tavern. The only problem was that he wasn't quite twenty-one years old yet, which didn't deter most underage college students from having a brew or two (or more) via the six pack route from the liquor store. As we walked into this dreary little establishment, it was readily visible that we were the only customers. It still felt cool being twenty one and able to drink, vote, and do all the other things adults were permitted to do. Somehow we decided Pat would order. That way, if the bartender asked for ID he'd probably ask me. Besides, Pat looked older than I did.

"How old are you?" he looked directly at Pat. "Do you have any proof that you're twenty-one?" I quickly stepped forward with my military ID, but our scheme unraveled. Not only did he refuse to serve my underage friend, but he also refused to serve me—a legal-aged soldier just back from Vietnam. It was somewhat amusing at the time, but what does a guy have to do to get a drink? I returned from Nam, after having been shot at twice while serving a country in which I couldn't vote merely five months prior. I had been too young to vote, yet I was old enough to be in a combat zone and possibly someday have my name on The Wall; that black marble memorial in D.C. that would eventually have the names of more than 58,000 boys and young men who weren't as lucky as me. Yet, despite all this, I was still deemed unworthy of a single beer.

* * *

Tuesday night. April 22, 1969. I got permission to use the family car. No Camaro yet. I picked up Pat, and rather than getting shot down by another bartender (I wasn't much of a drinker anyhow), we hung out at the local burger joint for a while. I had to get back fairly early, not only to return and park Pop's Chevy in front of that tiny Aztec gold home at 69 Lauder Avenue, but also because college boy McKenna had an exam to study for. This sucked. I had earned my thirty-day leave from Uncle Sam and hardly any of my friends were there to hang around with.

As I drove down Fortin Avenue (where most of my extended family lived), Paul was standing in front of his house. I stopped to chat briefly and tell him I was dropping Pat off and bringing the car home.

He asked, "Would you like to meet my girlfriend and talk about Saturday night?"

"Sure, I'll be right back." Finally, someone to hang around with.

Darkness had settled in as I walked from my house to his. Paul and I talked for a while in front of his house before he said, "Let's go downtown, I want to check out the shoe store on Main Street. Maybe you can meet my girlfriend after that. I'm picking her up after work."

We hopped into his Volkswagen Beetle and headed up Fortin Avenue. Paul took the turn onto Prospects Street a bit wide, and faster than he should have.

"You don't have to show off for me," I lectured him.

I figured Paul was trying to make up for his suspect military discharge by trying to be macho. Once in the shoe store, we walked around for a while until we ran into one of Benny O'Sullivan's younger sisters. (Benny, another neighborhood friend, was in the Army also, which he would make his career.) After speaking briefly with Eileen, we walked across Main Street and got back into Paul's VW. Little did I know the significance of that short walk.

As we continued up Main Street toward Columbus Avenue, a light rain fell from the sky. Shortly before reaching Newport Avenue, the rain turned to a drizzle, and rather than take a left turn onto Newport, Paul turned right. It was still much too early for Paul's girlfriend's shift at Hasbro to let out. (Hasbro was the toy factory where I worked full-time during my senior year of high school.)

As Paul drove down Newport, we passed Slater Park where we used to hang out, ice skate during the winter, and occasionally play baseball games in the Boys' Club League. This trip brought back old memories of a more innocent time in our lives.

We were approaching St. Theresa's Catholic Church (where I had been baptized, made my first communion, and confirmation), when Paul blurted out, "Watch how I can make it fishtail!" Paul immediately lost control as the Volkswagen slid toward the utility pole in the parking lot of my church. Within a split second in time, in the infinite mystery that is the universe, my life was forever changed. My only thought was—*my first accident.* Many people I knew had been in accidents, even our neighbor Mrs. Briden, although most were only fender benders. It was rare to hear news of serious accidents in quaint little Pawtucket.

I braced myself, placing my hands on the dashboard of the VW Beetle. It seemed as though Paul didn't, or couldn't, slow down. We slammed into the pole with a jolt. I remember Paul getting out and inspecting the front of his car. I couldn't move. My arms seemed to flail uncontrollably for an instant before dropping down and resting by my sides. Then my head began to slowly fall forward. I remained unable to move anything.

My chin rested on my chest as Paul shouted from in front of the vehicle, "Are you all right, Jack?"

* * *

As I lay motionless in the emergency room, I asked the attending nurse, "What's wrong with me?"

"You're probably in shock," was her reply.

"When will the doctor see me?"

"Soon" she said, as she left me alone on the hospital gurney.

A policeman came in next and asked, "What happened? How did the accident happen?"

"He lost control, and we just slid into the pole."

It never crossed my mind to give more exact details. Not only was my body numb, but so was my mind. I was scared, and my only concern was to have a doctor examine me. The policeman filled out his report and disappeared, just as the nurse had minutes earlier.

Mom came in sometime after and said, "I should have known *he* was involved," referring to Paul. Whatever negative opinion my mother had of Paul just multiplied astronomically. I can't even begin to imagine what Mom must have been going through as we waited in the emergency room. After twelve months worrying about her son in Vietnam, the relief of my return home lasted a mere five days.

My next recollection was of lying, still unable to feel or move my body, in a hospital bed. The rest of my family had gone home, but Mom was given special permission to stay with me—as if she would have left me there alone had she not been given permission. The nurse arranged for a more comfortable chair so that Mom could get some rest or sleep, as if that was even possible.

The nurse would reappear periodically with a urinal and ask if I could "void." My clothing, at least my favorite polo shirt, was removed from my body with scissors. Finally, someone was thinking this might be more than merely a patient in "shock."

There was an early morning ruckus as one of the doctors ordered someone to prepare something. He was holding x-rays.

"Who was the doctor on duty last night?" he demanded. "This man has a cervical fracture!"

He was obviously talking about me, and when he approached the bed, I asked, "Doc, what does that mean in English?"

"You have a broken neck!"

Chapter 6

The Never Ending Road to Recovery

Within an hour, holes were drilled into each side of my head and tongs were inserted. Weights were attached to the tongs in an effort to stabilize my neck. I was placed on an old wooden Foster frame. It was like being sandwiched between two stretchers. Every few hours the frame was flipped over and I would find myself being turned from my back to my stomach, and vice versa to prevent pressure sores on my now lifeless body. The weights were on some sort of swivel. I can only imagine what this contraption must have looked like, but from my vantage point I was either staring at the ceiling above or the floor below. The time spent lying on my stomach was like torture. I was totally paralyzed, and my dead weight pressed up against the frame beneath me. The straps and supports for my head and chin were the worst as the few places on my body that had any remaining feeling were soon aching from the pressure of the supports holding my head in place.

I was moved to a private room in the Intensive Care Unit (ICU) of Pawtucket Memorial Hospital. Ironically, I'd walked past the hospital many times as a youngster and teenager. It was about a mile from home, and walking was just one of the things I liked to do. I often walked over to the west side of Pawtucket either alone or with Bobby, and on occasion I walked the eight miles home after classes at Providence College.

Now, my walking consisted of sending messages from my brain to my no longer responding limbs. A popular song at that time was one by Motown soul singer Edwin Starr titled "25 Miles." That song danced in and out of my head as I lay on the Foster frame "exercising" my legs in a fruitless effort to get them to move.

It's twenty-five miles from home.
Girl, my feet are hurting mighty bad.
Now I've been walking a three day, two lonely nights.
You know that I'm mighty mad,
But I got a woman waiting for me
That's gonna make this trip worth while.
You see she's got the kind of lovin' and a kissing

A make a man go stone wild.
So I got to keep on walkin'.
I got to walk on...

I got fifteen miles to go now,
And I can hear my baby calling my name...
I got to keep on walking...
I got to walk on...

I spent countless hours alone at night spurred on by Edwin Starr's motivating words.

Visitors were allowed one at a time. Family and friends provided company and support, but it wasn't enough—not yet. I still had to make sense of everything that had happened. I'd lost that feeling of being on top of the world. I was supposed to be having a blast; an active social life with all the worries of Vietnam behind me. My mood went from euphoric to confused and depressed in a split second. I was paying the price for an idiot driver who did something stupid. I felt like the proverbial innocent man serving a life sentence for a crime he didn't commit.

I received a surprise visit from Bobby and Denise. After a year of "playing the field," as Bobby put it, he and Denise had gotten back together. Bobby had been drafted, as expected, and was headed off to boot camp. He had given Denise a Hope Chest as a symbol of his commitment to her. They were the typical made-for-each-other couple. Denise absolutely adored the freckle-faced kid with the toothy smile, while Bobby always said he would eventually get back together with the blue-eyed blonde who everyone knew was the girl he loved and respected.

After enduring seven weeks of hell and torture on this bizarre frame device designed to keep my neck immobilized, I remember fading into unconsciousness. Some type of infection had invaded my body's weakened immune system.

A phone call was made to Mom saying, "You should come to the hospital as soon as possible. We don't know if your son is going to make it." It was the first of two such calls my family would receive. I can't imagine the torment Mom went through—a year of worrying while her son was in Vietnam, the tragedy of my injury, and now being informed that I might not survive the night.

My next recollection was that of being in a regular bed, at least by hospital standards; there was no Foster frame or tongs connected to weights, but I was in isolation due to the dangerous infection. I had been given the Last Rites of the Catholic Church, and God had answered many prayers. My family gathered just outside my door. My nurses were now mostly Catholic nuns. Others would enter my room with hospital masks and gowns. I would remain here for another couple of weeks until the antibiotics drove the infection from my body and I could be transferred to the military hospital. Mom brought daily home-cooked meals and tomatoes and corn from Pop's garden in an effort to get me to eat. I had lost quite a bit of weight due to an inability to keep any food down, but even Mom's best efforts failed as my shocked system rejected even the most lovingly prepared meals from home. My paralyzed body continued to atrophy despite the best efforts of doctors, nurses, therapists, and my dedicated mother.

* * *

Chelsea Naval Hospital provided a stark contrast to my experience at Pawtucket Memorial. For one thing, the beds were aligned in a horseshoe fashion in the huge hospital ward. Many of my fellow patients were recent injuries from the ongoing war in Southeast Asia. I soon learned that four of the patients also suffered spinal cord injuries, while others suffered head injuries and had their bodies ravaged by bullets and shrapnel.

The heat of late June in the summer of '69 was at times unbearable. Despite the best efforts of the medical staff at Memorial, I had developed a huge pressure sore in my tailbone area. Once I had been taken off the Foster frame and placed in the standard hospital bed in isolation, turning my body from back to side to remove the pressure was no longer a priority, or so it seemed. I also had developed a nasty urethra fistula from the many weeks of having a Foley catheter inserted into my bladder for drainage purposes. Each problem further complicated my already compromised medical condition.

My weight had plummeted from the 152 pound high I had reached prior to going to Vietnam to a new low of 97 pounds. One cliché that is quickly learned in times like these is "no matter how bad you think you have it, just look around and you'll see someone who's got it worse than you." I did not have to look very far. Walter Fabian, the guy in the bed next to mine was one of those whose body was ravaged by shrapnel. He was in a comatose state that he was not expected to ever recover from. Fabian tipped the scales at a whopping 88 pounds.

The summer of '69 was famous for a couple historical events: Woodstock officially ushered in the era of "Free Love," while the moon landing would go down in history as one of mankind's most stunning accomplishments. I witnessed neither. I missed seeing the coverage of the lunar landing compliments of having to lay on my right side in bed with a special heat lamp focused on the gaping hole in my lower back. This summer of my own personal hell was about as far from Woodstock as my bed was from where Neil Armstrong took that "one small step for man, one giant leap for mankind."

But there were a few positive developments that summer. In addition to the pressure sore shrinking in size, two of the spinal cord injured patients literally walked out of the hospital, one paraplegic and one quadriplegic, leaving me with the added hope, no matter how remote, that one day I could do likewise. A couple of the doctors and nurses had alluded to that possibility since my injury was deemed a compression fracture and not a complete severance of the spinal cord. With each passing month, however, hope was fading. I often wondered if this was a realistic possibility or merely false hope fed to me to nourish my adjustment to the inevitability of living my life as a quadriplegic.

Another positive development took place shortly after my arrival at Chelsea Naval, a few of the patients and corpsmen (the Navy's equivalent to Army medics and those most responsible for our daily care), ordered pizza one night. Although I had no appetite and could barely eat, the smell of this nighttime snack served to open my heretofore dormant taste buds. A corpsman named Sanders offered me a slice of pizza. It was the first solid food I managed to eat and keep down. Despite the head nurse's ranting during morning rounds, the doctor was much more enthusiastic; telling her, "At least he was able to eat something."

* * *

Throughout my hospitalization, Mom would visit as often as possible, which was nearly every day. Mom and Pop and other family members would make the trip from Pawtucket to Chelsea on weekends, usually by bus. During the week, Mom would visit with my Aunt Catherine, or whoever volunteered to accompany her on the hour-long bus ride. During this time, my family formed a supportive relationship with some of the other families who visited their sons at Chelsea, but especially with Walter Fabian's family. The Fabian's were such decent, kind people, often going out of their way to make sure Mom and my other family members were taken to the most advantageous bus stops for their trip back to Pawtucket. The Fabian's held a constant prayer vigil for their son, despite being told he would never recover from his sadly vegetative state.

As the summer wore on, I began to show some progress. I was allowed once again to lie on my back during mealtimes. The therapists had provided me with a simple plastic device that would slip on my hand and have a fork or spoon inserted to help me self-feed. Since being a quad usually meant no independent hand or finger movement, this feeding device was used to help one be a bit more "independent." The first time I tried to feed myself, sitting up in bed with a hospital tray table in front of me, I was motivated by a small container of chocolate ice cream. The results were mixed. I could now move my paralyzed right arm somewhat, and was strong enough to touch my face with my hand—and that's just about what I managed to do; chocolate ice cream soon covered my chin. Within a week, however, I was feeding myself simple foods such as cereal, ice cream, and my new favorite: french fries. Although the Navy nurse would again complain that I barely touched my hospital food, the doctor was satisfied that I was, at least, eating something.

Sometime in August, about four months after my injury, I received a visit from a high ranking "lifer" (career military man). I was notified that the Army had listed me as AWOL from Fort Benning, GA. Despite having my family contact the American Red Cross, as we were instructed to do during Army orientation, somehow the Army hadn't been notified. Not only that, but Fort Benning had been axed in favor of Aberdeen Proving Ground during my Pentagon side-trip. The visit cleared up the confusion on my military status, and I would soon be eligible for transfer to a veteran's rehabilitation hospital. All I needed was a medical discharge from Uncle Sam's Army, and the unexpected visit from the high ranking sergeant would confirm I was no longer the mean, leaner than lean, fighting machine who had finished at the top of his class in basic training.

I received a bittersweet visit later that month from Mike and Bobby Taylor. Mike was finally home after putting in his year in Cu Chi, South Vietnam, while Bobby was on leave for another week before his tour of duty would begin. What must have been going through Mrs. Taylor's mind and heart, as well as the entire Taylor family's, as they welcomed one son home and prepared to say goodbye to the youngest? Mike had been awarded a Bronze Star for bravery during his tour as a simple supply clerk for his courage after being called upon to defend his unit; an act of bravery he never spoke of. Bobby was ticketed a nightmarish hell as an infantryman. I still remembered his words; “I’ll take my chances with the draft.”

I learned later that Bobby had confided in our friends, “I’m gonna come back in a pine box.” If those thoughts were in his head during the visit to see me at Chelsea, he did a good job keeping both our spirits up despite his true feelings.

As I contemplated the inevitable transfer (probably to the Spinal Cord Injury Center at West Roxbury) I was informed that the fistula at the base of my penis had reached the point that the indwelling catheter had to be removed. I was whisked away to a nearby linen closet where a doctor with an odd looking surgical tube poked a hole into my bladder through my lower abdomen just above the pubic bone. A supra pubic catheter was inserted, and the Foley catheter was removed. It happened so quickly I had no time for questions, but I would learn soon enough.

On a sunny September afternoon, the still comatose Fabian and I were shipped out of Chelsea Naval Hospital without any fanfare. The first stop by our ambulance was Jamaica Plains VA Hospital, where Fabian was to make his new home for many months to come. As expected, I was finally transferred to a spinal cord injury rehab center in West Roxbury, Massachusetts. By now, I had been paralyzed for five months; five long months with general care and minimal physical therapy—not the best scenario for a newly spinal cord injured patient.

* * *

Ward Three South would be my new home for the foreseeable future and beyond. The warden’s name was “Mother Mary,” as she was affectionately referred to by the patients. A no-nonsense but fair former Army nurse, Mary Arronson took one look at my improving lower back and ordered, “Side to side. And get this guy a Bye-Bye cushion.” (A Bye-Bye cushion, short for Bye-Bye Decubiti, was a simple inflatable rubber cushion, usually filled with air and water to weigh it down and keep it in place.) I was once again in a horseshoe shaped hospital ward; twenty-one beds and all occupied. The usual feeling of apprehension and temporary depression set in as I surveyed my new surroundings. I finally drifted off to sleep.

I was woken up at about 9:00 p.m. that night by a very inebriated Jim Toll ramming his motorized wheelchair into my bed.

"Hey rookie, new guy, take a look around. Everybody in here has a wheelchair. Did they tell you you're gonna walk someday?"

I tried to look at him, but from my position on my left side, he was behind me over my right shoulder. He was gone in a matter of minutes, but his words stayed with me for a long time.

Within a few weeks, I was transferred to an eight-bed sideward. Mother Mary thought that being in a room with younger patients, patients my own age, would boost my morale. She was right, as usual. The guys in the sideward were a mixture of Vietnam combat-injured, swimming and diving accident victims, and two others injured in auto accidents.

Ward Three North was an orthopedic ward; a sprinkling of Vietnam amputees and veterans of World War II, Korea, and some injured during peacetime. Both Wards Two North and Two South were also Spinal Cord Injury (SCI) wards, bringing the total number of SCI patients to over one hundred. While it appeared that most of the patients on Three South were older and more prone to be permanent residents or "homesteaders" of West Roxbury VA Hospital, there were a number of younger guys on the second floor. These men were the many wheeling reminders of the craziness taking place half way around the world.

Since I was still grounded (stuck in bed until my pressure sore healed completely) and most of the other guys were mobile, I'd be left alone in the sideward as soon as the *Newlywed* and *Dating Games* were over and everyone scattered off the ward to make appointments or look for something to fill the time. Sometimes there would be two or three TVs left on the ABC network and, like a few others, soon I was watching (or listening to, depending on my position in bed) *All My Children*, *General Hospital*, and *One Life To Live*.

As I settled into my new home and daily routine, I began making new friends. Stuttering Vinnie Nash was grounded for a while, so we got to communicate as best we could by shouting across the width of a few hospital beds. When Vinnie was up in his chair, he'd stop by and talk. Earl Annis, dubbed "Big Earl from Boston" by the guys because of his 6'5" stance and 260 pounds, was kind of an outcast from the core group of paraplegics on our ward who were mostly combat-injured Marines. Earl was Air Force. He rolled his car down in Florida attempting to make a ninety-degree turn at too high a rate of speed, or so he confessed. Earl would stop by to talk knowing that he had a captive audience—me. It was helpful to make new friends, especially since I'd been in bed for over five months.

About the only advantage to being grounded was that young female volunteers would often stop by to chat. Considering the circumstances, this was as close to a social life as I could expect. Many of these girls had brothers or friends in the military, some serving in Vietnam. Every weeknight one or two young women would help the nursing staff by refilling water pitchers, helping some of those more severely disabled with a nighttime snack, or merely pulling up a chair for a visit. They also would light an occasional cigarette or two for the patients.

I had started smoking again; a habit I picked up while stationed in Vietnam. Every morning, the lady pushing the canteen cart would stop by each room peddling everything from shampoo to cigarettes. At least we got the smokes at a reduced rate.

One of the volunteers who befriended me confided what they were told during their orientation from the recreation director, "Not to get involved with the patients on a personal level due to their many psychological problems." This infuriated me. The same guy, who acted like a concerned friend, was saying these things about us behind our backs.

From what I witnessed between some of the active paraplegics and some of the girls, it was obvious that many simply ignored the warning. Rumors of a cute sixteen-year-old girl being fired for slipping under the sheets of one of the guys on the second floor spread through the hospital. I never saw her after that.

While Vinnie and I were grounded we met two dental technicians. After initially treating us on the ward, Lynn and her friend returned about every lunch break to spend their time with us, talking and helping with our cigarettes. I got to know Lynn fairly well. The attractive twenty-year-old blonde with a sports car and surfboard had definitely caught my attention. Unfortunately, after a few weeks of having something to look forward to, the girls finished their VA assignment. Lynn promised to write, but I never heard from her again.

* * *

Whenever I saw Jim and Terry jump out of bed and into their wheelchairs so quickly and independently when some of the paras from the second floor stopped by to make a canteen run, I imagined myself as being a "super quad"—one of those totally independent, hard working quadriplegics who required little or no assistance. That was my goal. All hope, false or otherwise, of walking again faded over the months at West Roxbury. I dedicated myself to working as hard as possible whenever my physical therapist paid his daily visits; compliments from my therapist for putting in 110% made me want to work even harder.

Family visits were a Sunday ritual. Timid driver Pop finally took the freeway for the thirty-four mile drive from Pawtucket to West Roxbury. Not bad for the man who didn't obtain a driver's license until the age of fifty-seven. My family, at least on the surface, appeared to have accepted my life's happenstance. The care I received at the VA was far superior to my previous two stops, and with my condition now stabilized, we all felt more comfortable with the ironic hand life had dealt me.

Periodic mid-week visits from the guys, as well as frequent visits from my Uncle Charlie and Aunt Kay, who lived in nearby Canton, MA, also helped boost my morale.

* * *

In October, after almost six months in bed, Mother Mary informed me that my pressure sore had healed sufficiently for me to get out of bed and into a wheelchair. Sitting up in bed was surreal. Not only did I have the balance of a wet noodle, but the room soon turned dark as my blood pressure dropped like a rock with the sudden change of position. Daily doses of Ephedrine twenty minutes before sitting up solved that problem, although low blood pressure ran in the family—my new family, simply referred to as "Quads."

Within days I was pushing myself from one end of the ward to the other. Soon I was able to push myself down to physical therapy to visit Sam and Dave; not the Sam and Dave who made the contemporary song "*Soul Man*" a chart topping hit, but close enough. My reward for my afternoon workout was a solo return trip back up to Three South. My dream of becoming a "super quad" was finally looking like a possibility.

Early in 1970, SCI Chief Dr. Talbot and Dr. Watkins, our ward doctor, paid me a visit. It was time to attempt to repair the hole in my urethra caused by my long-gone indwelling catheter. Although I never got to see for myself, the wound was best described as similar to an inch-long hole in the bottom of a straw. If this wasn't fixed, nothing was ever going to pass from my bladder out of my urethra because of the gaping hole at the base. Comments were not very encouraging. It seemed like none of the medical staff had ever seen such a large fistula.

I was assured everything would go well; the VA had spared no expense by bringing in an outside urologist, Dr. Jeffery Talbot. Dr. Jeff just happened to be the son of our well-respected SCI chief.

A three-stage urethraplasty was proposed. After two months of being up and out of bed, I was now looking at an additional couple of months on bed rest to heal from this plumbing repair trilogy. The recent progress I'd made pushing around the ward in my first wheelchair, and the accompanying benefit to my already retarded therapy program would be put on hold yet again.

Stages one and two of this unusual repair job were completed in January and mid-February. I had now been at West Roxbury VA for five months. It had been close to ten months after the night I tried to forget, and I still had another health care hurdle in front of me: stage three. Add to the mix that I was still not medically discharged from the U.S. Army (thanks to a bureaucrat snafu), and my saga just kept getting worse. I didn't even qualify as a veteran yet.

As I lay in bed one evening staring at nothing, my eyes focused on a welcome sight: my friends and cousins Rich and Joe were joined by Pat McKenna. It was unusual to receive such a late night visit, especially on a cold mid-week night as the calendar was changing February to March, but my mood quickly perked up.

"Great to see you guys," I began, as they approached my bed. I sensed that something was amiss by the lifeless expressions on their faces.

Before I had a chance to think, Rich spoke up, "Bobby's been killed."

Chapter 7

Longing for Independence

The news of Bobby's death left me emotionally numb. The reality took days to sink in. I was given permission to attend the wake and funeral by an empathetic medical staff. Stage three of my unusual medical procedure would have to wait, and any possible damage to what had already been reconstructed didn't matter. Everyone understood.

Subconsciously, perhaps, I wasn't ready to accept that my close friend was forever gone. Memories of competing in basketball, baseball, football, and all around horseplay that bonded Bobby and I were running through my head. I remembered leisurely walks down Prospect Street past Memorial Hospital on our way downtown on Saturday afternoons in hopes of meeting girls, hanging out on the West Side with the girls from St. Mary's Parish, and double dating with Denise and her sister Eileen. I had so many fond memories; memories that would last a lifetime for me, but were stolen from my friend at only twenty years of age.

My only lasting memory of Bobby's wake was the disrespectful behavior of Ray and Stevie, a couple of the neighborhood guys who preferred monkeying around with cars rather than participating in sports. I remember attempting to squeeze along one side of the narrow hallway that led to the main room of the funeral parlor with those two idiots joking around as if they were leaving an auto workshop instead of a memorial service for a fallen friend.

I remained in my brother-in-law Alan's car for the funeral service. He was able to park close enough for us to be merely a few yards behind the crowd of mourners. Family, friends, and just about everyone from Bishop's Bend came to say goodbye to the first resident of our neighborhood to give his life in service to our country since World War II.

The tragically sad and solemn funeral service was punctuated with the crackle of the twenty-one gun salute that filled the cold morning air. The finality this military tradition signaled was too much for Denise, as she collapsed and was caught by Bobby's cousin. After composing herself, Denise walked over to Alan's car. We talked for a few minutes before Denise left and a few other friends stopped by to greet me. Ironically, Denise's sister Eileen, who once told me, "If you join the Army, I'll never speak to you again," was not among them.

After returning to my all-too-familiar bed at the VA hospital, a few more days passed. I was watching the Saturday afternoon college basketball game—a game in which Notre Dame defeated the seemingly invincible UCLA Bruins—when tears began to flow from my eyes like water pouring uncontrollably from leaky faucets. Reality finally thawed my previously numb emotions. Bobby Taylor was dead.

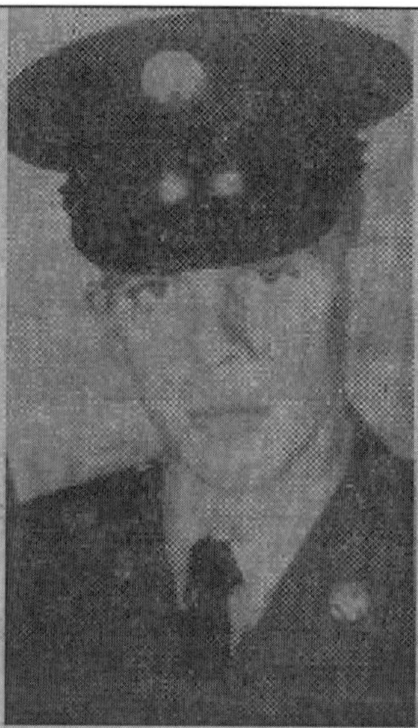

Pfc. Robert T. Taylor

Robert Taylor Of Pawtucket Dies in Action

Army Pfc. Robert T. Taylor, 20, of 33 Bishop St., Pawtucket, was killed in action in South Vietnam last Friday. He was the son of Joseph and Beatrice (Howe) Taylor.

Private Taylor, a member of the 196th Light Infantry Brigade assigned to the Central Highlands, had been in Vietnam since September. Full details of his death were not available last night.

A graduate of Tolman High School in 1967, he had worked for three years at Metallized Products Inc., Roosevelt Avenue, Central Falls. He was inducted into the Army last June.

Private Taylor, who had attended St. Teresa's Grammar School, was once a member of the Darlington Braves Little League team and the Monday Night Homemakers Lincoln Bowling Team.

Besides his parents, his survivors include four brothers, William Taylor with the Marine Corps in San Diego, Calif., John Taylor and Richard Taylor, both at home, and Sp-5 Michael with the Army in Alabama, and two sisters, Mrs. Allan Bistrick of St. Ann, Mo., and Mrs. Robert Hanley of Cumberland.

A military funeral will be held from the Cheetham Mortuary, 1012 Newport Ave., Pawtucket, with a requiem Mass in St. Teresa's Church, Newport Avenue. Burial will be in Mount St. Mary's Cemetery. Funeral arrangements will be completed when his body arrives from Saigon next week.

With the third stage of my urethraplasty completed, I was soon out of bed and back to my rehab pursuits. The anticipation of working on transfers—from my bed to my wheelchair and back, and eventually from my wheelchair to the car—had been the driving focus since Bobby's death. I was more determined than ever to succeed in becoming a super quad.

About this time, an ex-girlfriend of sorts contacted me. Sue and I had dated innocently off and on for about one year prior to my enlistment. Sue was three years younger than I, and her father was a cop, which, combined with her early curfew, probably explained why our relationship was so innocent.

Soon, Sue was a weekly visitor. I volunteered my sister Kathy to give Sue a ride whenever she came to visit. Kathy didn't seem to mind, and the two girls became fast friends.

I began receiving cards and letters of encouragement and affection on a daily basis. Whatever clerical skills Sue learned at Katherine Gibbs School, one must have been how to budget her time wisely so as to bombard a receptive veteran with everyday mail while still maintaining good grades. Along with the cards and notes from Sue came almost daily razzing from Jumping Jim the para. He was especially impressed with the picture of Sue I pasted inside of her birthday card and taped to my locker door, adding even more incentive to achieve my goal.

One Sunday afternoon, while Kathy and Sue insisted on pushing me from one end of the hospital grounds to the other, we passed an attractive young nurse who greeted me, "Hi, Jack."

Sue, who was doing the pushing at the time, replied, "He's spoken for."

* * *

With the warmer weather and my slow but steady progress, my parents and I agreed to make an addition to the family homestead at 69 Lauder Avenue. Pop's prized vegetable garden would be the victim of the extension, but Pop didn't mind—even though the son of a farmer, born in Norwich, Connecticut would have to sacrifice the soil that he enthusiastically planted seeds and seedlings in every spring since we moved there. Mom would soon have a larger house—but more importantly—her son home!

Spring was turning into summer and continued positive results from my oft-delayed plunge into spinal cord injury rehabilitation, my relationship with Sue, and groundbreaking for the addition to the house progressed. I decided that if Sue stood by me throughout the summer—resisting the temptation of going to the beach and hanging out with friends—that, in September, I would ask her to marry me.

It wasn't long until I was dealt another setback. Recent problems with profuse sweating were diagnosed as another kidney stone. Unlike my previous experience in Vietnam, this stone would require surgery.

A six-hour operation to remove pieces of stone from the large fragile one that had shattered inside my left kidney during the procedure doomed my summer. Much like the summer of '69, the summer of '70 found me on bed rest. Instead of a heat lamp focused on my lower back, another experimental procedure was ordered—a continual drip of antibiotics and saline were introduced through the (usual output) neuphostomy tube in an effort to flush these tiny fragments from my problem kidney.

Warmer weather in New England transformed the SCI patient parking lot into a weekend beer garden. With no therapy or appointments, most patients without passes to leave the hospital premises to visit family, take a day trip, or merely go anywhere, congregated there. It wasn't unusual to see a half dozen different brand names being generously shared with fellow inmates. From Narragansett to Black Label—if it was sold in the Boston area, it was consumed by someone at the West Roxbury VA "Weekend Beer Garden." Nobody from the hospital staff seemed to care; after all, beer was good for the kidneys, wasn't it?

My brief initiation to the weekend beer parties was now on hold as I was transferred to the urology ward. It was the first time I heard mention of trips West Roxbury patients had taken to Mexico—a place called Guadalajara. Loveland, Connelly, and Abe Nadel all had been there and talked of returning. Villa del Sol seemed to be where these wheelchair-bound quads and paras stayed.

At first, Sue continued to visit me weekly, but her visits soon become biweekly as the temptations of summer seduced her. It was difficult to face the fact that my girlfriend would rather hang out on the beach with friends—my friends, at that—than to visit her "spoken for" boyfriend who was laid up in a hospital bed with no shower and three weeks of facial hair awaiting her. I had the answer to my September surprise without even having to pop the question.

I managed to salvage the tail end of the summer of '70. Whenever my parents, family, or friends didn't drop by the VA to see me, I was where most of the guys hung out on the weekend. The fraternization and goofing off tended to have a therapeutic effect of sorts; probably why none of the staff cared about the alcohol consumption unless patients tried to bring their party favors into the hospital itself, which they often did.

Resuming therapy was more difficult this time. I seemed to hit a wall, one I could not break through or find a way around. How much did losing my girlfriend factor in to my stagnated recovery? What about my late start in rehab due to the various setbacks? Or had I achieved everything possible that was expected of a C6/C7 quadriplegic?

Progress on *my new house* adjacent to the family home was slow but steady. Kathy would take pictures to show me when she came to visit. Sue still visited, but not as often, and I'm not sure if her visits now had a positive or negative effect. I never told her how close we came to that big question. It was best to forget.

Winter weather slowed the progress of my "dream home." Although many of the guys who were injured about the same time that I was, and a number who came to West Roxbury after me, had already been discharged, no mention of an impending discharge was ever discussed with me. At least the construction company would have more time to build my future home to the specifications we discussed when the process began.

A routine IVP (Intravenous Pyelogram, an x-ray of the kidneys, ureters, and bladder) revealed the presence of another kidney stone in my left kidney. The doctors theorized that it probably formed from one of the tiny particles of stone that remained entrenched there despite their earlier efforts. A rather uneventful surgery was performed to remove this stone, and I was up and out of bed in eleven days.

The sound of someone opening a window in the dead of night woke me. The view from my end bed enabled me to see the entire eight-bed ward. A tall young nurse had opened it as quietly as she possibly could at the request of one of my roommates who, apparently, didn't mind the rush of the cold night air. The curtains were drawn partially around him as she reached into her left pocket and handed him a cigarette. It was of the roll-your-own variety. (The patient would later meet an untimely death, while the nurse would eventually marry another patient.)

Countdown to discharge began as I was informed that, upon completion of my new addition adjacent to the family home, I'd be a free man once again.

After twenty-three months and four days of hospitalization and rehabilitation, give or take a few hours, I was formally discharged from West Roxbury VA Hospital on my sister Diane's twenty-fourth birthday, March 26, 1971.

Returning to the newly renovated homestead was something I'd been looking forward to for many months. The year and a half spent at West Roxbury seemed like an eternity. When I thought about it—joining the Army in October '67, time served on active duty combined with almost two years of hospital/rehab time—I hadn't been a free civilian in almost three and a half years. I didn't know what the future had in store for me, but I was eager to find out.

It didn't take long. The bachelor pad I had envisioned adjacent to the existing dwelling was merely an addition. Nothing separated my part of the house from the twenty-five-by-thirty-two-foot former Aztec Gold home other than two doors; one that opened to the new hallway next to the kitchen and one that opened directly to the newly remodeled living room. Neither door had a lock. What had happened to my privacy? What about my independent living quarters? This was not how we drew up the plans so many months before.

The initial disappointment dampened the big homecoming, at least for me. Although I could access the house from the inclined driveway and ramp in the garage, there was absolutely no privacy. *Nada.*

The first few weeks at home were a non-stop visiting session. Outside of my immediate family, the vast majority of my uncles, aunts, and cousins lived within walking distance in the familiar surroundings of Bishop's Bend, not to mention all of my friends in this closely knit neighborhood. The adjustment to finally being home was facilitated by daily marathon-kitchen-table card games. As soon as someone announced that they would be leaving, another would take their place as other well-wishing visitors continued to look on and chat.

My parents had contracted a part-time caregiver for those things I was unable to tend to for myself. With an hour and a half of assistance (three mornings per week) from a former neighbor and nurse's aide named Ben, along with minimal help from Mom and Pop, I was able to get by at home. I would never ask any of my sisters for assistance, that would be too embarrassing and I didn't want to become a burden on my family. I didn't achieve super quad status, but months of rehab had allowed me to be fairly independent, at least within the confines of home.

That was the problem. After visits of well-wishers dwindled to a trickle, I asked myself over and over, "What am I gonna do with the rest of my life? What now? Create the next popular board game?" I went so far as to calculate the odds on any particular baseball player to strike-out, pop-up, ground-out (into a double play, if there was a runner on first base), hit a single, double, triple, or a home-run. I made up a formula involving dice and cards, and played the game myself a few times before getting bored with its simplicity. I gave up—just another exercise in futility.

Quiet afternoons were once again filled with watching *All My Children*, *General Hospital*, and *One Life to Live*. The soap operas that took away hours of boredom while stuck in bed at West Roxbury VA were now an addiction. After supper, which took place about 4:30 or 5:00 p.m., it was back to the boob tube for another night of TV viewing.

Daily family life consisted of having lunch with Mom. (Kathy had left the nest for her own apartment.) Pop and Debbie would join us for supper after work and school. On weekends, Kathy, Diane, and my little nephew David would stop by along with other visitors. Some of the guys might drop in during the evening, but visits were becoming less frequent.

One troubling aspect of Kathy's evening weeknight visits was that she and Sue remained close friends. I doubt if Kathy had a clue as to how difficult it was for me to see my ex-girlfriend stop by unexpectedly with my sister. My former girlfriend was now my sister's girlfriend, in a manner of speaking.

I had only been discharged from the VA for four months when I made an appointment for my first post-discharge check-up. After waiting for so long to get out of West Roxbury, I now found myself wanting to go back.

I learned that it was not unusual for individuals who spent significant time in an institutional environment to feel out of place in the "real world." I never imagined the real world would have been so cold, empty, and hopeless for me. The staff allowed me to remain at West Roxbury in order for me to tackle something I hadn't before—driver's education. It was the perfect excuse for me to climb back into the womb of familiarity that the hospital provided.

As with most other attempts at rehab, another roadblock appeared from nowhere. While doing strengthening exercises, I jarred loose yet another undetected kidney stone. Another IVP confirmed the obvious. The only surprise was that it was the right, rather than the left, kidney. The struggle began with chills and a high fever. I had to be placed on a water mat, a thin plastic mattress where cold water would be circulated under my body to keep my fever down. The nurses administered frequent alcohol baths, cold water mixed with alcohol, via constantly submerging wash cloths into this strange form of human antifreeze and wetting me down. I felt like I was in a meat locker and wanted more blankets. It was Friday night. I'd have to endure this torture over the weekend until surgery could be scheduled at the beginning of the week.

By the time it got to be the summer of '71, it felt like old times again. Vinnie was back in the hospital as well, talking about the eight months he'd just spent in Mexico. The patient's parking lot had again been transformed into a giant beer garden; I knew where I'd be as soon as I recuperated from my third kidney stone operation in a year and a half. It was as if I had never left the hospital.

"Jack, you gotta try Guadalajara," stuttered Vinnie. "You can live like a king on $500 a month. You can go just about anywhere, and if you come across any steps, just say: 'hey kid, you want to make a peso?' There's always someone around who's willing to help you out."

Vinnie's account was the most detailed of anything I'd heard about Mexico.

"As soon as I'm out of here I'm going back," he informed me. "I met this girl and we got married, but her family is trying to break us up. I gotta get back down there."

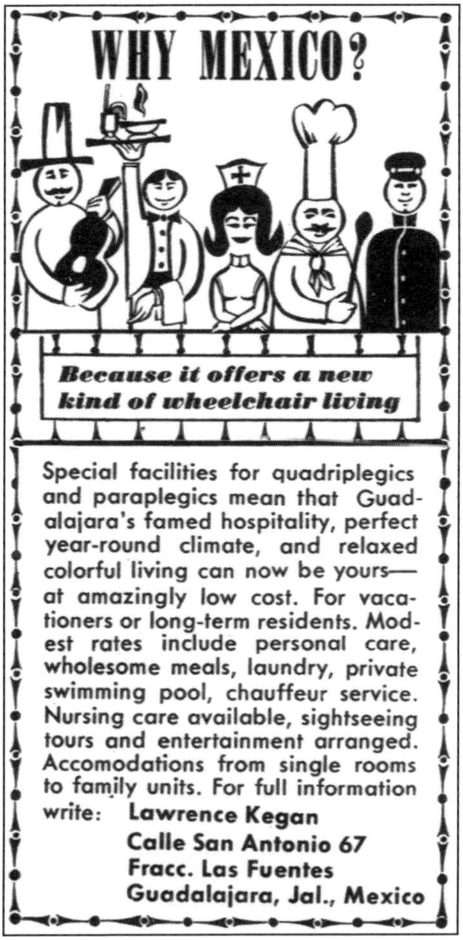
WHY MEXICO?
Because it offers a new kind of wheelchair living
Special facilities for quadriplegics and paraplegics mean that Guadalajara's famed hospitality, perfect year-round climate, and relaxed colorful living can now be yours— at amazingly low cost. For vacationers or long-term residents. Modest rates include personal care, wholesome meals, laundry, private swimming pool, chauffeur service. Nursing care available, sightseeing tours and entertainment arranged. Accomodations from single rooms to family units. For full information write: Lawrence Kegan
Calle San Antonio 67
Fracc. Las Fuentes
Guadalajara, Jal., Mexico

I wasn't sold on the idea of visiting Guadalajara, but at times it seemed like an intriguing idea. My goal now was to learn how to drive and transfer independently from wheelchair to car and back. It had been difficult, but seeing some of my fellow quads driving and getting in and out of their vehicles on their own encouraged me.

Summer faded to fall as my renewed hopes of becoming that independent quad who could do it all faded also. Again I hit that invisible wall, part physical and part psychological, that was signaling me to move on. After four months in the safe confines of my Massachusetts home-away-from-home, I left West Roxbury minus one kidney stone and up one certificate stating I'd passed Driver's Ed.

Settling in again at home wasn't such a transition this time. The daily routine was punctuated by frequent visits from Big Earl. Weather permitting; Earl would drive from his Danvers, MA wheelchair-accessible home to mine. When we weren't engaged in battle across the chessboard, Earl and I would talk about travel. We had been given a two-week pass for travel from the hospital early in '71. We had promptly taken our first airline trip as wheelchair travelers to Las Vegas. We talked often about making a second journey to "Sin City." Before I could get the words out of my mouth, my new attendant Bob readily agreed to accompany Big Earl and me to the gambling capital of the world.

* * *

After having an unprofitable stay at the Thunderbird Hotel on our first visit, Earl made reservations at the Union Plaza for our second attempt to conquer Vegas. We each paid our mutual attendant the agreed upon amount. Even though Earl was a self-sufficient paraplegic, he didn't mind sweetening the pot to assure we had an attendant to accompany us on the flight and assist me while there.

Both Earl and I, an SCI version of Laurel and Hardy because of our fat man/skinny man contrast, had gone to bed after a rather long day of traveling and gambling. Bob, however, had decided to return to the casino and the temptation that was a mere elevator's stop below.

While we slept, our attendant managed to stay up most of the night; not a difficult feat to accomplish given the allure of the casino. By morning, our fuzzy-headed helper proclaimed, "I'm going back. If you guys want to stay I'll get the number of the visiting nurses." We couldn't believe what Bob had just informed us.

"Are you sure?" I inquired. There was no way that idea would work.

How could an eagerly anticipated trip to Las Vegas turn in to such a debacle? Had Bob spent his first night in Las Vegas gambling and over-consuming "free" drinks? Did he spend his money on a call girl? Or was it some combination thereof? He never said anything other than stating he was broke after the first night. "I just want to get out of here," was the best answer he'd provide.

I felt responsible for ruining Earl's vacation. Bob was my attendant. And what about Mom? What could I possibly tell her about the newly acquired attendant's bombshell announcement? How could he possibly continue to help me after this?

I persuaded my soon-to-be-fired attendant to stay another day.

I'd called home and told Mom that Earl had some sort of medical emergency. She'd bought it. In the interim, Bob agreed to help me for another two weeks at home, giving me time to look for a replacement.

On the morning of our flight back to Boston, I decided to take a chance at roulette. I had lost $400 on our abbreviated trip and wanted one last chance to break even. I hadn't come all this way, and experienced such disappointment, to leave like this. I wanted action.

I pushed up to the quiet roulette table with the thought of playing the color red on the betting option in front of me. As I removed the four crisp $100 bills from my wallet, my thoughts drifted. I was trying to break even, right? I shifted the bills to the betting area marked "Even."

The dealer announced, "Place your bets. Any more bets?" Seeing none, he spun the black, red, and green horizontal wheel and dropped the ball. We watched it bounce to its temporary resting place.

"Number three, red," he proclaimed, as I contemplated one of the worst gambling decisions I could possibly have made. Instead of sticking to my original plan and partially salvaging something from this travel nightmare, I compounded it by second guessing myself. Instead of breaking even, I went from being behind $400 to losing $800 in seconds. My only consolation: having something else to fume about besides Bob's unexpected renege. I would fume about each for the entire flight home and thereafter.

* * *

Winter, spring, summer, fall—it didn't matter—was spent in my room watching television. Visitors would occasionally break up the daily monotony of my new life as a shut-in. After supper I would make an evening appearance in the adjacent living room to watch TV with the family. If I was "fortunate," I'd manage to get out of the house once a month. Even then, however, I'd stay in the car. I was petrified of going out in public for fear that someone I knew before my injury might see me; not as the former basketball hooping, cross-country running, Army soldier, but as "the guy in the wheelchair."

Earl and I kept in touch by phone or an infrequent visit. Our friendly chess matches fizzled as we each lost interest. One thing Big Earl never lost interest in was travel. One day he called.

"Jack, would you be interested in a trip to Hawaii in the fall?"

"I'll think about it, Earl," I said. The thought of a trip to Hawaii was intriguing, but it seemed impractical.

The summer of '72 was another disappointment. As many of my friends were enjoying summer vacation and the outdoor activities that went well with warmer weather, my routine remained the same. Occasional spur-of-the-moment invites to see a Red Sox game in Boston or to go camping in New Hampshire were made more out of politeness than practicality. Maybe if I was that "super quad"…

Depression had taken grip of my life. I was no longer the newly rehabilitated quadriplegic afraid to leave the VA hospital, but rather a seasoned shut-in afraid to go outside the house. I would lash out, from time to time, at those closest to me. Poor Mom bore the brunt of, if not all of, my frustration.

Finally, one day I picked up the phone.

"Earl, how would you like to take a trip to Mexico instead of Hawaii? We can always go to Hawaii later." While I thought about my travel buddy's earlier suggestion, Vinnie's stories of "living like a king on $500 a month" in this place called Guadalajara still lingered in my mind. What did I have to lose: sitting around all day thinking of what I could make of my life?

A reluctant Earl offered, "Let me check out a couple of places in the *Paraplegia News*."

Within weeks we were on our way to Casa de Vida Nueva in Guadalajara, Mexico. All I knew was that the guy who ran the place spoke English and we'd each have an English-speaking attendant for a measly $50 per month. While Big Earl was less than enthusiastic, I knew I had made the right decision.

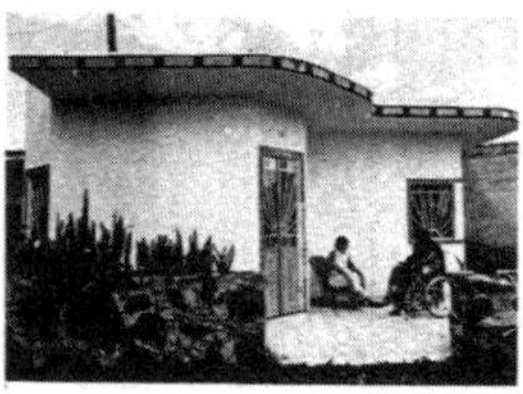

Retire or Vacation in

BEAUTIFUL GUADALAJARA at

CASA de VIDA NUEVA

A luxury resort for the retired and disabled. Monthly rates ranging from $200 - $300 include private room, 3 meals a day, medical care, laundry service, "ship-shape" clubhouse for dining and recreation, 100-ft. swimming pool, and weekly trips.

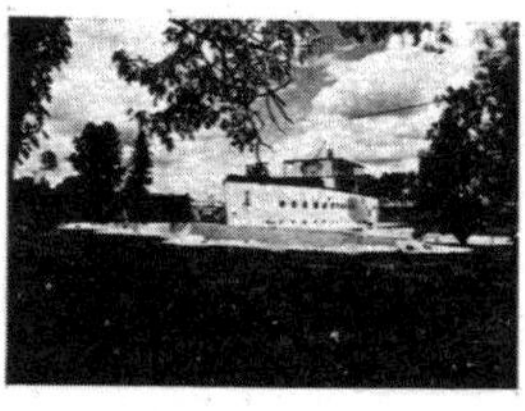

Call: (213) 439-4856 or
Write: Ralph Gambin - Mike Moore
Casa de Vida Nueva
Dr. R. Michel, #725
Guadalajara, Jalisco, Mexico

Part Three

Finding a Home South of the Border

Chapter 8

Casa de Vida Nueva

October 14, 1972. I met Earl at Boston's Logan Airport for our flight to Guadalajara. In addition to the nervousness, there was a definite excitement because I'd been waiting to check out Mexico for over a year and a half.

Earl was a mountain of a man, 6'5" and now close to 300 pounds. It was a wonder his wheelchair didn't collapse beneath him from all that weight. We made quite a pair as I only tipped the scales at about 125 pounds. Earl's little brother, Chris, would accompany us as our attendant for the flight. Like Earl, Chris was close to 6'5", but he was a slender high school basketball player.

After changing planes in New York, we were finally on our way. The Air France flight from New York to Guadalajara would take about five and a half hours. I thought a lot about what Vinnie had told me about Mexico: how a quad could get a full-time attendant for $50 a month, how accessible the city of Guadalajara was, and how one could live like a king on $500 a month.

Our destination in Guadalajara was a place called Casa de Vida Nueva, or House of New Life. We had selected this particular "gimp-camp" (as the guys so affectionately referred to them) at random from *The Paraplegia News* (*PN*), the official publication of the Paralyzed Veterans of America (PVA). There were half a dozen places in Guadalajara that regularly ran classified ads in the *PN*. They all tended to sound alike: 365 days of sunshine, skilled personal care attendants, American-style food, beautiful gardens, etc.

Earl had made the reservations reluctantly, since he had wanted to go to Hawaii. We had taken two previous trips together, both times to Las Vegas, but somehow I convinced Earl we should try Mexico. I just had to see for myself what Vinnie and some of the other guys from West Roxbury were so excited about. Little did I realize that I was about to enter into a special place in time.

* * *

At some point in the history of this intriguing Mexican city, someone cutely gave it a nickname which—at the time—seemed quite appropriate. By replacing the letter "G" with the letter "Q," Guadalajara became Quadalajara. Advertisements that appeared in the *Paraplegia News* and elsewhere made Quadalajara seem like an attractive alternative to U.S. institutional living or living as a virtual shut-in with ones' own family for newly injured quadriplegics and paraplegics—victims of auto mishaps, swimming and diving accidents, and those whose lives were permanent reminders of the horrors of war.

* * *

The sun had already begun to disappear beyond the horizon as the plane touched down at the airport. To my horror, I discovered we would have to be carried—wheelchairs and all—down a deep flight of some twenty stairs to get to Customs and Immigration on the ground floor level. Three or four uniformed men came to help us. I took a deep breath; if they could get Big Earl down those stairs, they would not have a problem with me.

After clearing customs, and getting our tourist visas, we were greeted by our driver from Casa de Vida Nueva. The man spoke English and, as we piled into his red station wagon, he and Earl began to talk about Pele, the famous Brazilian soccer player. This guy was a real soccer fan. (We soon found out that in Latin America it was "*fútbol*," not soccer—soccer is what *gringos* called it.)

The drive to Quadalajara from the airport took longer than I expected. As Earl and the driver talked about *fútbol*, I stared out the window at the darkening landscape. We passed cornfield after cornfield where adobe houses were spread out here and there, all the way into the city. My expectations began to drop as the reality was sinking in—we were in a poor, third world country.

We arrived at our vacation destination, and after that my enthusiasm was dampened even more: this place was depressing. The October night air had turned cooler as Gabino greeted us while we unloaded the station wagon. Like the driver, Gabino also spoke English; he was the head honcho in charge of directing the other attendants and running the place.

Casa de Vida Nueva was like some strange ghost town. There were a series of individual bungalows arranged in a circular shape. At one end of the property there stood a building in the shape of a boat. Rumor had it that Casa de Vida Nueva, or "the Boat" as most gringos referred to it, was a former dance hall/bordello. That might explain the group of bungalows located on the property. The silence that hung in the air added to the eerie feeling that was eating at me inside. Gabino tilted my chair back and pushed me across the grass to my quarters as Chris helped his brother. Once inside, the slender Mexican disappeared into the night, leaving us alone inside my bungalow. It was the first time Big Earl and I had had a chance to talk and compare notes. I had a feeling he wasn't very impressed either. The wall in the living room was covered with mosquitoes and a variety of other insects. Earl just shook his head, "This place is depressing." *Where had I heard those words before?*

Gabino suddenly reappeared with a short young man.

"Jose Luis is going to be your attendant," he informed me, as he began to blast the walls with some concoction of insect spray. It was the first positive thing that had happened since we safely made it down the stairs at the airport. Maybe I was judging this place a bit too prematurely.

After getting some fresh air and gazing at the stars on this cool Mexican night, it was time to turn in. There were a few voices in the darkness, and some of the bungalow's lights were still on. It had been a very long day; I had already been up for fifteen hours. I said good night to Earl and Chris as they made their way to Earl's bungalow. Chris still had to help his brother unpack and be back to the airport by midnight for his return trip to Boston.

Little did I know I was about to be hit with another series of unwanted surprises. As Gabino helped Jose Luis unpack my stuff and put me to bed, I found out that the stocky young man who was to be my attendant didn't speak a word of English, as advertised, and didn't have *any* experience.

I lay in bed watching the two Mexicans unpack my things and felt a cold draft pass over my left shoulder. The window was broken; jagged-edged glass protruded all the way around the cement wall, which served as its frame. As I turned my head to examine further, I noticed what looked like blood smeared on the flimsy, flowered curtains. I didn't want to speculate on how it got there.

Gabino listened to my complaints. How was I going to communicate with Jose Luis? What about the broken window? And this certainly wasn't a hospital bed; wasn't I paying an extra $44 a month for that?

"I'll talk to Sergio in the morning," Gabino replied.

I asked, "Who is Sergio?"

"Sergio is the lawyer who owns Casa de Vida Nueva," I was

informed.

Figures, I thought to myself. *I'm getting ripped off by a Mexican lawyer.* My roller-coaster day was headed back down again. What else could go wrong?

As Jose Luis and I tried to communicate with the few words I remembered from high school Spanish, Gabino reappeared with a list of commonly used expressions with their English translations. "*Ah, quiero un vaso de agua.*"[1] I remembered that one. As my attendant left the room, fulfilling my first request of him, Big Earl came rolling in with Chris and another man behind him, carrying bags.

"I'm getting out of here," Earl stated. "This place is a dump. I've got a taxi waiting; we still have time to make it to the airport by midnight."

"Damn it, Earl! There's no way I could possibly get dressed and packed in time," I said in frustration. Besides, I had waited a year and a half to come to Mexico. I was at least going to stay until the sun came up.

After finally drifting off to sleep, I heard a familiar, distinctive voice wake me around 2:00 a.m. I was never so glad to hear anyone's voice in my life. It was Vinnie Nash from the West Roxbury VA. His unmistakable stutter was like music to my ears.

It was only fitting that the person most instrumental in my coming to Quadalajara would be my temporary savior. Vinnie was a real character, and it wouldn't have surprised me in the least for him to be roaming the streets of Quadalajara at 2:00 a.m.

With Vinnie was his attendant, Salvador. As I watched Vinnie and Salvador communicate, I wondered how he had become so fluent in Spanish in such a short period of time—well, at least what seemed fluent to me.

I asked him if Salvador could turn me from my back onto my side. It was reassuring to know there was someone around with the experience to help me. Vinnie and I talked for a while longer. He told me he heard through the grapevine that two gringos from the Boston area would be arriving at Casa de Vida Nueva. We made plans for the next day. Vinnie and Salvador would pick me up in a taxi, and we would go to a drive-in Mexican restaurant. Finally, things had taken a turn for the better.

---

[1] Oh, I want a glass of water.

With the dawn of the day, I was assigned another personal care attendant. Armando spoke some English and would have been Earl's attendant had he stayed. Vinnie and Salvador arrived around 1:00 in the afternoon with a taxi, as promised. Salvador picked me up and carried me to the back seat of the taxi. Armando, although familiar with English, had little or no experience with quads.

Valencia Restaurant was a curious combination of old and new Mexico. You could eat curbside in your vehicle, dine on the patio, or eat indoors. But the thing that really distinguished this restaurant was the monkey cage on the sidewalk in front of the patio. On one occasion, as my attendant assisted me into the back seat of the taxi Vinnie and I had rented, the mischievous hairy primate managed to wrap his tail around the handle of my E&J and pull it up against his cage. Curious onlookers got a kick out of the show put on as my helper attempted to convince the little guy that I needed the wheelchair more than he needed his newfound toy. It took about one minute to persuade the would-be thief there was no way he could get the E&J into his cage and away from my attendant.

* * *

After five days at Casa de Vida Nueva, I met a gentleman named Charlie Gilliam. It was early Saturday afternoon, and Charlie and his attendant, Timateo, were visiting. Charlie was a former resident of this unusual place; a bald-headed ex-bartender from Tennessee who was what the rest of us quads referred to as a "blinker." Charlie had a high level injury and was virtually paralyzed from the neck down with no movement of any limbs whatsoever. Señor Gilliam was like many quads; with a happy-go-lucky personality most able-bodied people would have difficulty understanding.

It was a comfortable sunny day, typical for Quadalajara, and one of the main attractions that brought so many otherwise institutionalized veterans to this wonderful city. On the lap board where Charlie rested his arms was a copy of the *Colony Reporter*. Since this was all new to me, he asked if I would like to read it. After we chatted for a while, Charlie told me about a package deal. One of the guys was experiencing kidney problems and had to return to the States to live near a hospital facility. The rent was only five hundred pesos a month for a three bedroom house with a wheelchair accessible bathroom and one of the few residential phones available in Quadalajara in 1972. The package included the entire house full of furniture with the asking price of $1200 (which Vinnie and I agreed to split), and would be available in less than two weeks.

The following Sunday, Jack Lastor, the gentleman who had to return to the States, invited Vinnie and myself to dinner at The American Legion Hall. Big Jack, as he was called, was also a quad and a former WWII pilot. He was a tall, stocky man, although not as huge as Earl, and dwarfed his tiny wife and helper, Teresa.

What a difference a few days made. Things were taking a positive turn, and I loved this city more and more with each passing day.

Little did I know this house would be the first of a number of houses I would rent in my newly adopted Mexican home-away-from-home. After seventeen days as a resident of Casa de Vida Nueva, Vinnie and I were reunited in our new, five hundred pesos a month home; complete with furniture, telephone, and someone to share the rent with—a whopping $40 a month.

October 31, 1972, exactly five *long* years after Mike, Charlie, Paul, and I entered Uncle Sam's Army, I was embarking on a very different adventure in a very different Third World Country. The seventeen days spent at Casa de Vida Nueva would soon fade to memories. My new home was now 1715 Siete Colinas (seven hills), Colonia Independencia. One of my reasons for leaving home was to recapture my independence and never be a burden to my family. Here I was, situated on another "hill" in the colony of "independence."

* * *

October brought in the end of the monsoon season. Winter nights would get colder and colder, but the days in Quadalajara were as advertised: 365 days of sunshine, or as close to it as one could hope to find. This mile high city, 620 miles south of Laredo, Texas, was like paradise, with the notable exception that the cement block homes had no central heat. I now understood why hundreds of paralyzed and otherwise disabled wheelchair users decided to leave behind the security of shut-in and institutional living for the adventure into this city of beautiful fountains and historic cathedrals. An attraction that began in the mid-50s with its lure of sunshine, accessibility, low cost of living, pretty señoritas, and friendly southern neighbors who welcomed us gringos with open arms—at least the vast majority did—would endure throughout the '60s, '70s, and into the early-80s.

Vinnie and I soon became acquainted with some of our Mexican neighbors. The Familia Flores lived directly across the street, and the Familia Tomas lived on the south side. The north side of these strange common wall dwellings was an infirmary run for the poorest of the poor by Catholic nuns and volunteer doctors. Little Daniel Flores and La Señora de Tomas were the first to welcome and accept their newest visitors from the North.

The title *Daniel el Travieso* (the Spanish version of *Dennis the Menace*) fit this friendly *muchacho* perfectly. Whenever Vinnie and I were outside in the carport enjoying another sunny day in paradise or pushing down to the corner store, Daniel would seem to appear from nowhere, joking around and eager to help in any way. He became a good runner whenever Vinnie ran out of cigarettes, or when one of us needed something from *la tienda*. Daniel just loved to go to the store for us. Of course, a peso or so once in a while never hurt when dealing with a wide-eyed eight-year-old.

Besides Daniel, the Familia Flores was composed of two or three older brothers, an older sister, Elizabeth, and a shy younger girl they called Nena. It wasn't long before eighteen-year-old Elizabeth and her best friend, Veronica, started coming by to visit. Elizabeth had a *novio*, but Veronica didn't have a boyfriend. Veronica and I seemed to connect right away. It's not hard to communicate in any language when there's a boy/girl attraction. I didn't need Vinnie to do any translating by now. I had studied all the English/Spanish phrases from the paper Gabino had given me at Casa de Vida Nueva, and my high school Spanish seemed to come back to me even faster than before whenever this raven-haired señorita stopped by to visit and chat.

La Señora de Tomas was, outside of Vinnie himself, one of the truest characters I met on my first Quadalajara trip. She was always joking, always kidding around, and always wanting to speak English with us. La Señora's *esposo* (husband) was fluent in English, and she could more than hold her own whenever she had an opportunity to use her acquired English speaking skills with us. She was also the first person to teach me to cuss in Spanish—this from my jovial neighbor lady with two daughters of her own. Teresa was a serious medical student. Gloria was a curious little girl, who besides hanging around with shy Nena from across the street, giggled a lot and liked to show us the baby lizards she caught in their flower garden.

It didn't take Vinnie and me long to meet some of the other gringo inhabitants of Quadalajara. Bill and Gil lived up the hill. Actually, it was up the next street (Kilimanjaro), but still a steep climb from Siete Colinas. There were three poker games every week: Tuesday and Thursday were of the penny ante variety, while Saturday was the "Big Game" with table stakes/pot limit, just like the game at the Club (I would later become quite familiar with this favorite hangout). Guys would go to Bill Fausnight's house on these days to play poker and eat some of cook Margarita's American-style cooking. Bill was a retired Army mess hall sergeant, so having his willing cook whip up familiar food for only eight or so poker-playing guests was like cooking for himself alone. Bill loved getting compliments on the food he taught Margarita to prepare, especially his beef stew. It was worth a drive across town just to chip in five pesos (40¢ at the time) for that tasty dish.

Gil Turetsky was an amputee with Multiple Sclerosis. He rented a room from Bill. It was not uncommon for people to share these reasonably accessible houses. Even those of the most meager means were able to live quite well in Quadalajara by pooling their resources to pay for rent, food, utilities, and even attendant/domestic help. Gil was another happy-go-lucky guy who, after getting to know him, would make one forget he had any type of disability. He and Bill made quite an odd duo, and Gil had to hold back his poker-time laughter—especially if his landlord was losing.

Quadalajara was home to many, but the vast majority of wheelchair-bound gringos were quadriplegic and paraplegic veterans from both wartime and peacetime. Close to a hundred veterans from World War II, Korea, and Vietnam, as well as many who served their country ready to sacrifice if called upon, belonged to the Club. The Club was just how everyone referred to the gathering point for The Mexico Chapter, Paralyzed Veterans of America (PVA). The Mexico PVA was, at that time, one of only two officially established chapters of the PVA's thirty-three chapters located outside the country, the other being in Puerto Rico. Founded and nationally chartered in June 1964, the Mexico PVA was one of the most active and influential veteran's service organizations in Quadalajara, rivaled only by its better known cousin, the American Legion.

* * *

Although it took Vinnie and I a while to get settled, and for me to feel like part of the American community, we finally made our way out to Ciudad Granja and the Club. The taxi ride went smoothly enough until we reached the *La Granja* (or farm). Our driver had never been to the PVA Clubhouse before, and following Vinnie's directions didn't help. Quadalajara seemed to disappear behind us as we trampled our way over dusty, bumpy dirt paths bordered on either side by wire fences to keep the animals in and intruders out. I hadn't seen anything remotely like this since my first night's ride into the city from the Quadalajara airport; only this time I wasn't looking out over the landscape, but rather I was smack-dab in the middle of it. Brick shacks and small houses were everywhere. After going in circles around some of Ciudad Granja's mini-*glorietas*, we finally found ourselves bouncing down Avenita Las Palmas, the cobblestone street that led to the Club.

Vinnie had warned me about the Big Game; the same type of game of poker played on Saturday at Bill's house. He mentioned you needed about $100 just to get a seat, which was actually only $24, or three hundred pesos. As we strolled by the poker room, I glanced in. There were seven or eight men, some seriously studying their cards with black, light blue, and yellow poker chips stacked neatly or piled loosely in front of them. I had never seen anything other than the standard red, white, and blue plastic variety. I recognized Gerry and Fred from the penny ante games I'd played in up on Kilimanjaro with Bill and Gil and the guys. We continued down the hallway until we entered the back hall. It was huge; too many tables of BINGO players to count.

We settled in at one of the tables closest to the doorway. On the far end of this spacious Clubhouse was a four-foot high stage with a long, steep ramp leading up to it. The stage was set up with a BINGO cage and balls ready for the caller to bark out numbers through a microphone next to the table. We were soon approached by the most attractive Mexican señorita I'd seen since my arrival at Casa de Vida Nueva. She even made Veronica look average, and Vero was hardly unattractive. I was surprised when she spoke—her English was probably better than mine. I don't remember exactly what flirtatious comment I made, but Vinnie quickly informed me that Maria was Pete's wife. I hadn't met anyone named Pete yet, but he sure seemed to have won the lottery with this extremely attractive señora.

* * *

Christmas was rapidly approaching, and I was now settled in to the Quadalajara lifestyle many gringo newcomers fell so much in love with. There was a poker game every day of the week. If not at the Club or Bill's house, someone had a game going on somewhere. There were restaurants everywhere in and out of town, and a cheap taxi ride could get you to one whenever the need or desire arose. For Vinnie and I, this was just about every day that we didn't eat at Bill's or the Club.

Quadalajara, like most large cities (second only in population within Mexico to Mexico City itself), also had its nightlife. The nightlife activities many young men—finally out of a hospital, rehab center, or shut-in situation (which, in my case, was "only" three and a half years)—enjoyed most were that of the old wine, women, and song variety. I'd already been to a few cantinas, or dance halls, within wheelchair pushing distance of the Boat, as well as those downtown close to *La Plaza de Los Mariachis* (Mariachi Square). Some were clubs and some were nothing more than bordellos, while still others were populated with girls willing to leave with the right customer for the right price. Being a gringo with dollars only served to attract more female attention.

In late December, I was forced to alter my active Quadalajara lifestyle. All those days of basking in the sun and playing poker, coupled with the ever-tempting nightlife and staying up later than my body was accustomed to, had finally taken their toll. I was developing a menacing red area on my backside that I knew could spell serious trouble. I had been fortunate up until that time, except for the initial bedsore on my tailbone, to have avoided one of the pitfalls of paralysis: developing a decubitus ulcer. The thought of those five long months I had to remain in bed, five months that set my rehab back and led to some of my other initial health concerns, was enough. I'd have to stay in bed and keep pressure off that area. But how? I couldn't imagine being in the back bedroom alone while there was an adventure a day just outside my front door.

Daily visits from Veronica were the best therapy for this gringo. I don't know if she completely understood that she was helping me just by visiting, but she would sit on the side of my bed and keep me company. That meant a lot to me. Vero and Elizabeth were into selling Avon-like products to residents of Colonia Independencia within walking distance of their homes. I received my first Christmas present from Veronica, a fancy bottle of cologne. I hadn't even thought about Christmas in Quadalajara, or of getting something for my favorite señorita. I was bored and frustrated and had made a January 20 reservation to fly back home. The lonely hours by myself made me realize I missed my family. Hopefully, the trouble spot on my bottom would be healthy enough for the return flight to Rhode Island and bed-rest at home.

The relationship with Veronica was moving slower than I expected. Although she seemed quite comfortable with her first American boyfriend—if that's what I was—and continually sat closer to me in bed, a hug when she arrived and another when she left was the extent of our intimacy. I thought about trying to steal a kiss, but I respected my first "Mexican girlfriend." My gut instinct was that she wasn't ready. I knew Mexican customs dictated that good girls didn't, and I had never met any of Vero's family, with the exception of her sister, America. Was there a protective older brother or two who wouldn't appreciate such a relationship? Was she warned by family members not to get too close to me? Maybe some family members were aware that many of us frequented Quadalajara's night spots. Maybe Veronica didn't trust me. After all, I was leaving for the States soon, and she may have wondered if I would return.

As January 20 approached, I was ready to get out of bed and give my improving backside a test. A simple change of cushions, from the easy-to-transfer from foam, to the unsteady water cushion Mother Mary first introduced me to on day one in the West Roxbury VA, was all I needed. Within a week of my departure date, I was almost completely healed. Although I now needed more assistance getting in and out of bed, at least my thoughts of another extended stay on bed-rest or in the rehab facility had vanished with it.

About the time of my newly regained freedom, I seemed to have lost Veronica, as her visits were becoming less frequent. Somehow, the tradeoff didn't bother me. I preferred getting out and about town more than ever, if that was possible, especially after spending a couple of weeks in bed. And I met the perfect person to help jump-start my activities: Joe Anderson. I knew Joe from the poker games at Bill's house and the PVA. He was a retired photographer from Omaha who still kept his studio open years after first arriving in Quadalajara in the mid-60s. He injured himself while swimming underwater in a Nebraska lake. The cloudy water deceived Joe with a submerged log lying in wait as he held his breath for an underwater swimming attempt to break a personal record. Joe's underwater mishap left him an incomplete quad. He was still able to stand and, while his left side was much like that of a stroke victim, Joe was lucky to have maintained almost normal use of his right side and some convenient internal body functions (like a few other quadriplegics I'd met). After Joe lost his lawsuit, he met and married an attractive telephone operator, who he sweet-talked into a date, never mentioning the fact he was disabled. Confident Joe seemed to get all the women he went after.

(Joe's American wife soon tired of Quadalajara, and a handshake divorce pretty much ended that marriage after Joe decided to make this interesting city his winter home.)

One sunny Quadalajara day, Joe stopped by the house with an attractive Mexican girl named Alida and her two-year-old son. For Vinnie, it was instant love. Vinnie immediately let Joe know he'd hire the job-seeking young lady. After a lengthy conversation in Joe's Oldsmobile, Alida stayed behind to talk with Vinnie, while my attendant and I hopped into Joe's car.

"She really wanted to work for you," Joe informed me. "She said that you were *guapo* (handsome), and did not want anything to do with Vicente." *Must have been my hippie long hair*, I thought. "She liked your long hair," he followed.

"Can we run down a few blocks? I want to drive by Veronica's house," I asked.

Elizabeth had told me where Veronica lived, and I was anxious to take a quick look for myself. As we approached the address, there was a young woman standing by the front gate. Since I'd met America once before, I was comfortable talking to her.

"*¿Hola, està tu hermana aquí?*"[2]

"*No, se fué con un primo,*"[3] Vero's sister informed me.

I remember Veronica mentioning something about her cousin a week or two before. As Joe was turning left back up toward Siete Colinas, I spotted something that took me aback. There was my Veronica embracing and kissing some guy under a tree. *Some cousin*, I thought. *What a friendly family.* I don't know if I was more shocked, jealous, or angry, but it certainly explained Veronica's reluctance to get closer.

Joe laughed at my surprise, "All these Mexican girls are alike; they're jealous as hell, but always have a novio waiting on the corner."

While Vinnie was making, or trying to make, friends with Alida, Joe and I were establishing our own rapport.

"Any idea when you'll be back, Jack? I'm leaving for Nebraska in April for six months. If you want to rent out my place while I'm gone, the rent is dirt cheap; only nine hundred pesos per month."

"I'll probably be back, Joe, but I have no idea how long I'll stay in Rhode Island." I didn't bother to tell Joe I was only paying $20 per month, splitting the five hundred peso rent with Vinnie; 900 pesos

---

[2] Hi, is your sister here?

[3] No, she left with a cousin.

was $72, but still quite reasonable for a three bedroom house in 1973.

After driving around Quadalajara in the front seat of a roomy American automobile, as opposed to my usual seat in the back of a taxi, I had Anderson drop me off at the house as Alida was waiting for her ride with Joe.

"I'm gonna hire that girl," Vinnie gleefully stuttered. I was leaving in a few days, so Vinnie's announcement meant little. My mind was still on what I witnessed earlier under that tree.

The next day Vinnie's attendant Rafael offered us a joint from his pocket. Rafael had replaced Salvador after he and Vinnie had a falling out, Armando had a difficult time staying sober and lasted less than a week after the move to Siete Colinas. Vinnie simply raided Casa de Vida Nueva, first for Sergio E. who replaced Armando, then for Rafael.

It was mid-afternoon and the four of us were seated at the kitchen table discussing my upcoming trip back to Rhode Island. Rafael was to accompany me, while Sergio E. was to help Vinnie until we returned.

My only experience with marijuana was when Lee showed me how to smoke it in Bangkok. Rafael handed his joint to Sergio E. who lit it and took the first hit. It was now my turn. Inhale, hold it in, and then exhale. Vinnie passed, which surprised me, and Rafael also passed, which surprised me even more.

Within a few minutes my head was all messed up. I seemed to be seeing double, or triple. Sergio E. took off running up the street, and Rafael was acting suspiciously. Soon a young doctor appeared from the clinic next door. He began asking me questions and examining me. Someone—I don't know if it was Vinnie, Rafael, or myself—told him that I had taken valium and had a few beers. This was true, I had taken my prescribed 5 mg of valium at 2 p.m., and I had drank a beer or two, but the doctor heard no mention of the suspicious funny cigarette that came from Rafael's pocket.

The fuzzy feeling seemed to last for a couple of days. I later learned that a friend of Rafael's had given him the suspect marijuana. Rafael confessed that his friend had laced the joint with a white powder. Recounting the story sometime later, I was told that the powder was probably angel dust.

It didn't matter to me what the substance was, I made a promise to God that if he cleared my head I would never smoke pot again, much less use any other illegal substance. It was an easy promise to keep. My brief experimentation with marijuana was history. The question of whether to blame Rafael, or his friend—or to thank them—was irrelevant. It was the best thing that could have happened to me.

I was still feeling fuzzyheaded the following day, but I was improving. La Señora de Tomas came over to talk with us outside in the carport. She'd hardly stopped by lately; maybe because of my time stuck in the house, or maybe because she knew that I'd rather talk to Veronica? Maybe it was improper for a married woman, no matter how friendly our conversations in front of the house were, to visit someone in his bedroom? She already knew about Veronica and her "cousin."

The always jovial neighbor lady then inquired, "How old did Veronica say she was?"

I had never asked, assuming she was about Elizabeth's age.

"*Tiene catorce años*," she informed me.

I had been flirting with a fourteen-year-old girl! I was again stunned. I actually wanted to kiss this "innocent" señorita who was ten years younger than me. Maybe it *was* time to leave Quadalajara.

"Before you leave, Jack, I want to tell you both something. I may not be here when you return," she stated in a somber tone. "The doctors told me I don't have much time to live. I have cancer."

Chapter 9

Maria, Maria

The flight back to Rhode Island began uneventfully. Rafael was eagerly anticipating this adventure. Sergio E. stayed behind to assist Vinnie. This switch of helpers was probably best for all four of us, at least temporarily.

Rafael had no trouble getting a passport, and I had no problem obtaining a tourist visa for him from Guadalajara's United States Consulate. On the way to the airport, my formerly excited travel companion asked nervously, "*¿Qué tan seguido caen aviones?*"[4] I assured Rafael that planes don't just "fall out of the sky," and that air travel was probably the safest mode of transportation to get someone to their destination, but he wasn't convinced. The closer we got to the airport and the flight itself, the more nervous he became.

As the flight from Quadalajara to Houston was taking off, I observed my usual ritual; I braced myself, closed my eyes, and prayed to God to protect us all on our journey through earth's sky blue heavens. Rafael was not the only nervous traveler. When I opened my eyes, to my amazement, my Mexican friend was looking out the window like some wide-eyed child on his first trip to Disneyland.

The Houston airport was huge and confusing. We had to take a shuttle from the terminal where we arrived to another for our continuing flight into Boston's Logan Airport. It was then that I learned—to my shock and dismay—that we seemed to have a small problem.

"This flight is no longer in existence," explained the gentleman at the ticket counter. "It was discontinued two weeks ago."

"*¡Dos semanas!*" exclaimed Rafael.

Apparently, what little English he had studied before the trip had paid off, but the poor young Mexican thought the agent was explaining that we would have to wait in the airport for two weeks before another flight. After some reassurance and an exchange of tickets, we were finally on our way home—home sweet home for me and another couple of months in unfamiliar surroundings for the young

---

[4] How often do planes crash?

man from Mexico City.

The four-hour flight from Houston to Boston gave me a chance to get better acquainted with my new helper. Outside of the fact that Rafael was from El Distrito Federal (Mexico City), I knew very little about Vinnie's helper of the past month.

"*Había una muchacha bonita siempre esperando el camión*,"[5] he began, as he told me the story of how he came to Quadalajara. He told me he finally got up the courage to approach her, and seized the opportunity when a seat beside her on the bus became vacant.

Rafael was good at seizing opportunities, as he explained, "*Hicimos novios*."[6] After dating his pretty new girlfriend for a few months he got some unwelcome news. "*Me dijo que estaba embarazada*," he confided, "*tenía miedo y fui a Guadalajara con un amigo*."[7] Now I knew how this strong young Mexican lad had come to work here. He was running away from his now-pregnant girlfriend in Mexico's capital city. And, intentionally or not, was distancing himself even further by accompanying me to Rhode Island.

After the group welcome I received from my family, Mom asked quizzically, "You're not planning on going back to Mexico, are you?" I guess some mothers are reluctant to see their children leave the nest. In my case, I knew Mom was a worrier, and Mexico seemed like a different world to her. She felt like her vulnerable disabled son would be much safer living at home with the family. What she didn't realize was that a whole new world of opportunities and adventure had opened up to me like some blooming flower. It was the springtime of my life and I wanted to explore it—finally on my own.

The six week visit home only served to reinforce my decision to give Quadalajara another shot. Memories of my former routine—of watching *All My Children, General Hospital,* and *One Life to Live* on a daily basis—invaded. The two-hour break of lying down after the shows and getting back into my wheelchair for 5:00 p.m. family dinnertime was followed by more TV watching in the evening. As difficult as it was to find Veronica kissing her "cousin" under that tree, it still beat watching the damn TV. Infrequent visits from my friends, those not away at college or serving their country, occasionally broke up the all-too familiar routine, not to mention Rafael asking Kathy what

---

[5] There was a pretty girl always waiting for the bus.
[6] We became boyfriend and girlfriend.
[7] She told me that she was pregnant. I was afraid and left for Guadalajara with a friend.

certain words meant. (Vinnie could make many a sailor blush, and Rafael was now applying some of what he had learned to try to score points with my sister.)

As much as I loved my family, I missed Quadalajara even more. Besides, I had just barely left home after eleven straight months of living the life of a shut-in. I knew there was more out there waiting for me, and Mexico was where I wanted to experience it. By early March 1973, I was once again taking a journey into uncertainty, but this time I embraced it wholeheartedly.

* * *

Returning to Quadalajara to find my mattress reeking from the smell of urine marked a turning point in my relationship with Vinnie. The guy most responsible for influencing my decision to check out Quadalajara, and the same guy who saved my butt that first night at Casa de Vida Nueva, had managed to convince Alida to stay with him. And stay is exactly what she did. Vinnie and Alida were now a couple. My former helper, Sergio E., was long gone, having been replaced by Alida's son, "little" Sergio, and his new puppy. Obviously one, or both, had found my bed comfortable for more than merely sleeping.

Joe Anderson came by a few days later with the offer of staying at his place for six months. It was now much more appealing. I quickly accepted, and was scheduled to move in to my temporary new home in a few weeks.

In the meantime, Rafael and I couldn't stop arguing.

"*Dame un vaso de agua,*"[8] I requested of him.

"*Dime, por favor,*"[9] he demanded.

"*Por dinero,*"[10] I reminded him. I wasn't about to say please to my paid helper every time I wanted water or needed something. Rafael agreed to stay in Quadalajara for a few days while I asked around for a new attendant. Somehow, the six weeks spent in Rhode Island had made him homesick. Or was it the letters he had received from his family? My gut instinct told me he was ready to face up to his responsibilities. Maybe he missed that attractive girl he'd first met on the bus. I never found out; in two days he was gone, never to be heard from again.

---

[8] Give me a glass of water.

[9] Say please.

[10] For money.

One advantage to living in Quadalajara, where so many quads in similar circumstances now resided, was finding help. As soon as word got out that I needed a new helper, Sergio S. appeared at the door. Although Sergio S. had little experience, he was willing to learn. He spoke perfect English, having been adopted and raised in Chicago most of his life. He was now a permanent resident of Quadalajara, married with children, and living in Ciudad Granja, just down the street from the PVA Club. The only drawback was that he was unavailable to spend the night, preferring to be with his wife and young children. Alida would assist me at night, with water and my 10:00 p.m. muscle relaxant, Valium. Sergio would come to work around 9:00 a.m. and Alida would help me to bed. This temporary arrangement was acceptable to everyone, and I'd tip Alida for her minimal assistance.

The first night with Alida as my fill-in helper made me think back to what Anderson had told me a couple of months before, "This girl thinks you're guapo. She wants to work for you." Alida re-entered my room with a glass of water wearing a sexy nightgown. Joe was a breast man. He had commented on Alida's well-developed chest earlier, "This girl is stacked like a brick ____house!" I hadn't seen that much cleavage in my life. She got as close as needed, closer, cupped her hand behind my head and gave me my medication and water. She remained hovering over me.

"*¿Necesitas algo más?*"[11] she inquired.

"*No, estoy bien, gracias,*"[12] I hesitantly replied. This awkward moment reminded me of my cute little temptress in Bangkok, with the notable exception that I would not have hesitated back then.

A few days later Vinnie confronted me, "Are you fooling around with Alida? She doesn't want to do anything with me."

Persistent Joe solved everything with his next visit. He showed up with another extremely attractive young woman. Joe's reputation of being a magnet for good-looking women was well deserved. Maria was as attractive as any girl I'd met in my short time in Mexico. She rivaled Pete's wife in that category. But there was an obvious problem—she had to be at least six months pregnant. The next day I packed my belongings and moved into Joe's house.

Maria's history with Joe dated back about a year. She was his girl, but since she had a young daughter, Anderson decided not to take her to Omaha with him for his annual April to October visit. Joe took

---

[11] Do you need anything else?

[12] No, I'm fine, thanks.

one of his former girlfriends, while Maria began dating a Mexican-American blowhard whose parents were yearly visitors to one of the local trailer parks. He soon took Maria back to California with him, stopping in Tijuana to leave the baby girl with Maria's father and stepmother. Mr. Macho's promise of marriage was as empty as his soul. Once he found out he had impregnated his bride-to-be, he brought Maria back to Quadalajara and left her to fend for herself. She eventually showed up at Joe's house looking for work and a place to stay. It was the missing piece to the puzzle. Anderson now had the perfect solution for himself, as well as his new friend from Rhode Island.

The first few days staying with Joe were awkward. Maria didn't seem comfortable with me, not even bringing a glass of water into the room. It was as if she was incapable of trusting a man. Being in her third trimester didn't help either. It was beneficial that Joe's girl, Sofia, was willing to assist me after Sergio left for the night. I first met Sofia before I flew back to Rhode Island. She was a few years older than most of the other girls, more serious, and didn't fit the usual Anderson Girl stereotype. She was divorced and had three children. Joe constantly raved about her work ethic, but they didn't seem right for each other. Maybe his experience with taking one of his former girlfriends to Nebraska the previous year had caused him to rethink his priorities? Whatever the case, it was reassuring to know that Sofia would be available until Anderson's mid-April departure date.

As the month of March wore on, I was getting accustomed to my new routine. Sergio agreed to stay at Joe's a couple nights a week. This allowed Joe to give Sofia extra time to spend with her kids before the trip to the States. The arrangement also got Joe something else he wanted—use of a male attendant to help him enjoy Quadalajara's nightlife. I didn't mind, and Anderson certainly knew Quadalajara at night as well as any. When we didn't go downtown, there were always the poker games at Bill's house and the Big Game at the Club.

I had become attracted to Maria, pregnancy and all, but she was obviously not interested. The closer I tried to get, the farther away she would move. Maria didn't seem to like the fact that Joe was emerging as my new mentor. She'd been down this road before, and wasn't interested in getting involved with any more *mujeriegos* (ladies men). Late night poker games and nights downtown were becoming the norm.

It was after one of these Friday night games at the Club that Sofia informed us, "*Maria fué al hospital para tener a su bebé.*"[13] It was around 1:00 in the morning when we pulled up to the house. Joe's usual beep on the horn was always followed by Sofia's appearing at the front door, unlocking the gate to the driveway, and helping each of us out of Anderson's Oldsmobile. It wasn't until we got into the house that it dawned on me. Friday night had given way to Saturday morning; it was now April 1st—my twenty-fifth birthday.

Within twenty-four hours, Maria had gone into labor, had her child, was discharged from the Hospital Civil (where many poor women gave birth), and returned home with her baby boy. I saw Armando for the first time on my birthday. "My girl" had just come home from the hospital on my twenty-fifth birthday with a new son—only Maria was not *my* girl.

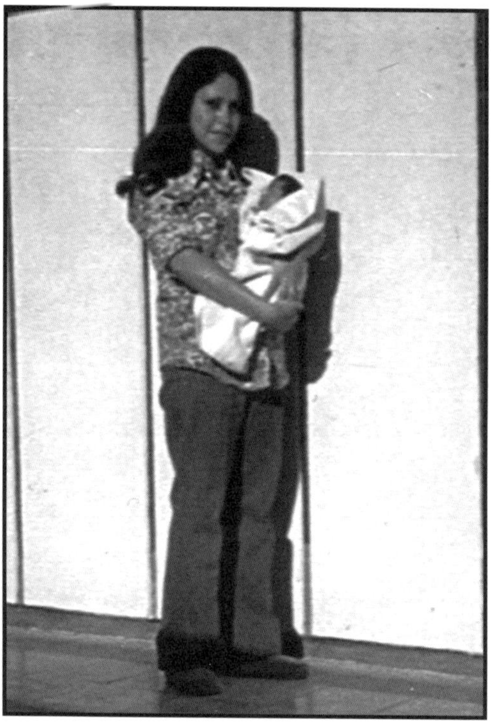

Maria with Armando in her arms
Quadalajara, May 1973

---

[13] Maria went to the hospital to have her baby.

The final weeks before Anderson's trip back to Nebraska were frantic. Joe desperately wanted to bring home a girl he met in one of the cantinas. He kept giving Sofia more time off, while Sergio didn't mind picking up a little extra cash for helping Joe on our nocturnal adventures. Joe was determined to take this girl out of the bar; one last fling before his six-month stay in Omaha. Sofia seemed oblivious to what he was up to, and Maria knew not to say anything. I had found a girl I'd liked at least well enough to bring back to the house. When we got home, the house was dark. Maria and Armando were asleep in the middle bedroom. Sergio helped us out of the car, put me to bed, and then took his customary place on the living room sofa for whatever sleep this night would allow him. All week long Joe kept thinking about this night, and wondering if he'd be able to perform. The anxiety was wearing on him as the time drew nearer. Since my date was also one of the better looking girls in the bar, Anderson and I hatched a plan.

At about 2:00 a.m. I'd find an excuse to send my girl to Joe's bedroom, while Joe was to have his girl bring me a cigarette. I didn't smoke. At the agreed upon time, I sent my companion to Joe's room. His girl appeared shortly thereafter with my cigarette, but fully clothed. The two bar girls stayed another hour or so before taking a taxi to wherever. Before they left, I could hear one of the girls talking to Maria. I didn't think much of it. Maria knew Joe quite well and probably didn't get much sleep anyway. By the time I got up and talked to him, it was early afternoon. He was quite satisfied with the two-for-one companion swap. I, on the other hand, felt somewhat cheated, but it was a stupid idea to begin with. At least Anderson could leave for home with memories of this night.

* * *

A few days after Joe and Sofia departed for Nebraska, Maria came into my room after Sergio had helped me to bed. Besides my water and medication, Maria brought with her a look of emotional vulnerability. She had always seemed indifferent toward me, but something had changed. I couldn't read her. I thought that since we were spending more time alone together in the house that maybe Maria's previous lukewarm reception was changing. She did help me in the mornings now, before Sergio came to work, and even brought Armando into the room in his tiny blue bassinette. She would also set him down beside me in bed whenever she needed to make a quick trip to the *farmacia* around the corner.

But this night was different.

"*¿Puedo sentarme?*"[14] she inquired.

"*Sí, esta bien,*"[15] I agreed. I recognized her look as one of desperation.

"*Me dijo una de las muchachas que usted le ofreció trabajo.*"[16]

"*¿Cuál muchacha?*"[17] I inquired. I had never asked any girl to work for me. Did she think I wanted to ditch her as Joe and Armando's biological father had? I had no idea what she was talking about.

"*Una de las muchachas de la noche que usted y Jose trajeron a la casa me dijo,*"[18] Maria explained. Now it all made sense. Maria was afraid I was going to replace her with one of the girls who came back to the house with Joe and me. It wasn't jealousy that was upsetting her, as I would have preferred, but the fear that yet another gringo was contemplating putting her out on the street, baby and all.

My reassurance significantly lowered Maria's apprehension and stress level. It also marked a turning point in our relationship. She appeared more relaxed around me now. Had I been afforded a new respect, or maybe it was simply Maria finally being able to trust a man again? Whatever the case, my attraction to her and fondness for both Maria and Armando grew stronger.

* * *

I was awoken one night by the sound of Mariachi music just outside my window. Apparently, the neighbor from across the street was attempting to woo his way back into his home. Sam was the quintessential mujeriego. Although married with four attractive young daughters (one of whom would blossom a few years later and go on to represent the state of Jalisco in the Miss Mexico beauty pageant), Sam was constantly being asked to leave due to his marital infidelity. This desperate attempt at romance was just his latest ploy to win back his wife's affection.

The sound of the music on this warm May night had surely caught the attention of a number of Sam's neighbors. Although many

---

[14] May I sit?

[15] Yeah, it's okay.

[16] One of the girls told me that you offered her a job.

[17] Which girl?

[18] One of the girls that you and Jose brought to the house that night told me.

young (and not so young) men in Mexico would serenade their novias in this fashion, it happened so infrequently that the intriguing blend of the string and horn instruments would at first startle and then soothe one's mood—unless someone had to get up early in the morning.

I had one of the best spots for this midnight concert. The window was already slightly open, and my bed was close enough to the wall that I was able to push the curtain aside to view the entire show. Another of the Samuel's neighbors came into my room for a closer look at the talented musicians. Maria, although somewhat sleepy, didn't seem at all annoyed and was quite interested in watching the musicians from my window.

The serenade may or may not have helped Sam temporarily win back his wife's affection, but the fallout from this romantic night did succeed in bringing two lovers together. The next morning, Maria moved into my room.

It was two months after my return to Quadalajara, and I now felt like a married man with an instant family. I had never shared my bed (for more than two nights) with anyone before. The comfort and security Maria and I felt in each other's arms was something I had never imagined possible after that night in April 1969. There weren't many days I ever thought I could feel like I did now; a complete man with his loving woman and son.

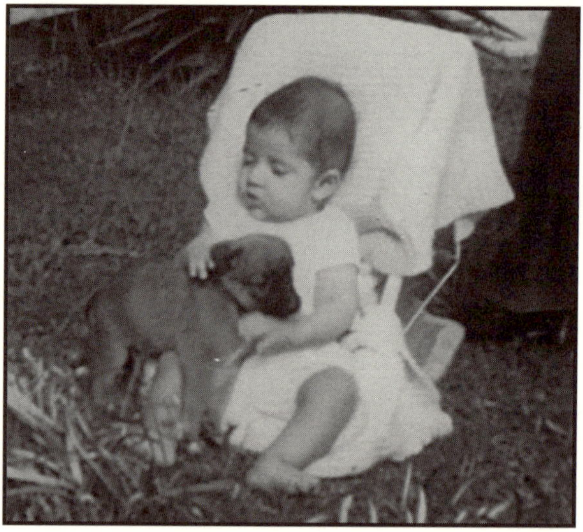

Armando with his new friend
Quadalajara, 1973

My union with Maria opened the door for Joe Anderson's best friend, Bill Christensen to move into the house. Bill had recently returned from South Dakota with his girlfriend and her baby daughter. I had met "Chris" briefly one Saturday at the poker game at Bill and Gil's place. Apparently Joe had a "Plan B" in case I turned down his house-sitting offer. Or was Chris "Plan A" and I merely "Plan B?" Anderson always seemed to have had things covered.

Chris and I hit it off right away. He was a very easy-going and decent man who was respected by everyone who knew him. Bill Christensen was truly an officer and a gentleman. Well, at least a gentleman. His officer days came to an abrupt end years earlier after a diving accident left him a quadriplegic. Lorena and Maria became fast friends as well. There was always something about babies that universally drew women closer. Anna was four months older than Armando, and the two young Mexican mothers had much to offer each other. Their constant cooing over the babies didn't faze me one bit. I was now a family man enjoying sharing Joe's house with the Christensen family.

An experienced attendant named Alberto soon occupied the now-vacant middle bedroom, once home to Maria and Armando. Chris first met Alberto when the shy Mexican man accompanied another Quadalajara veteran to Hines VA hospital where Chris received his rehab. They came to know one another through mutual friends after Chris decided to give Quadalajara a trial visit in the mid-60s. Alberto would free Lorena to concentrate more on Anna and the daily domestic chores that came with being a mother and sharing the running of the household with Maria. It also took some of the burden off Sergio, as Chris and I did about everything together. When we weren't going to the poker games or visiting other gringos, our two "families" would go places and do things together. Quadalajara's many daytime attractions were suited for family fun: parks, beer gardens, Mariachi plazas, heated pools and swimming spots, and drives to Jalisco's famous Lake Chapala. My new best friend was a more positive influence on this relative newcomer to Quadalajara. I was enjoying hanging around with the Christensen's in a totally different way than my time spent with either Vinnie or Joe, and I knew Maria was finally happy again. The realization that I was no longer Anderson's protégé served to bring us closer together as a couple, and I was as happy and fulfilled as at any time since becoming a quad.

Chapter 10

Adios, My Pretty Señorita

Over the next couple of months things began to change. Although Maria and Lorena were like inseparable sisters most of the time, they began to bicker more and more frequently. Whenever things heated up between the two, each would go to their respective corners; Lorena to tell Chris her side of whatever they were fighting about, and Maria to mine. This put a strain on my friendship with my new friend from South Dakota. The Christensen's were planning to return to Sioux Falls shortly, and the thought of having the house to my new family and me was becoming more appealing.

In addition to girls acting like sisters one day and squabbling the next, both Chris and I were hearing troubling stories about Sergio's behavior toward the girls, especially toward Lorena. He apparently was "accidentally" brushing up against them in the kitchen while Chris and I were still in bed and Alberto was busy doing other chores. Alberto had always been respectful of Maria. They had known one another since she was an Anderson Girl. The same was true of Lorena, but probably more so out of respect for Chris. I learned over time that many of the *mozos,* or helpers, resented the treatment they received from some of the Mexican women who married or dated gringos. Suddenly, women from the same lower socio-economic class felt superior due to their elevated status as wives and girlfriends of Americans. This definitely didn't sit well in Mexico's macho culture.

One particular morning, Maria and Lorena came into my room.

Lorena had a complaint, "*Sergio trató de meter su dedo en mis shorts*."[19] Maria wasn't witness to whatever happened in the kitchen earlier, but if Sergio had indeed become so bold as to attempt to slide his finger under Lorena's shorts, he was way beyond the boundary of simple horsing around. Sergio denied that anything close to that had taken place, and Chris seemed to let it slide. Whether he thought his girlfriend was exaggerating, or if he just didn't say anything because they were a few days away from returning stateside, I don't know. But I did feel uneasy and in an awkward position since Sergio worked for me. Whatever the case, things blew over quickly and everything

[19] Sergio tried to stick his finger in my shorts.

returned to normal—whatever normal was in my constantly changing stay in Quadalajara.

In a matter of a few days after Bill, Lorena, and Anna left for South Dakota, I was confronted by a more serious concern.

"*Sergio se bajó el pantalón en la cocina.*"[20] Maria confided to me. The thought that Sergio had exposed himself to Maria was disturbing, to say the least, and I needed to talk to someone before confronting Sergio when he came to work in the morning.

I was able to contact Reverend Paul Hunter in the morning and explain what had taken place. Reverend Hunter was a well-known member of Quadalajara's American community, and the unofficial chaplain of the Mexico PVA. I first met him at Casa de Vida Nueva on the same sunny Saturday I met Charlie Gilliam and got my first glimpse of *The Colony Reporter.* Reverend Hunter arrived shortly before Sergio came to work.

"Jack," advised the clergyman, "Don't be confrontational. When you feel the time is right, just thank him for having helped you and wish him well. I'm sure he'll know why you are letting him go, and probably appreciate being informed in that way rather than by any further accusations."

Sergio must have known something was amiss, and didn't seem at all surprised or upset when I thanked him for the months he had been my attendant and informed him that his services were no longer required.

The next day I hired Alberto. (It never took long to find help in Quadalajara.) I now had a full-time live-in attendant who had a mutually respectful friendship with my girlfriend.

Just another day in paradise...

* * *

It was around this time I became more acquainted with Mexico PVA President Jack Black. (He once won a 100 peso bet at the poker game by merely showing his driver's license; one of the other players didn't believe anyone could actually be named Jack Black.) Jack lived only a few blocks from Joe's house and would push himself around the corner and down the street to pop in for an impromptu visit a couple of times a week. Since I was becoming more of a regular at the Big Game, Jack tried to interest me in becoming involved with the Mexico PVA. It

---

[20] Sergio pulled down his pants in the kitchen.

was standard practice to recruit new blood in most organizations, and the Mexico Chapter PVA was no different.

When Jack learned I was a former novice bridge player, our new partnership evolved. Soon, Jack and Jack were fixtures at the Quadalajara Duplicate Bridge Club. We would be assigned the stationary end table; Jack always played the North Hand, I the South. I had never before played duplicate bridge, much less tournament competition, and I soon became hooked on this afternoon pastime. I also relented and agreed to do some odd jobs for the Club, most noticeably as part of a four man kitchen rotation. Frank Stoppiello, Ray Clifford, Jack, and I would alternate doing the shopping, running the kitchen, and collecting the cash and receipts after each night the kitchen was open. This could be as many as three or four days per week, depending on Wednesday and Friday BINGO nights mixed in with chess club, an occasional Sunday fiesta, and membership and Board of Directors meetings. We each were responsible for the entire week before handing money and receipts to the treasurer and passing the baton on to the next person. Having Alberto as my attendant was a plus since he was respected and well known by most of the guys.

Family life was becoming routine. I would get up in the afternoon, and Maria would have my meal prepared. Then it was off to the PVA or bridge club. Jack and I were bumped up from the beginners bridge tournament after a week or two, dominated in the intermediary level tournaments for another five or six weeks, and soon made it to the big time, playing against Quadalajara's best and most experienced tournament players—even masters and grand masters. The "how-to" books I had picked up when Jack and I first began playing together were paying off, as we quickly adapted to one another's game and were now placing among the leaders from time to time and earning IMPs (International Match Points).

Nights with Maria would bring comfort and intimacy. Although our previous nightly encounters had become a two or three times per week routine, we were happy and completed one another's lives. Armando continued to grow from that tiny bundle of joy that made all the women coo, to an even cuter little person who still was the center of attention whenever I brought him and his mom to BINGO at the PVA Club.

But Armando wasn't the only attraction at Friday PVA BINGO nights. One of little Daniel Flores older brothers seemed all too eager to volunteer to drive my old buddy Vinnie to BINGO—seems like Maria had a secret admirer. I never thought much about it since I trusted

Maria. It was only after Maria would visit Alida at Vinnie's house, directly across the street from La Familia Flores, on a more frequent basis that any red flags were raised. But I wasn't concerned since the Flores kid was two or three years Maria's junior and she was still as jealous as any Mexican woman could be. I wrote it off as an innocent attraction.

* * *

As Quadalajara's monsoon season was winding down and the evenings once again became chillier, most of the "snowbirds" (winter visitors) would soon be returning from their six month stateside visits. The monsoon season, which basically extended from June to October, was in fact, quite refreshing. The almost daily afternoon downpour served to cool this fascinating Mexican city from the oppressive May to early June heat. A sunny afternoon would be interrupted by a torrential rain similar to what I witnessed in Vietnam. After the clouds emptied their contents on the earth below, the sunny skies would return. Although there were some not so unexpected evening rains, it didn't take long to adjust to the season. Keeping candles in the house, though, was a must.

Among the returning "snowbirds" were Joe and Sofia. Maria wasn't thrilled with Joe's return home. And I knew why. My former mentor would surely tempt me to return to my bachelor ways. It was about this time when Maria brought up the idea of marriage. We had never spoken about a permanent commitment before, and the suggestion caught me by surprise. It was the '70s in Mexico, too, and the post-sexual revolution arrangement of "shacking up" was becoming a societal norm. The thought of marriage made me feel uneasy. I had witnessed a number of guys marry their Mexican sweethearts, only to find themselves trapped, some happily, others not, with a caregiver wife and lost freedom. The next inevitable change was to get rid of the attendant "to cut down on expenses." I was definitely not willing to give up my new-found freedom. And did I really want to marry my first Mexican girlfriend? I was still in my rookie season as a resident of Quadalajara. I wished she hadn't asked.

A few weeks after Anderson's return to Quadalajara, Joe informed me he overheard part of a phone conversation between my girl and some Mexican guy. Apparently, Maria was telling him I'd be leaving at a certain time the next day to fulfill my new responsibilities with the Mexico PVA. I didn't know if Joe, with his less-than-perfect command of the Spanish language, had understood correctly, had exaggerated what he thought he heard, or if he had heard correctly that something was indeed going on. Why would Maria be pushing the marriage thing if she was messing around? But then I thought back to what Joe had told me months earlier, that "these women were as jealous as they get while having a novio waiting around the corner," made me think back to my earlier experience with Veronica and her "cousin."

Friday night was the big BINGO night at the PVA Club. I found myself in the front room, the meeting room, talking to Tom Kirch. Tom was a fellow quad, fifteen years my senior, as were many of my close friends. Tom and I had formed a close friendship a couple of months earlier when Maria had made an emergency trip to Tijuana due to family problems, and Tom's wife, JoAnn, was visiting family back in Minnesota. This particular game night cost both of us a seat in the Big Game because we each arrived after the poker game was full. It was first come, first served. Always. The best either of us could hope for was for one of the big winners or big losers to leave early and open up a seat at the popular game. At any rate, it beat hanging out in the main hall, the BINGO room, or as some of the local populace referred to it, "El Casino" PVA.

While Maria and JoAnn were playing BINGO and socializing with the mostly female crowd, Tom and I were joined by the sister of one of the original founders of the Mexico PVA. Chuckie was Bill Bailey's sister. Bill, co-founder and first president of the Mexico Chapter in 1964, was that night's BINGO caller. Bill's wife, Maria Elena, who acted as a kind of first lady of the Club, came from a big family, and a good portion of the BINGO crowd, including the waitresses, were members of the Bailey clan.

Chuckie knew Tom from an earlier trip Tom had taken with the Baileys to visit family in Oregon and Idaho. That was back in Tom's bachelor days, and I had a feeling that the two old friends could have been more than just friends if Tom had not met and married JoAnn a couple of years earlier. Tom seemed uncomfortable with the attractive sister of one of his close friends cozying up to him while his wife was only a few rooms away. He excused himself just as break time for the diehard BINGO fanatics approached. I was left alone in the front room with the blonde gringa for a short time. Very short. Chuckie and I had yet to begin much of a conversation when Maria walked in, Armando safely in her arms. I had never seen such a jealous stare and look of betrayal as I did when Maria walked in on her man and this attractive American blonde.

In a matter of minutes I was sitting in a taxi ordering the driver to "*Sigue este taxi.*"[21] There was no time to wait for a ride home from Joe, as Maria's taxi led mine in a mad dash back to Joe's house. It was like something out of a movie; taxi chasing taxi on this memorable Quadalajara night. Upon reaching our destination, Maria's taxi pulled away from the curb, as Alberto help me out of my taxi and into the house. Maria fainted just as I entered. I had seen her do this one other time when we had had a fight and I had decided to spend the night in Joe's empty bedroom. Maria burst in about 2:00 a.m., expecting to find me with another woman. She crumpled to the floor with a thud, and Alberto was there to help her up and compose herself. This night was no different, as Alberto once again helped Maria to her feet, except that Vinnie's volunteer driver had somehow gotten into the house just before me. As he walked out he muttered to me, "*No te disgustes con ella.*"[22] Whether I was upset, which I wasn't, or simply dumbfounded by what had just transpired was none of this kid's business. But his unexpected appearance at the house just served to make a bizarre night even more so.

I had been in Quadalajara since early March, and as the year drew to a close, I had a decision to make. I wanted to return to Rhode Island to visit my family. I knew Mom liked the idea that Maria and I were a couple and that Armando completed our little family. Maybe Mom harbored the same wish as Maria that we would marry.

My other option did not include Maria or Armando. I could visit my family taking Alberto along as my attendant. I wasn't sure how long my relationship with Maria would last, but for now marriage was not in my plans. I thought constantly about what would be best, not for me and not for Maria, but for Armando. I was definitely more concerned with the eight-and-a-half-month-old boy than either his mother or myself. I also thought that maybe what would be best for Armando and Maria would be to reunite them both with Maria's daughter Elizabeth. I had only met Elizabeth briefly when Maria's father brought her to Quadalajara looking for his own daughter.

The inquisitive then two-and-a-half-year-old asked me, "*¿Tio Jass, dónde compró su bicicleta?*"[23] I guess that to a toddler, there wasn't all that much difference between a wheelchair and a bicycle. Maybe she understood that better than most grownups.

---

[21] Follow that taxi.

[22] Don't be upset with her.

[23] Uncle Jazz, where did you buy your bicycle?

I again asked Reverend Hunter to stop by the house. I was certain he would give me good counsel, even though I was aware of his reputation for playing cupid and encouraging many quads to opt for the ready-made family.

As things turned out, Reverend Hunter and I were on the same page. He pointed out that obtaining a visa for Maria and two children would be next to impossible. We agreed that reuniting her family, at some point, would be best for them all. He didn't push the ready-made family option, probably being able to read me better than I realized.

Maria made my decision even easier. Shortly before Christmas, she disappeared on her way back from visiting Alida.

I called the house and inquired of my old buddy Vinnie, "Was Maria there this afternoon?"

He hesitated and then stuttered, "Yeah, but she left around 4:00."

"Was that neighbor kid there?" I grilled my friend. Alida was talking to Vinnie in the background.

"Yeah, but he left about twenty minutes later." I knew better. That story was one of the worst stories I had ever heard. Vinnie and Alida were definitely covering something up. Neither seemed at all concerned that Maria and Armando left their house five hours earlier and hadn't returned to Joe's yet.

I waited as the hours passed, pushing back the curtain periodically or whenever I thought I heard the sound of an automobile break the nighttime silence. Around 3 a.m., a distinctively restored colorful antique Ford drove by the house. The car belonged to another of the older neighborhood boys. I couldn't see who was driving, but it was no coincidence that this particular vehicle just happened to pass by the house—twice. Once at 3:00 a.m. and again around 5:00.

Maria finally came home around 8:00.

"*Me quedé dormida en la casa de Alida*,"[24] she attempted to explain, as if I was going to believe she fell asleep at Vinnie and Alida's. We continued to sleep in the same bed for another week or so. Maria tried to initiate intimacy one last time. I was awakened by my former lover's attempt to arouse me. Her behavior was that of a desperate partner taking one last shot at proving something, but my failure to respond signed an end to our relationship.

January 2, 1974. I took Maria and Armando to the bus station for a one way trip back to Tijuana—back to her family and her

---

[24] I fell asleep at Alida's house.

daughter Elizabeth. Although I was still in denial and refused to believe the rumors and gossip, I said goodbye to my pretty señorita in a similar fashion to the condition she was in when I first laid eyes on her back in March.

Compliments of Vinnie's part-time driver, Maria gave birth to her second son seven months later.

Chapter 11

Finding My Niche: The Mexico PVA

The Mexico Chapter, Paralyzed Veterans of America (PVA) would become my new mistress, the focus of my passion and energy. My neighbor and current chapter president, Jack Black, had already started the grooming process by recruiting me for kitchen duties. What would come next? Every organization needed workers, members to become actively involved in carrying out the numerous responsibilities and tasks that most of the membership took for granted. The Mexico PVA was no exception. An infusion of new blood was constantly needed to replace older members who were burned out from being over-worked and under-appreciated, those returning stateside, and those who had passed on, making Quadalajara their final resting place.

The Mexico Chapter PVA was approaching the tenth anniversary of its founding. It officially became the first PVA chapter on foreign soil on June 17, 1964, when the national organization of the Paralyzed Veterans of America voted in favor of accepting the group of nineteen wheelchair-bound paralyzed veterans living in Quadalajara to represent its newest chapter.

This particular week was my turn with kitchen duty. Black had warned me there would be an unusually large turnout for our regular membership meeting. The topic of the meeting would be the future of the PVA Clubhouse itself; it would be the only chapter business that mattered on this day. With membership stagnant and fewer members involved in the daily running of Mexico PVA affairs, the Clubhouse itself had become an albatross to some members, Jack Black among them.

I left the house early, and Alberto and I made the usual four or five stops to pick up supplies; everything from hot dogs and hamburgers to ice cream and ice. This was my first turn of weekly kitchen duty that coincided with the Mexico Chapter's monthly membership meeting. I wanted to get to the Clubhouse as early as possible to ensure the kitchen ran smoothly on my watch. I took my PVA duties seriously.

As the 5:00 p.m. meeting time drew closer, more and more

members arrived. I leaned up against the wall of the ceramic tile bar adjacent to the kitchen door. From this spot I had a clear view of the ample meeting room and of the head table where the chapter officers sat. Seated at the front table were President Jack Black, Vice-President and Secretary Frank Stoppiello, and Treasurer Ray Clifford.

Just before the meeting was to begin, a cigar smoking "old timer" had his helper wheel him directly in front of me and park his ass there, obscuring my view. I muttered to myself some not-so-friendly words as Black rapped the gavel signaling the beginning of this historic event.

The Clubhouse had been bought and renovated in 1967—merely three years after the Paralyzed Veterans of America had sanctioned the Mexico Chapter. The chapter and Clubhouse had grown to be inseparable. Many of our members were under the illusion that they belonged to a club, the PVA Club, without fully understanding that the Mexico PVA was a fully accredited veteran's service organization. The Clubhouse was also considered to be the chapter itself. It was a monument to the hard work and dedication of that small band of early Quadalajara Pioneers who originally petitioned our national office for membership status ten years earlier. For many, it was sacrilege to suggest selling the Clubhouse; that would be like disbanding the chapter itself. The large turnout, which included many of the old-timers no longer active in Mexico PVA affairs, soon turned on the chapter president. After a lengthy heated debate, the votes of the members present were taken. Stoppiello had recently signed me as a PVA life member ($100 for lifetime membership, instead of the $8 annual fee) and I was about to cast my first vote as a Mexico PVA member. The members overwhelmingly voted in favor of keeping the Clubhouse. Since this was all new to me and in fairness to those involved and those who were among the original movers and shakers of the Mexico PVA, my first official vote was cast. I abstained, the only member to do so.

I don't know if my friend, neighbor, bridge playing partner, and PVA mentor considered my abstention a cop-out, but Black had little time to reflect on his defeat. Within seconds of the gavel signaling the meeting's end, the cigar smoking old timer had his attendant push him up to the front table directly facing Black. He sat there stunned as the now red-faced man verbally tore him apart. I couldn't hear what was said, but by the pale expression on Black's face, it must have been more than Jack could possibly have expected, even from a gathering and a vote he knew would not be popular.

After the meeting ended, I learned that the cigar smoking old timer was not just any old timer—he was Bill Bailey. He had been a resident of Quadalajara since 1958. Bailey and some of the other long time residents of Quadalajara were especially less fond of the relative newcomer Black than his suggestion to sell what would become a sort of shrine to the founding fathers of the chapter for years to come.

The fallout from the Clubhouse meeting continued as Bailey and his compadre Luis paid Black an unexpected home visit. Jack Black was a post-polio para known to carry a small caliber pistol for protection, while Bill Bailey, a high level quad, carried his signature cigar; half of it deeply imbedded in his oral cavity, the rest constantly needing to be re-lit due to his tendency to chomp on the cigar as much as smoke it. Luis, an intimidating para for those who only knew him from his reputation as sort of a loner you didn't want to cross, was with Bailey for more than just moral support during his visit; he was his bodyguard.

The sometimes emotional PVA president let it be known that the visit by Bailey and "bodyguard" Luis was taken as a death threat. He soon announced that he himself had taken the precaution of contracting his own protection in the event that anything happened to him.

This was my initiation to Mexico PVA and chapter politics. It was interesting, if nothing else.

* * *

I had decided to run for Mexico PVA Board of Directors (BOD) for fiscal year '75, which ran from June '74 through June '75. I was now a mainstay at the Club, attending the Big Game, membership meetings, and kitchen duty. The disaster caused by the Clubhouse proposal claimed a few of our chapter's officers, Black and Stoppiello among them. The Mexico PVA was in need of new blood and the coaxing of some burned out former workers to come out of temporary retirement in order to help it survive. I was elected to the BOD in June of '74, merely six months after separating from Maria.

My old friend and current landlord, Joe Anderson, would be returning from Nebraska soon, and I had made up my mind to find my own place in Quadalajara. With my further commitment to living in Mexico, a house of my own would be a necessity, as would finding new friends to hang around with.

I had become good friends with many of the PVA regulars by

now, including Tom Kirch. Tom was a true friend, always willing and eager to help out in any way he could. If a poll was taken of those who knew Tom well, he would be at or near the top of everyone's list of friends—he was that kind of human being. He and JoAnn, who was "disabled" with Muscular Dystrophy, were one of the most respected couples in the Quadalajara community, which says a lot about them considering all the wonderful people I came to know.

Ray Clifford, Frank Stoppiello, and Jimmy Lietz were some of the other Vietnam veterans I met through my association with the Mexico PVA. The difference between us was that each of them had been disabled on the battlefield; Ray and Frank were paralyzed from the waist down, while Jimmy was a low-level quadriplegic with good upper body strength and some use of his hands. Jimmy's injuries happened when the APC he was in, or armored personnel carrier, got hit. Ray was a Navy corpsman who patched up wounded marines on the battlefield. The cross he wore indicated, according to the Geneva Convention, that he was a non-combat participant only there to tend to the wounded. Apparently, this served as a more convenient target for the enemy. To my knowledge, Frank never spoke of his injury, and most respected the silence of others and wouldn't inquire. That was just the way it was.

I often felt uncomfortable when people assumed that I too was some sort of battlefield hero who was injured protecting the Free World from communism. It may have played a small part in my desire to join PVA. I wanted to give something of myself, as most volunteers do. I wanted to help other disabled vets and the community at-large. There was always that underlying guilt like I was some type of fraud receiving basically the same benefits, even though my injury had nothing to do with Vietnam or combat.

* * *

With my initiation into the PVA and all it had to offer, Tom Kirch, Jimmy Lietz, and I soon began hanging around together. Tom and I were close friends by now. Jimmy and Tom got along well, probably because Tom wouldn't allow the moody Vietnam vet to get down on life. Jimmy also had a great respect for Tom. Jimmy and I were beginning a friendship that was still awkward at times, but the three of us developed a unique bond. Tom was the glue that held our friendship together. Tom was also one of those people who hated to waste many days sitting around Quadalajara just talking. There was a whole lot of Mexico, especially the area surrounding Quadalajara that begged to be investigated and explored. Maybe the quad from rural Minnesota was what city slickers Jimmy (from Washington, DC) and I needed to prompt us to make an excursion to the countryside.

Zapotlanejo, Arenal, and the famous town of Tequila were a few of the country towns within easy driving distance of the city. I had already made a nighttime trip with Anderson to the small town of Arenal, some ten miles west of Quadalajara. I'd gotten the "privilege" of sitting alone in Joe's Oldsmobile while Alberto pushed Joe down the street and into one of Arenal's popular whorehouses. While Anderson was searching for a young beauty he had noticed on an earlier visit, I sat in Joe's car, under a streetlight, praying the group of young Mexican men who had gathered behind me were there just to shoot the bull; I was too young to die on this dirt road in a town whose name I hadn't even heard of. Fortunately, Alberto brought Anderson back without incident, but also without the object of Joe's desires for the evening. You win some, you lose some.

On this sunny afternoon in late May, Tom convinced Lietz and me that a ride out to the town of Tequila would make for an interesting day. We could escape the hustle and bustle of Mexico's second largest city while enjoying a cold beer in the town known for its own famous beverage: Tequila. Tequila was west of Quadalajara, about another three or four miles past the town I had no desire to revisit.

Alberto and I stopped by Tom and JoAnn's house to pick up their '70 Chevy Impala. The roomy trunk could easily accommodate three wheelchairs. The former bachelor had informed his bride before their marriage that he'd remain faithful, but that he still intended to look whenever a pretty girl walked by. Such romantic honesty.

Having loaded the two quads and placed their respective wheelchairs into the trunk of JoAnn's car, Alberto drove back to neighboring Jardines Alcalde to pick up Jimmy and his attendant, Miguel. This mini day trip was merely an innocent afternoon drive, not at all like my nocturnal excursion to Arenal with Anderson. It was impossible to gauge how many earlier residents of Quadalajara had made similar trips to the small towns outside of Quadalajara, or the purity or intentions of their visits, but this was a first for Jimmy and me. I had a feeling that Alberto, and then-bachelor Tom, had been to these towns before. As for Jimmy's helper, Miguel, I couldn't offer a guess as Miguel had worked almost exclusively for Jimmy since 1969.

By the time we arrived in the town of Tequila, it became apparent that Jimmy and I were suffering from the early symptoms of heat exhaustion. We unloaded from JoAnn's Impala and into a still open, but empty house of ill repute. Miguel helped Jimmy inside and came back to assist Alberto with Tom and me. Tom's attendant was off for this afternoon, as two attendants could easily handle three quads. The inviting ceiling fans and cold beer in the thin brown bottle all three of us quads could easily handle, would surely spell relief after our out-of-town drive under the hot afternoon sun.

Unfortunately, the slow moving ceiling fan seemed to be circulating nothing but warm air, and the effects of the alcohol only served to sap my strength even more. Before long, Jimmy signaled Miguel that he felt weak and needed to lie down. The proprietor was both understanding and accommodating. He led Jimmy and Miguel to an empty room. Soon, Alberto was helping me into bed in another downstairs room. This time, the combination of the ceiling fan above the bed and a wet towel from the car did the trick.

While Alberto went to check on Tom, I looked around the room in amazement. Was this the private quarters of some innocent girl who lived here, or was this the room a Mexican working girl used to "entertain" gentlemen callers in? The room was immaculate, but I knew that whoever lived, stayed, or worked here was no saint. Later in the evening there would be a coupling of men and young women exchanging money for sex. Above the bed was a crucifix. Among other religious figures was a small statue of the Virgin Mary by the bed and Rosary Beads hung by the statue. It wasn't what one would expect to see in the room of a working girl. I wondered about its inhabitant. Was she a poor single mom from an even poorer rural village doing this out of desperation? Had she been forced or enticed into a lifestyle that seemed so incongruous with the sanctuary she inhabited? I would never know.

Alberto returned a few minutes later.

"*¿Comó està Tomas?*"[25] I inquired of my attendant.

"*El està bien, y Jaime se està levantando ahorita,*" Alberto informed me. "*Dice Tomas, que si usted està bien, mejor regresamos a la casa.*"[26]

With Tom doing okay and Jimmy getting back up already, it was time to head home. The heat was not as much of a factor by late afternoon, and it was time to put a punctuation mark on this failed,

---

[25] How is Tom?

[26] He's fine, and Jimmy is getting up now. Tom says that if you're okay, it's better that we head back home.

strange mini adventure in paradise.

* * *

I received a call from Jimmy Lietz one Sunday afternoon.

"Jack, do you want to go over to Bill Bailey's house?" he inquired. I had never spoken to Bailey, had never forgotten the incident at the meeting, and felt uncomfortable with the idea.

"I can't, Jim. Alberto is off today so I'm kind of stuck here."

"Miguel can put you into the car and help you out. It's better than staying home and doing nothing," Jimmy added. "Besides, they're always doing something over there on Sundays and enjoy having company."

Lietz talked me into it, and as Miguel drove Jimmy's red and white Plymouth Satellite toward Bill Bailey's house, I couldn't shake the feeling of discomfort within me to meet the red-faced cigar-chomping man who had torn into Jack Black merely weeks before.

Jimmy was right on all accounts. Yes, there was a penny ante family type card game going on and, yes, both Bill and Maria Elena Bailey were genuinely happy we stopped by to visit. The apprehension I felt melted away within minutes as I was made to feel at home in their home. The expression "*mi casa es su casa*"[27] must have been coined with the Baileys in mind.

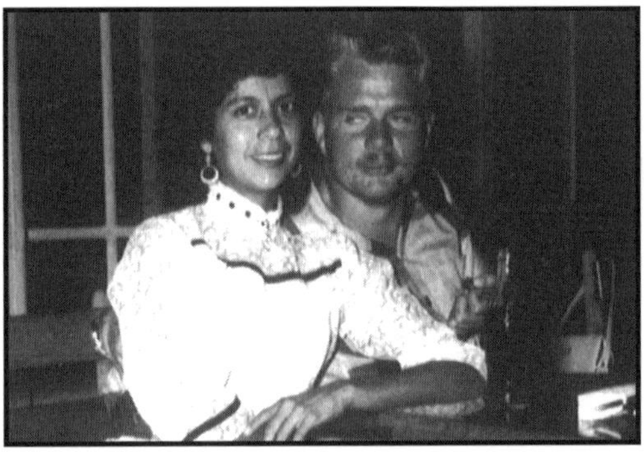

Quadalajara's first Pioneer couple Bill and Maria Elena Bailey, newlyweds Quadalajara, October 1958

[27] My home is your home.

After spending a few relaxing hours playing cards on this particular Sunday afternoon, the subject of housing was brought up. As soon as Maria Elena heard I was looking for a house to rent, she mentioned, "*Hay una casa en la cuadra en renta. La casa tiene un escalón enfrente, pero creo que usted si puede arreglar algo con la dueña. ¿Si quieres, yo hablaré con ella mañana y pregunto?*"[28]

If La Señora Bailey thought the house would be convenient and was willing to inquire for me, then just maybe I'd found a place of my own—finally.

Joe Anderson had returned from the States with his most recent girlfriend, sixteen-year-old Esperanza. Well, she was sixteen when my forty-four-year-old friend and landlord got her a passport and tourist visa using an older sister's birth certificate. I razzed Joe a number of times before he took Esperanza to Nebraska, but Joe was totally unfazed by it. He had that "what, me, worry?" attitude about everything. Joe had convinced a confused and broken-hearted Sofia to continue working for whoever rented his house. Sofia's *esperanza* (hope) was that Anderson would tire of his teenaged "bride," and that she would reclaim her place by his side and in his heart. It didn't happen.

Sofia had been a more than adequate temporary helper: neat, responsible, dependable, easy going. Things had been awkward at Joe's ever since his recent return from Omaha. He never really told Sofia of his intentions, and the fact that tiny Esperanza was still sleeping in Joe's room while Sofia was commuting by bus from home to work and back, spoke louder than what Joe didn't say.

As Sofia helped Alberto pack my belongings for the move to my own place on Monte Olimpo 1046, Colonia Independencia, I noticed that she also cleared out what little she had at Anderson's house. Not a word was spoken by Joe, Sofia, or me, but it was apparent that my temporary housekeeper was now my regular housekeeper. I said nothing. It worked for everyone concerned from a practical standpoint, but not on an emotional level for the heartbroken Sofia.

---

[28] There's a house down the block for rent. The house has a step in front, but I believe you could work something out with the landlady. If you want, I will talk to her tomorrow and ask?

Bill Bailey had lived on Calle Monte Olimpo since he first settled in Quadalajara in 1958. The man, who spent his youth in Lewiston, Idaho and Baker, Oregon, met and married Maria Elena in October 1958. Son Samuel and daughter Lucy would round out the family a few years later. Don Guillermo, as most of the neighbors called him, was well known and respected by his Mexican neighbors. Bailey was accepted as one of their own in his chosen home-away-from-home. Both he and Maria Elena Cruz de Bailey were known for their charitable and neighborly endeavors.

Maria Elena Cruz came from a family of six children, and husband Bill encouraged and helped his new in-laws to learn a trade that would bode well in the future, encouraging Gabriel, Jorge, and Luis to study jewelry making.

I soon became an unofficial member of the extended Bailey clan. The only person who disliked the idea seemed to be Jack Black.

"Black can't believe you moved onto the same street as Bailey," Anderson remarked.

As my friendship with Bill Bailey grew, I became persona non grata in the eyes of my old friend Jack Black, who would soon be moving back stateside.

A routine quickly developed that had me joining Bailey and his family regularly for dinner, outings, trips to the PVA's unofficial favorite *playa* (beach), Manzanillo, playing Gin Rummy (and every other card game imaginable), or enjoying a game of chess outside in Quadalajara's sunshine. I continued visiting my other friends, but less frequently. Other days were spent at the Clubhouse on PVA business or playing poker with the high rollers.

There were other fringe benefits of hanging around with Bailey. One was named Teresa. Teresa was Bill and Maria Elena's oldest niece. She appeared to be Maria Elena's favorite. Due to the fact that Teresa was an infant when the then-childless couple first met, Maria Elena had gladly babysat her niece while sister-in-law, Angelina, was expecting her second child, Suzanna. I had seen both girls, now sixteen and fifteen years of age, whenever they waitressed at the Club a year or so earlier.

The first mini excursion outside of Quadalajara I was invited on was to the swimming pools of Los Camachos, a few miles out of town on the road toward Zacatecas. Alberto had driven me there once before with Maria and Armando. Los Camachos was a simple, calm, family locale, at least until Tio Guillermo, another of Quadalajara's occasional instigators, decided to spice things up. While Maria Elena,

Suzy, Samuel, and little Lucy played in the pool, Bill and I enjoyed some of Mexico's finest beer. Teresa, who was sunning herself in a red bikini, was an easy mark for the former Marine sharpshooter and favorite teasing uncle, Tio Guillermo.

"Joaquin," he called me by my new nickname, "Call La Prieta over here. But don't call her Teresa, call her Prieta." (Prieta meaning someone with a dark complexion.)

My Spanish vocabulary hadn't yet included the word *prieta*, so I asked, "Okay, how much trouble are you getting me into? What does prieta mean?" Bailey had a uniquely contagious laugh. Whether from childhood or something that evolved over years of laughing with half of a cigar stuck in his mouth, it sounded like Santa's "Ho, Ho, Ho," but in reverse and with a bit of a cackle.

I followed orders, "*Prieta, ven aca, por favor.*"[29]

Teresa was very outgoing with a great personality, and she readily came over knowing that Tio Guillermo was instigating something. She was about to be teased, but seemed to enjoy getting the attention. The girl who I knew would grow up someday to be a real cutie approached us. As Teresa walked toward us in her red bikini, it quickly became apparent; the dark complexioned Mexican girl was indeed already a cutie. The seed had been planted. From that point on, every time I saw or joked around with my neighbor's blossoming niece, my harmless crush on Teresa would intensify.

* * *

Since Bill Bailey was one of the first of the quadriplegics and paraplegics to explore this fascinating city in the heart of Mexico, it was always interesting to listen whenever he spoke of the early years. I would kid around with him whenever he mentioned coming down to Quadalajara in 1958. I was ten years old and in the fourth grade at that time. Much of what Bailey talked about confirmed things Joe Anderson had mentioned a couple of years prior. Many of the same names and interesting stories were brought up, although Bailey had some seven years in Quadalajara before Anderson arrived from Omaha with his American wife. Many of the names of the original Quadalajara Pioneers that Bailey mentioned were unknown to me.

---

[29] Prieta, come over here please.

My duties at the Mexico Chapter PVA continued to increase, as I began taking minutes of chapter meetings whenever the chapter secretary was ill or traveling stateside. I ran for, and was elected chapter secretary after serving one year on the Board of Directors. I quickly discovered that what had seemed to be a clique only a few years earlier was really a few dedicated, hard-working men who kept the Mexico Chapter functioning as smoothly as possible.

The Mexico PVA, in addition to being a veteran's service organization, was an integral part of the Quadalajara community. It was much more than a BINGO hall and high stakes poker game, although coupled with the generosity of its members, BINGO nights and money "dragged" from the poker game (a few pesos per poker hand were set aside by whoever was responsible for banking the game, i.e., collecting the money and handing out the chips), were the main sources of revenue.

El Sombrero News July 1979:

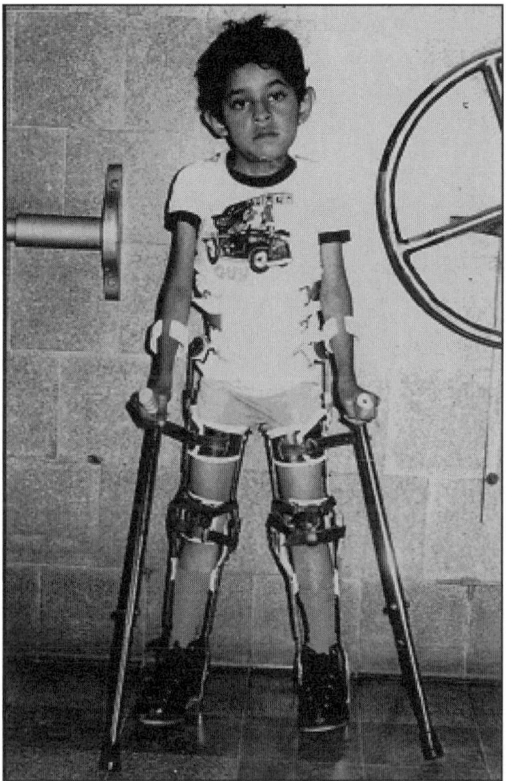

This young man is 13 year old Jose Pierros. He had polio when he was an infant. "Pesos for Braces" thanks each one of you for your generous donation. A child will walk because you cared enough to help him.

Sally Holmes
"PESOS FOR BRACES"

PVA funds collected throughout the fiscal year (June through June) were used for Clubhouse and chapter expenses. Being a non-profit organization, the Mexico PVA would award end-of-the-year donations of remaining funds to a number of local charities, as well as U.S. national organizations. The Mexican Red Cross, Quadalajara's School for Blind Girls, and Pesos for Braces (an organization our chaplain, Reverend Paul Hunter, was deeply involved in used donations to buy braces and other prosthetic equipment for disabled children in the Quadalajara area). Other worthy causes, such as Asociación de Lisiados de Jalisco A.C. (ALJAC), which modeled itself after PVA as a service organization for all of Jalisco residents with disabilities, also received cash donations, wheelchairs, and equipment collected by the Mexico Chapter. Often, this equipment was donated by widows and families of chapter members who passed away in Quadalajara. Well-known organizations such as the "Make-a-Wish Foundation," and others not as well known, were yearly recipients of the efforts and generosity of the Mexico PVA and its members.

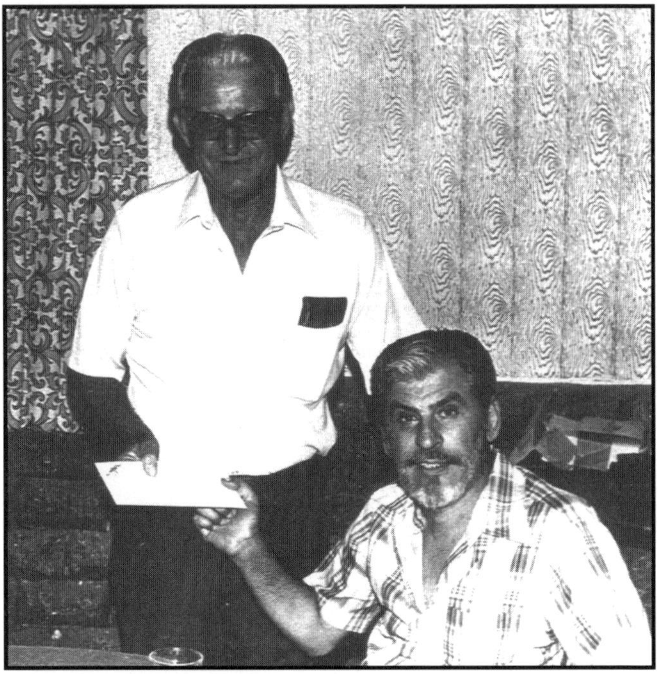

Eddie Lucier, on behalf of the Mexico PVA, presents a donation to Reverend Paul Hunter for the organization Pesos for Braces

Mexico PVA also sponsored Christmas parties every year for the children who attended some of Quadalajara's poorer grade schools. Since the PVA Clubhouse itself was located on the outskirts of Quadalajara, in the agricultural town of Ciudad Granja, there was no shortage of deserving schools and smiling children worthy of a brighter Christmas. Three schools, usually two of which were located in the Ciudad Granja area, were selected by the chapter members each year.

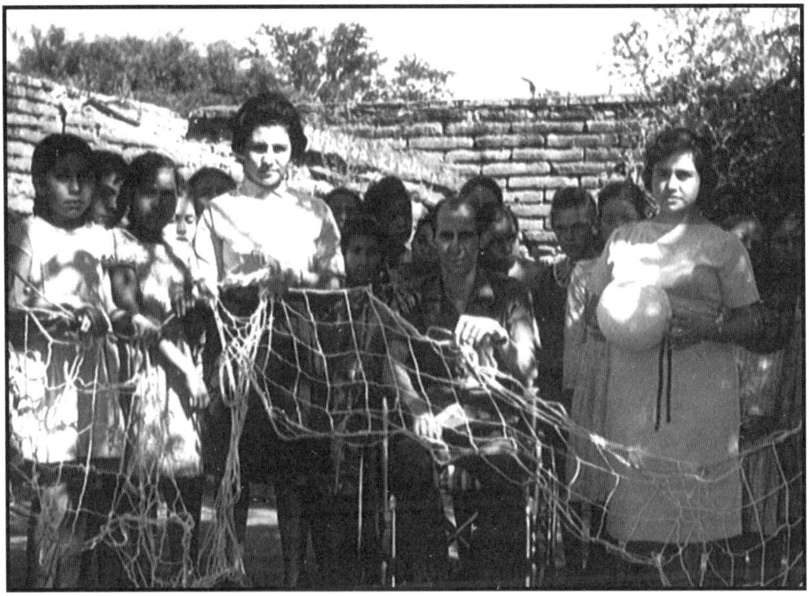

Maria and Ray Foland with teacher and students of Santa Cruz de las Flores Jalisco, Mexico, December 1965

Separate donations were solicited from the membership and friends of PVA for the purchase of piñatas, candy, fruit, and playground equipment, as well as notebooks, pencils, and other school supplies. The generosity of PVA members brought many smiles from the school children who watched as the chapter president, flanked by other chapter officers and members' wives, handed the goodies and school supplies to the teachers of their respective classes. All members were invited to attend these *posadas*—and many did—while the curious children looked at these differently-abled men and women, mostly seated in stainless steel Everest & Jenning wheelchairs. Many had never seen an American citizen before. Few had ever seen a wheelchair before. Shortly thereafter, these little angels became regular kids in pursuit of the bounty that spilled from the donated piñatas. This Christmas tradition, which sprang from the early years prior to the founding of the Mexico Chapter PVA, continued every year for twenty years until the chapter folded in the early-80s.

In addition to end-of-the-year donations, the annual June membership meeting also served as the awards and installation of chapter officers gathering. Invited guests included United States Consulate officials, representatives of other local American organizations, officials from the Hospital Mexico-Americano, our ALJAC counterparts and friends, as well as local Mexican dignitaries.

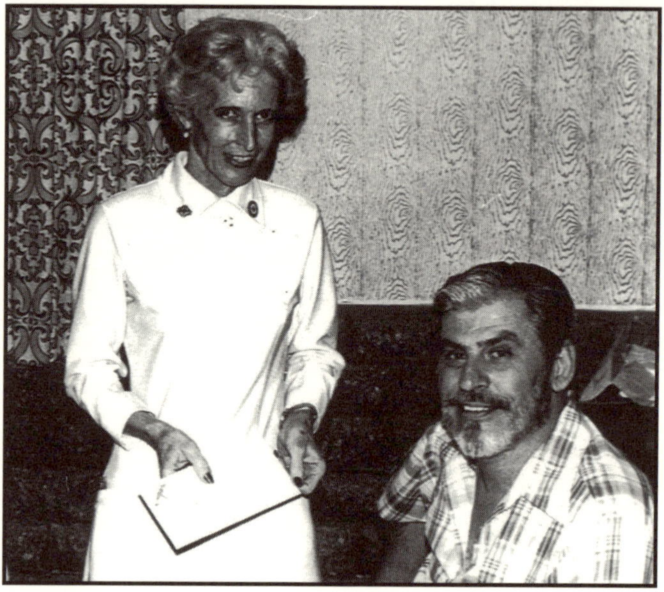

Eddie Lucier, on behalf of the Mexico PVA, presents a donation to Mrs. Lillian Cartlidge for the Mexican Red Cross

It was the time of year when the Mexico PVA helped those in need. The George E. Ray Award was presented to individuals who the membership voted to be the "Outstanding Member" and "Outstanding Non-member" for services rendered to the Mexico Chapter, Paralyzed Veterans of America during the year. (George Ray passed away before I arrived in Mexico, but no matter who served in the capacity of chapter president, vice-president, secretary, or treasurer in the early years, George Ray was the man most responsible for rounding up a handful of Quadalajara's early settlers and successfully petitioning National PVA for a sanctioned PVA chapter south of the border.)

The evolution of the Mexico Chapter PVA from its inception was remarkable. What began as a small number of mostly quadriplegics from the Long Beach VA Hospital, who braved all—leaving behind family, friends, and loved ones (not to mention a projected post-injury life expectancy of seven to fifteen years) to explore this intriguing Mexican city, gradually grew to a few hundred men and women, veterans and non-veterans, from all over North America and beyond.

The rowdy group, who first came to Quadalajara for its ideal climate, low cost of living, pretty señoritas, beer, tequila, card games, and a second chance at life, had matured. While all of these things attracted most to this unique city in that unique period in time, the founding of the Mexico PVA provided the vehicle that enabled so many shut-ins and social outcasts to touch the lives of countless others in a positive way.

Part Four

The Elite History of Quadalajara: In Search of Utopia

Chapter 12
The Explorers

According to the Paralyzed Veterans of America:

> *Prior to World War II, Americans who suffered a spinal cord injury (SCI) faced a bleak future and a life expectancy averaging about eighteen months. But veterans who sustained a spinal cord injury during the war years received the first ray of hope for a fuller life ahead—the development of antibiotics, modern medicine, and new techniques which added significantly to their life span. Because of this medical progress, for the first time, spinal cord injured veterans could leave the confines of the VA or military hospital, return home to work or rejoin society. Unfortunately, much of society proved to be unwilling, unable, or ill-prepared to accommodate the needs of paralyzed veterans.*
>
> *In 1946, paralyzed veterans from across the country joined together to form an organization to deal with the unique problems and challenges facing them. The organization they formed, the Paralyzed Veterans of America, is an organization of veterans who have served honorably in the armed forces and who have incurred an injury or disease affecting the spinal cord, causing paraplegia or quadriplegia.*

(An excellent reference point for a better understanding of the evolution of SCI post-injury life can be found in the 1950 movie, *The Men*, which just happened to be Marlon Brando's first Hollywood role.)

Paraplegics and quadriplegics who were fortunate enough to leave their institutional environment had a second chance at life, one radically different than before SCI, but they faced a new problem—where to go and what to do? There was no blueprint to follow. A small percentage was able to find employment, and another small percentage was able to pursue educational goals. Some were fortunate to live in, or relocate to, areas of the country where getting out and about in a wheelchair was possible. Many discharged SCI veterans were able to modify their homes and make them reasonably wheelchair accessible, but once home, many never left—unable to overcome architectural barriers, inclement weather, or a fear of leaving home. Many others, out of necessity or unwillingness to face the outside world, simply lived out their lives in institutions.

Steady progress was being made, spearheaded by the Paralyzed Veterans of America. The clout of the newly formed organization of paralyzed veterans helped secure legislation that enabled members to purchase automobiles with the special equipment necessary for them to drive, as well as financial grants to help purchase or renovate homes for wheelchair accessibility.

PVA's monthly periodical, the *Paraplegic News* (*PN*), went to print in 1946. The publication united paralyzed veterans from chapters initially formed in VA hospitals from New York to California. Information ranging from legislation, adaptive equipment, individual chapter news, and travel tips for those who were able and willing could be read by every PVA member or periodical subscriber who opened its pages.

One interesting article, complete with travel tips, was penned by active member James E. Seybold (Vaughn Chapter PVA, Hines VA/Chicago area) and appeared in the November 1954 issue of *PN.* Not content to push his wheelchair through the snow or sit around for another long cold winter, Mr. Seybold drove his hand controlled automobile 2,500 miles from Wisconsin to California by himself.

"It's not such a great problem after all," he reported. "I would like to enumerate a few of the main difficulties which may arise, and how to face them: Your car should be in A-1 shape. Good tires, and a well-lubricated engine and chassis for a safe comfortable drive. Pack your car so that the things you intend to use while traveling are easily accessible. Recognize your handicap and don't knock yourself out by seeing how far you can drive in one day...Try to plan your trip so you will reach a certain destination for a decent place to eat or sleep at a certain time. Toward the middle of the afternoon start looking for a place to sack out...When you stop, inquire before you get out if the bathroom is large enough to accommodate a wheelchair." He goes on to mention the necessity of water while crossing the desert and checking brakes before mountain driving. "Never hesitate to ask for help when you need it. You don't have to go into details about your condition...I have found people only too glad to assist in all instances where I needed help."

Jim Seybold was probably not the first active para, or possibly quad, to make such a trip, but his detailed report in the *Paraplegic News* appears to be a first. His journey would not end there.

Travel tales appeared regularly in the *PN.* Group travel, to and from about every European country where SCI survivors lived, was becoming commonplace. A late-40s letter, which gave kudos to the *PN* magazine editor, came from a PVA member living in Brazil. Our neighbors to the north also made the *PN* pages. The only conspicuous absence of travel news came from our neighbors to the south. Some adventurous para or quad must have explored Mexico, with the exception of anyone who may only have been shopping or looking for mischief in one of Mexico's infamous border towns.

Hernan Cortes and the Spanish Conquistadores certainly were fascinated by their new find. Cortes and his followers explored practically every inch of this enchanting territory resting on our southern border.

Who were the first to explore Mexico, not on horseback like Cortes, but using an E&J wheelchair to travel and explore a whole new world of adventure? The many unconfirmed reports of a paraplegic or quadriplegic having visited or moved to some city or town in Mexico's interior were just that—rumors.

* * *

Countless PVA members were surely mesmerized while turning their May 1955 issue of the *Paraplegia News* to page four: "*Mexico, a Paradise for Paraplegics*," by James E Seybold.

"Did you have a hard and trying winter?" the article begins. "And you Californians; did the smog and fog drive you to distraction? Your worries are now over, for here, in Mexico City, is the *ideal retreat*...Until you have actually seen it, it is hard to realize how beautifully modern, and how far ahead in architectural design Mexico, D.F. is." Seybold touts the "spring-like climate" and states that "the city was once the bottom of a lake" accounting for its wheelchair-friendly level landscape.

His article continues with detailed travel tips for adventurers like himself, who wished to drive down and explore Mexico's capital city. Seybold explains the advantages of services provided by the American Automobile Association, including obtaining Mexican auto insurance, arranging accommodations, and planning scenic routes while driving within Mexico. He cautions about highway conditions and the dangerous mountain stretches absent of guardrails.

Once there, Seybold notes, "Mexican drivers are the worst I've ever seen. Every day is like the Indianapolis '500' to them...The Mexican people are, in general, a happy, carefree race. Their exotic music grows on you and virtually becomes part of you. Speaking of exotic things, I must say a word in behalf of the lovely señoritas—WOW!" Seybold was not the first, and would not be the last, to discover one of Mexico's most beautiful natural resources.

"Activities are numerous; from bullfights to Jai-Lai and soccer to visiting such nearby places as Maxmillian's Castle in Chapultepec Park, the Shrine of Guadalupe and the Aztec pyramids. As Mexico City is centrally located it can be used as a base of operations from which these side trips can be made. Some of these points of interest are Vera-Cruz, Acapulco, Puebla, Cuernavaca, Guadalajara, and Taxco."

This interesting and informative article must certainly have served to pique the interest of a number of institutionalized SCI veterans and discharged shut-ins. The question is—how many curious adventurers, if any, were motivated to act?

James Seybold returned to Mexico City in the winter of 1956 and again sent his "*Report from Mexico City (The El Dorado of the Western Hemisphere)*," which appeared in the February 1957 issue of the *PN*:

"Did you just pick up your *Paraplegia News* after pushing your cold-rimmed wheelchair through a snow bank? Why not get away from it all? Visit Sunny Mexico!"

The article is a basic follow-up of his previous visit, with updates on the Mexican peso, highway conditions/improvements, new traffic lights in parts of the city, and a reiteration of "the magnificent architecture of Mexico, both the modern "hotels of Mexico City and Acapulco," and the ancient "beautiful cathedrals, like the one I visited yesterday in Taxco."

Seybold concludes his article, "All in all, I'm delighted to be away from the cold and the winter. The only Spanish I know, to some up how I feel about Mexico is *Pura Vida*, which literally translated means, *This is the Life*."

While James Seybold was marveling at the magnificent architecture, climate, accessibility, and lovely señoritas in and around Mexico City, another PVA member was crisscrossing the same terrain. Harold E. Doolittle "has been roaming around Mexico for the past several years looking for the most likely spot to live. He has settled on

Cuernavaca because of its climate and its location. Doolittle speaks fluent Spanish," according to an article in the April 1960 *PN*.

Mr. Doolittle had indeed been exploring Mexico himself since the mid-50s, something that would be verified in a future article in the August 1961 *PN*. His plan was to "arrange a set-up in Mexico where U.S. paras and quads can vacation or live on a permanent basis." Cuernavaca was where Doolittle envisioned renting a place that would become a co-op to house men and women with any type of disability, as well as their children. The city is "50 miles south of Mexico City" and has schools for children of all ages. "This is because of the large American colony in Cuernavaca…There are many, many things to see and do in Mexico."

Doolittle's article, which was intended to ascertain the number of paras and quads interested in his venture, concludes with a mailing address for Harold Doolittle at the VA hospital in Coral Gables, Florida. Apparently his dream did not become a reality.

* * *

At approximately the same time as Seybold and Doolittle were exploring areas in and around the hub of Mexico City, there was talk of Señor Roberto, an American para named Bob, who was renting rooms to fellow paras and quads in his four bedroom home up the road a ways—in Quadalajara.

Chapter 13

The Pioneers

Maria Elena Cruz was a single, 26-year-old woman when she was hired by George Ray as his all around "Girl Friday" and to help a nurse named Cory care for disabled American residents in his small group home in Guadalajara, Jalisco, Mexico. The year was 1957.

"What year did George Ray first rent rooms to other wheelchair Gringos?" Maria Elena was asked.

"*No sé*,"[30] she replied, "*El lugar perteneció al Señor Roberto antes*."[31]

"Was Señor Roberto Mexican or American," was the next question.

"*El era Americano en silla de ruedas también, su nombre era Bob*."[32]

"How long had Señor Bob been renting rooms?"

"*No sé eso*,"[33] Maria Elena responded.

George Ray was a self-sufficient paraplegic paralyzed from the waist down. His residents were, for the most part, paraplegics and quadriplegics in need of personal care. There were four wheelchair users residing at "George Ray's Place," as it came to be known. The men were World War II and Korean War era veterans who ventured outside the safe confines of the Long Beach Veterans Hospital in search of something different. The men wanted an alternative to institutional living. They found it in Quadalajara.

George Ray was one of the earliest Pioneers to explore the wonders of this glorious city of fountains and cathedrals, not to mention the fabulous sunny weather, the low cost of living, and Quadalajara's fame for having some of Mexico's prettiest señoritas. It was here that Maria Elena Cruz met some of Quadalajara's other wheelchair-bound American residents: Bill Macleary, Joe Miller, and a

---

[30] I don't know.

[31] The place belonged to Señor Robert before.

[32] He was American in wheelchair also, his name was Bob.

[33] I don't know that.

young man named Brad. Maria Elena would later recount the day she showed up for work to find George Ray and Mexican ambulance personnel talking outside the home on Avenida Españas, Colonia Moderna. Brad had taken ill the night before and passed away by the morning of December 8, 1957. Brad was one of the first of the Pioneers to pass away in this enticing Mexican city. He would not be the last.

Earlier that year, Joe Miller and Ray had parted company. Miller had rented a place near Quadalajara's soccer stadium in Colonia Independencia and was soon renting rooms to his own adventurous Pioneers. Maria Elena recalled that, "*Los primeros que llegaron venián del Hospital de Veteranos de Long Beach, California.*"[34]

One of Joe Miller's earliest roommates was Ray "Doc" Foland. The skinny quad straight out of the Long Beach VA in 1957 was joined by Ralph Nelson in Miller's four bedroom house in Colonia Independencia. "Doc," as he came to be known in Quadalajara, was one of the friendliest and most helpful to those who would follow.

In March of 1958, Bill Macleary returned to George Ray's Place from a visit to the Long Beach VA with two other young men willing to leave behind family and friends in search of a better life. Patrick Wolf and Bill Bailey were now part of a slowly expanding community of disabled American veterans inflicted with spinal cord injuries. They joined, or were soon joined by, George Small, Marion Fuget, Tatsumi Aragaki (a.k.a. "Gato," for his Japanese-American "cat eyes"), Charlie Reno, Tony Gomez, Bill Coe, Foland, and countless forgotten others.

---

[34] The first to arrive came from the Veteran's Hospital in Long Beach, California.

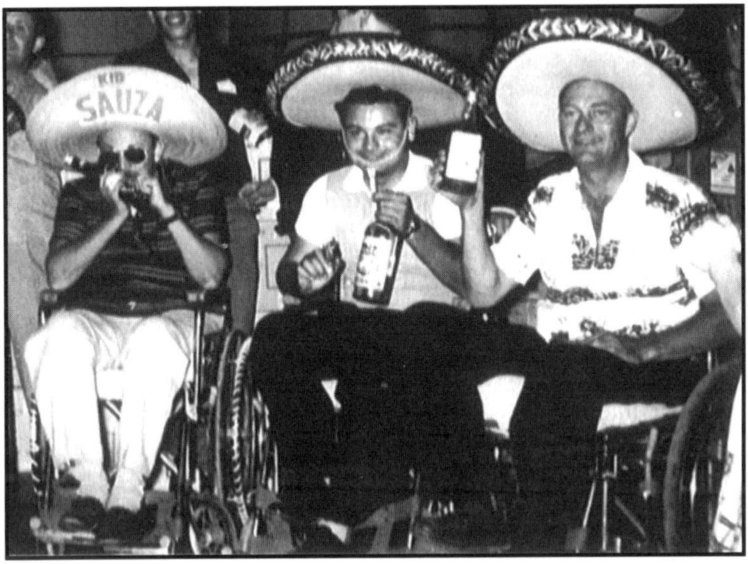

Bill Coe, Tony Gomez, George Ray (left to right)
At Tequila Sauza Factory, late-50s

When asked about the ease and availability of young women made famous in a 1972 *Los Angeles Times* article about paralyzed veterans living in Quadalajara, and further perpetuated by Ron Kovic's book (later to become the Oliver Stone movie, *Born On The Fourth Of July*), Maria Elena replied, "*George Ray no permitía eso en su casa. Quien sabe que harían cuando salían en su carro, pero casi siempre George llevaba los muchachos a cenar a algún restaurant. Fué cuando empezaron a venir de Chicago, y otros de quien sabe donde, cuando se portaron más locos,*" she explained. "*George Ray era muy listo y escribió cartas a muchas partes de Los Estados Unidos acerca de Guadalajara.*"[35]

On October 23, 1958, Maria Elena Cruz officially became Maria Elena Cruz de Bailey. Bill Bailey, the young Marine from Lewiston, Idaho who was injured in 1951 at the age of seventeen, and Maria Elena Cruz became the first wheelchair-bound American and

---

[35] George Ray didn't allow that in his house. Who knows what they did when they went out in his car, but he usually took the boys to dinner at some restaurant. It's when they began to arrive from Chicago, and who knows where else, that they started acting crazy. George Ray was very smart and sent letters to many places in the United States about Guadalajara.

Mexican señorita to marry in Quadalajara.

When asked how many wheelchair gringos were residing in Quadalajara at the time of their October 1958 wedding, Maria Elena answered, "*No me va a creer, pero como unos veinte.*"[36]

Shortly after newlyweds Bill and Maria Elena Bailey left George Ray's Place for a house of their own, George Ray and Bill Macleary went their separate ways. Macleary opened his own place on the southern outskirts of the city in the suburb of Las Fuentes. Ray moved his place to Colonia Chapalita on Avenida Cubiltete in an upscale part of Quadalajara. Within the next two years other gimp camps (as they were often referred to by members of the disabled community) opened in Colonia Independencia, Las Fuentes, and other parts of Quadalajara. Joe Miller moved his place from the soccer stadium neighborhood to a new locale that accommodated eight wheelchair users. Other residents began to rent houses on their own, sharing the expenses two, three, or four ways. Macleary would subsequently lose his Las Fuentes establishment, as well as his Mexican novia, to Bill Coe.

Bill and Maria Elena Bailey welcomed Charlie Whestine and his nurse/girlfriend into their home. Charlie and his fiancée eventually found their own home to rent and moved out on their own. The Whestines soon wed and moved to Los Angeles some six months later, becoming one of Quadalajara's first American wheeler and Mexican bride to do so.

George Ray's efforts to tout the many benefits Quadalajara possessed for wheelchair-bound veterans in need of personal attendant care, as well as presenting the aforementioned advantages that life in Quadalajara offered, would soon attract many curious visitors to this utopian mile high city. Not all wheelchair users were veterans, or men for that matter, and not everyone who visited this intriguing city would remain to call it home. Nevertheless, word-of-mouth spread and the trickle of curious newcomers continued.

* * *

George Ray envisioned a resort in Mexico that would cater to the specific needs of quads and paras. In 1959 he teamed up with Paul J. De Lecour to open just such a resort in the picturesque countryside some ten minutes from Quadalajara. San Jose del Tajo, designed by

[36] You won't believe it, but only about twenty.

Ray for the convenience of fellow wheelers and built by De Lecour, a retired building contractor from Minnesota, opened with much fanfare. The April 1959 article in the *PN* boldly announced its opening like no classified ad could possibly have done:

A PARAPLEGIC PARADISE NOW OPEN IN MEXICO

by George E. Ray

I have been living in Mexico for the past year and a half. During that time I have had but one dream: a place where paraplegics and quadriplegics could stay and receive personal services. That dream has been realized.

A vacation and retirement spot especially designed for the para and quad is now open and operating at Guadalajara, Mexico. It is a modern motel equipped with every modern convenience: comfortable bedrooms, convenient bathrooms, large dining-room particularly adapted to wheelchairs, beautiful lounge and a swimming pool.

It was built by Mr. Paul J. De Lecour, a retired building contractor from Minnesota, at the suggestion of this writer.

The San Jose del Tajo has 24-hour service for the ones who need help with personal services, getting in and out of bed and in and out of cars.

Guadalajara was chosen because of its year-round temperate climate. It is never too hot or too cold for the para or quad with circulation or perspiration problems.

San Jose del Tajo is located ten minutes from the city. It is modern, clean and boasts a population of over a half million. The motel is only 30 minutes from the world renowned Lake Chapala, the largest lake in Mexico, and the picturesque artist colonies of Ajijiic and Jocotepec.

Paras and Quads Only

San Jose del Tajo is closed to the general public; catering only to paraplegics, quadriplegics and their families. No expense has been spared to make a home-like, happy atmosphere for the person who wishes to spend a vacation in colorful Mexico.

For the paraplegic who is self-sufficient cost is $120 per month (room, three American cooked meals of the highest quality, and laundry). The monthly cost to the quadriplegic is

$180. He receives all that the para does, plus the 24-hour service (bladder and bowel care and medication).

For detailed information, write to: Mr. Paul J. De Lecour, San Jose del Tajo, Guadalajara, Mexico.

Is there truth in the saying, "There is no such thing as bad publicity?" A negative report from one Florida quad made its way to the top echelon on the Paralyzed Veterans of America. PVA President Harry A. Schweikert dispatched an emissary from New Jersey, Robert Lawrence, to personally investigate this mysterious resort built outside this newfound utopia, in the heart of Mexico.

The "he said, he said" follow-up article in the July 1959 issue of the *PN* served to reinforce the claims made by visionary Pioneer George Ray. As more and more curious *PN* readers contemplated the farfetched notion of leaving their secure institutions, complete with round-the-clock care, doctors, nurses, and specialists to handle whatever emergency might arise—a brave few gambled with uncertainty.

Maria Elena, when asked if she remembered a place named San Jose del Tajo, replied, "*Si, el dueño era un señor que se llamaba Paul. Hicieron muy buenas fiestas allí. El señor no estaba en silla de ruedas, era socio de Jorge* (George Ray). *Era muy, muy bonito lugar. Nosotros fuimos dos o tres veces a unas fiestas. Algo paso entre Jorge y Paul, no sé, Guillermo me dijo.*"[37]

When asked if she remembered who some of those were who stayed at San Jose del Tajo, Maria Elena replied, "*No sé, eran tantos, tantos.*"[38]

In a December 1959 issue of the *PN*, Quadalajara resident Zoeth Skinner wrote: "There are supposed to be, according to reports, about 40 paraplegics living in Guadalajara, Mexico. Ever since the closing of San Jose del Tajo, the fellows have been moving into the city…Two, three, and four bedroom houses are available for rent, furnished or unfurnished. A two bedroom house rents for $24 per month unfurnished, or $45 per month furnished."

---

[37] Yes, the owner was a man named Paul. They had some really good fiestas there. The man wasn't a wheelchair user, he was George's business partner. It was a very, very beautiful place. We went to two or three of the fiestas. Something happened between George and Paul, I don't know, (husband) Bill told me.

[38] I don't know, there were many, many.

George Ray's dream of a resort in this Mexican paradise, which catered solely to quads and paras, was short-lived. A dispute between George Ray and his business partner led to the closing of San Jose del Tajo within months of its well-publicized opening. According to Maria Elena, "*Ellos* (George Ray and some of the renters) *regresaron a* (Colonia) *Chapalita*."[39] The De Lecour family moved back to the States.

In the March 1960 *PN*, Skinner again reminded readers that San Jose del Tajo had closed, "There are numerous things in Guadalajara to keep one entertained. Five first-class movie houses show first-runs, a drive-in, a bullfight ring, and a cockpit also provide entertainment…the restaurants, bars, etc. accommodate wheelchairs…Very few people are bored here."

"Mr. Skinner," the article continues, "has leased a large home and will rent to paras with or without board. His charges are $75 per month without attendant. Single paras or quads who desire to stay less than six months obtain accommodations for $120 per month for the former and $180 per month for the latter. This includes attendant, food, and incidentals."

Ironically, the address for information from Skinner's December 1959 *PN* article was on the same street in Quadalajara, Monte Olimpo, where Bill and Maria Elena Bailey had made their home since marrying in October 1958. To her knowledge, had Skinner actually renter rooms in his Colonia Independencia home? "*Skinner nunca rentó cuartos. El se casó con una Mexicana y ellos se fueron a vivir a Los Estados Unidos.*"[40]

[39] They moved back to Chapalita.

[40] Skinner never rented rooms. He married a Mexican woman and they left to live in the United States.

The following article appeared in PVA's May 1961 issue of the *Paraplegia News*:

PERTINENT INFORMATION ON VACATIONING IN GUADALAJARO, MEXICO

At the request of Zoeth Skinner of Guadalajara, a seacoast resort in Mexico, we are printing information on the situation as an aid to our readers. Mr. Skinner says there has been a great deal of misunderstanding and that some paraplegics have even arrived unannounced.

Here is the information provided by Mr. Skinner:

¶There is no hotel, motel or other organization there with special facilities for the handicapped.

¶Disabled females cannot be cared for.

¶Any person capable of living with a companion or attendant in a home in the U.S. will have no trouble there.

¶At least 24 paras and quads living there now, some with attendants, some married to Mexican girls.

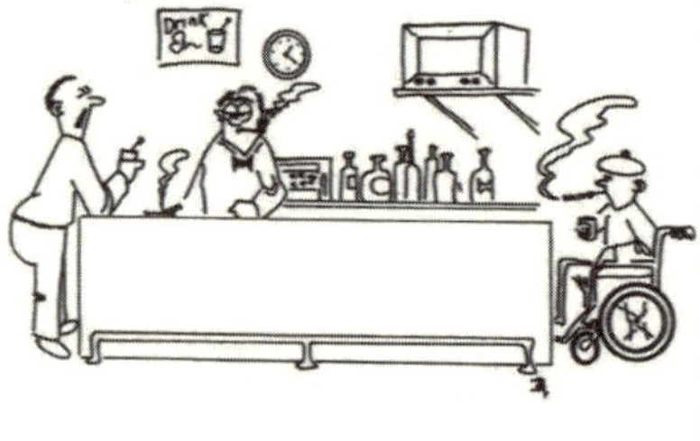

WHO'S THE SHORT GUY AT THE END OF THE BAR,—TOULOUSE LAUTREC

¶Attendants can be located by getting one from a returning para, or by securing a relative of another attendant.

¶Some knowledge of Spanish is important —elementary course is $8.

¶Attendant fee: $24 per mo. for 6-day week; female cook and housekeeper: $12.

Houses Available

¶Houses available, furnished or unfurnished; rent $16 per mo. up for unfurnished.

¶Water in taps unsafe; bottled water is delivered in 6-gallon glass jugs at 13¢.

¶Meals in restaurants are cheaper than in U.S.; meals begin at 72¢.

¶Excellent doctors in Guadalajara, and SC veterans can get out-patient care by applying through the U.S. Consulate there.

¶Entertainment: bullfights, cockfights, boxing, wrestling, football, cabarets, visiting points of interest, movies.

¶Guadalajara served by plane, train and bus or auto; Mexico City (more expensive and very heavy traffic) is eight or nine hours north.

¶In driving: tourist cards for six months, car permits for three and renewable, at border towns. Mexican insurance for car, and carry container of water and gas can.

¶In other travel: Mexican Consuls and tourist cards at border; proof of citizenship: passport, birth certificate or discharge from Armed Forces.

¶Permissable to bring radios. TV, wheelchairs and any special equipment necessary. Bring urinals, catheters, etc.

For complete board, private rooms or double, servants, meals, etc. cntact George Ray, Cubilete 147, Colonia Chapalita Sur, Guadalajara, Jalisco, Mexico.

Unfortunately, the article inaccurately describes Quadalajara as a "seacoast resort," and also, Mexico City is southeast, not "north" of Quadalajara.

* * *

Whether by design or accident, this eye-catching and interesting *Paraplegia News* article, which every PVA member and countless non-members might have read, further served to heighten curiosity about Quadalajara. It also provided more potential renters for the ever-expanding and now nine-bed, customer friendly gimp camp known as George Ray's Place.

* * *

Bob Beilsmith was nineteen years old when he became a quadriplegic in 1952. Beilsmith, originally from St. Louis, spent eight of his first ten post-injury years in the Hines VA (two were spent rooming with a fellow quad in the Chicago area). Bob Beilsmith asked for, and received a discharge from the Hines VA hospital in 1962 and headed south. He soon rented a three-bedroom house in Colonia Chapalita with fellow Chicago newcomer Donald "Cookie" Meinberg and Frank Vertinelli.

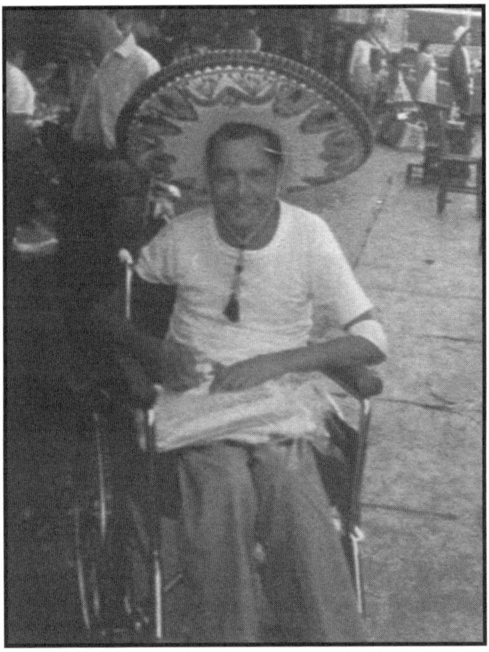

Bob Beilsmith
Quadalajara, early-60s

Such was the life of a spinal cord injured person post World War II. Whereas few paraplegics and quadriplegics survived the catastrophic injuries they incurred years earlier, "modern" medicine now enabled most to live for a limited number of years. Incomplete injuries, such as when the afflicted individual's spinal cord was only partially damaged, stood a better chance at longevity and quality of life. Few were fortunate enough to find educational opportunities or employment in a world not yet ready for them physically, psychologically, or socially.

This was the life that surviving SCI veterans and civilian disabled people faced for decades; decades of slow change in the field of medicine, in rehabilitation, and especially in society's view of "crippled" people who were spotted in their wheelchairs on those rare occasions they ventured outside their institutional environment. This was the life that Bill Bailey, Bob Beilsmith, and others faced for many of their priceless post-injury years—until they heard of a special place somewhere in Mexico, a place that promised the opportunity for a radically different life for those Pioneers willing to take that chance.

Bill Bailey and Bob Beilsmith had much in common besides their initials and the fact that each was injured in his teen years. The two high level quads (both had injuries at cervical 4/5, simply referred to as C 4/5) required attendant care practically twenty-four-seven. Both were avid card players. Name the game and they played it, and played it well. The Long Beach boy and the Chicago guy forged a friendship that would last for years, interrupted briefly years later when Bailey lost his quaint "little" restaurant to Beilsmith on the turn of a card.

* * *

Soon, ads were appearing regularly in the Paralyzed Veterans of America's monthly *Paraplegia News* and elsewhere:

> **WINE, WOMEN, MARIACHIS**
> **This may not be the reason you come to GUADALAJARA, but this is why you will stay.**
> **Write to LaMorada for brochure on the longest established center for men in wheelchairs. (Formerly George Ray's place). Unmatched advantages — location, special nightman, total facilities under one roof. Cubilete 147, Guadalajara 5, Jal., Mex.**

The new residents and visitors to Quadalajara were presented with a unique challenge: how to replace twenty-four hours of monotonous and, at times, depressing institutional or shut-in living with twenty-four hours of living in their new-found paradise. For most,

Mexico's version of wine, women, and song—*tequila, señoritas, y mariachis*—was more than one could possibly have imagined or ever hoped for merely a year or so earlier. Just being able to get around outdoors in the sunshine of a new day in Quadalajara was a blessing.

Unfortunately for some, however, overindulging in what their new lives had to offer was a problem. Young men on their own, some for the first time since joining the military or being drafted into serving their country, had very little experience in the "real world." It was a time for them to discover life and, in many cases, to mature in this foreign land and in a foreign body that even the medical profession had yet to gain an understanding of.

Having unstructured free time and extra spending money led some to consume more beer and tequila than the human body should. Spending more time in one's wheelchair than accustomed to or recommended, especially sitting on a simple '50s or '60s foam rubber cushion, was a bedsore waiting to happen. Most bed/pressure sores in the spinal cord injured population actually happened while the paralyzed person was *not* in bed.

The additional problem of urinary tract infections, which up until World War II and the evolution of antibiotics claimed the lives of most spinal cord injured, was another serious problem the early Pioneers faced.

The death of a few of Quadalajara's earliest explorers (including one who bled to death as a result of a punctured bladder wall incurred during a complicated catheter change), coupled with others returning to the Long Beach VA with horrific pressure sores and urinary tract problems, served to confirm what some of the chief medical staff had preached: "You're only going down there to die." But what alternatives did many of these young men have? With no social life, no job opportunities, and institutional living with a limited post injury life expectancy of seven to however many years, venturing into the uncertainty of living in Mexico provided an intriguing option.

Quadalajara's Pioneers pushed forward, and most who decided to take advantage of a second chance at life were soon returning from stateside visits with their own transportation. George Ray would encourage and assist other transportationally challenged newcomers wanting to make Quadalajara their new home by driving and accompanying them to the border, where his friend and local contact would make the arrangements for the purchase of a new automobile. A side trip to the commissary at the military base would allow them an opportunity to stock up on sheets, bedding, and some of life's necessities that were otherwise difficult to obtain in Mexico.

With more hand-control driven automobiles came more opportunities. Besides visits with new friends in other parts of the city and easier access to Quadalajara-after-dark, increased transportation meant increased opportunity to venture outside the already familiar in pursuit of other interests.

Trips to Mexican seaports like Puerto Vallarta, Barra de Navidad, and Manzanillo became more frequent. Many of the Pioneers had previously traveled by or stayed in Guaymus and Mazatlan, but guys like Tony Gomez, Doc Foland, George Ray, Joe Miller, Manny Trujillo, Steve Wilson, Vern Thorsen, Gato, Carroll Stodgel, and Jerry Fesenmyer, found the fishing port of Manzanillo more to their liking. It became common for groups of Quadalajara's earliest wheelers to pile into a mini caravan of three or four cars and head for their favorite fishing hole, Manzanillo. Once there, one or two fishing boats were rented, while the captain and mates would look on curiously as their newest clients were carefully transferred by their Mexican attendants—wheelchairs and all—safely on to the deck. A few hours of drinking cerveza and catching fish, while getting too much sun on a hopefully calm day at sea, was usually the norm. A tradition that began early on in the Quadalajara era would continue for many years to follow.

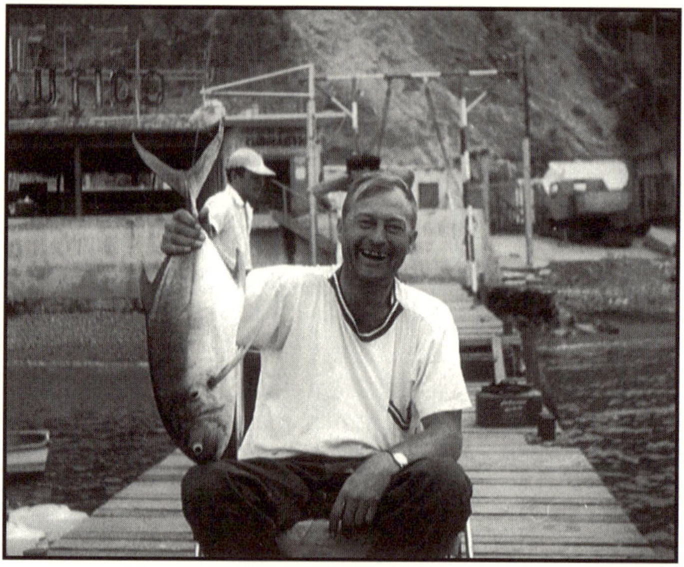

George Ray
Manzanillo, Mexico

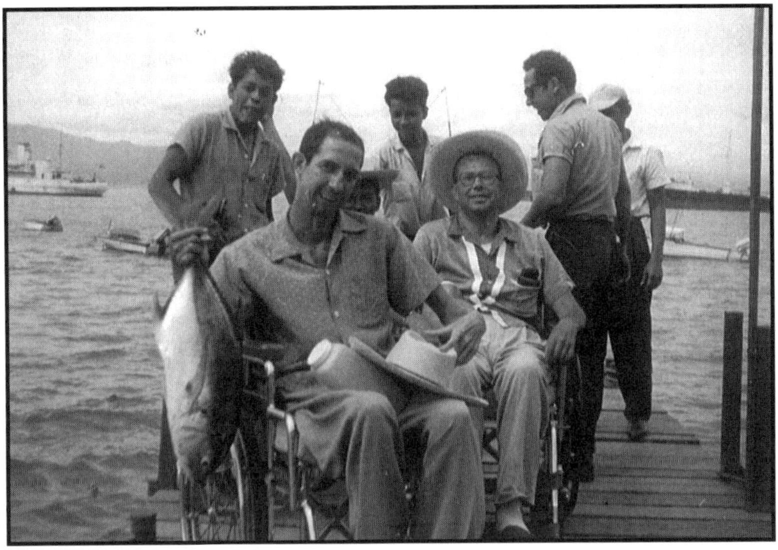

Ray Foland and friends
Manzanillo, Mexico

As Quadalajara's population grew, many of the newcomers came from the Hines VA. Whether these were indeed the wild bunch ("*De locos*") that Maria Elena spoke of or not, one thing was a given: the sunshiny weather and accessibility of this recently discovered utopia were important factors for all those migrating from the cold climate and inaccessible cities in the midwestern, northern, and northeastern areas of the United States. The boys from Southern California may have arrived first, but those from "*Chicago y otros de quien sabe donde*,"[41] as Maria Elena recalled, found Quadalajara just as intriguing.

In December 1963, a number of Quadalajara's quadriplegic and paraplegic American residents united in a historic effort to brighten Christmas for hundreds of children at the state-run Hospicio Cabañas orphanage. The newly formed "Alliance for Compassion" would be the foundation for future endeavors by Quadalajara's newest residents as they pushed forward into un-chartered territory.

This effort was described by John Reese in the June 1964 *PN* as the same "incorrigible bunch of American quadriplegics and paraplegics" who gave the big Christmas party at the orphanage. The Alliance for Compassion "took three hundred of the kids for an all-day

[41] Chicago, and others from who knows where else.

picnic and swim at one of the newest and most beautiful resorts here, Los Camachos, in the spectacular setting of the wild Barrancas."

Wheelers throw king-size party for orphans

by John Reese

GUADALAJARA, MEXICO—Those guys are at it again.

The same incorribigle bunch of American quadriplegics and paraplegics who gave the big Christmas party at the state orphanage took 300 of the kids for an all-day picnic and swim at one of the newest and most beautiful resorts here, Los Camachos, in the spectacular setting of the wild Barrancas.

This was an even more ambitious project than the Christmas posada. It meant transporting everyone but the nursery babies 15 miles out into the country, feeding them all day, providing lifeguard protection in an acre of clear mountain water in a blue-tile pool, and getting them all back, exhausted but happy and safe, that night.

3,200 persons raised

The paraplegics' "Alliance for Compassion," as they now call it here, raised 3,200 pesos in one of the quietest fund drives in money-raising history.

What baffles everyone in the big American colony here is that nobody seems to want any credit, nobody wants his name in the local papers, nobody even wants to admit he was a part of it.

Nevertheless, although only 18 contributors showed up to see their money at work, it is known that "around 30 or 40" donors contributed.

The picnic was unprecedented in the 177-year-old history of the Hospicio de Cabanas, the State orphanage. The kids drank 900 bottles of soft drinks and ate three-quarters of a ton of food. They kept the pool filled in relays, some of them wearing swim-suits paid for out of the paraplegics' money.

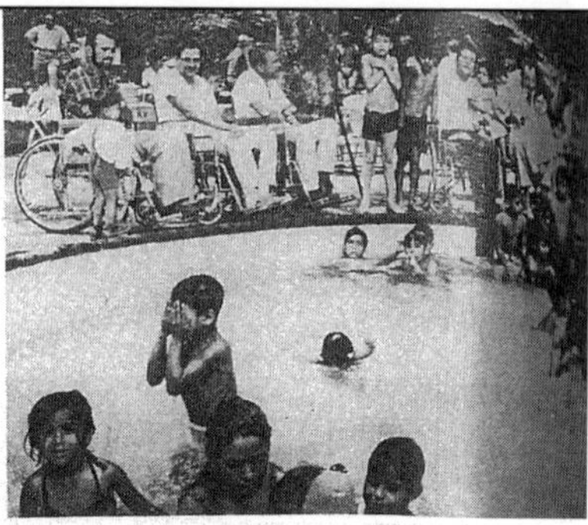

A few of the "Alliance for Compassion" boys watch their picnic guests from poolside. (L to R) Marion Fuget, Ernie Chavez, Bill Bailey, Larry Kegan, George Small (chairman of the group) Bill Coe, and Jose Miller.

Record in foreign aid

When you figure that the cost per kid was only about 10 pesos — that's 80 cents U.S. — you're getting pretty close to a new economy record in Foreign Aid It couldn't be done, but they did it.

The attention this "impossible" act of charity drew makes the American paraplegics one of the most influential groups in the big American colony here. From now on, their support is going to count heavily.

After the success of the Christmas party, it was relatively easy to line up help for this. The American School and the Municipal Police contributed the buses. State and Highway police detailed men to help handle the kids. A big brewery brought in folding tables and chairs, set them up, and hauled them away afterwards.

Early in 1964 George Ray and some of the residents of Quadalajara began to toy with the idea of a Paralyzed Veterans of America chapter in Mexico. Many of the Alliance for Compassion boys had been living in Quadalajara for a number of years, while still maintaining membership in their chapters back home. California PVA for the Long Beach crowd and Vaughn Chapter PVA for the boys from Chicago, with a sprinkling of PVAers from other chapters; a PVA chapter in Quadalajara would serve to unite all who wished to participate. In addition to helping the kids at the orphanage, it would be helpful to have a functioning veteran's service organization in Quadalajara to better serve those specifically disabled with spinal cord injuries who chose to visit or make Mexico their new home. It would also add clout and purpose to this ragtag group of gringo neighbors from the North who some locals still viewed as nothing but a bunch of drunks and womanizers.

On April 21, 1964, eighteen paraplegics and quadriplegics met at George Ray's Place to discuss forming a PVA chapter in Quadalajara. The *Paraplegia News*, July 1964:

> **2 new chapters seek PVA affiliation**
>
> Mexico and the Great Northwest join the growing list of areas wishing to establish their own PVA chapter.
>
> On April 21, 18 paraplegic and quadriplegic veterans met in Chapalita, a suburb of Guadalajara, to form the nucleus of a Mexico Chapter of the PVA.
>
> At the initial meeting, a slate of officers was elected: William M. Bailey, president; Charles J. Miller, vice-president; and George C. Ray, secretary treasurer. Named to the board of directors were Charles J. Ceska, Lee Schlyer, Stanley Pruncal, and Donald Evans.
>
> The new group adopted the by-laws suggested in the booklet "How to Run a PVA Chapter," and have applied for affiliation with the Paralyzed Veterans of America.

In an April 24 letter to National PVA Vice President Harold Stone, George Ray reported:

> *All eighteen were very enthusiastic about the prospect and all have pledged membership as soon as we can get a charter.*
>
> *The following officers were elected until the end of the*

fiscal year ending June 30: President, William M. Bailey; Vice President, Charles J. Miller; Secretary-Treasurer, George Ray; Board of Directors appointed Charles J. Ceska, Lee Schyler, Stanley Prucnal, and Donald Evans.

The pledged members were: Bill Bailey, Charles "Joe" Miller, Robert Krekeler, George E. Ray, Edward G. Lucier, Donald Evans, Carroll Stodgel, Lee Schlyer, John P. Nichol, Stanley Prucnal, Charles Ceska, Bob Barrett, Bob Beske, Chuck Derevjanik, Robert Enge, Ken Perry, George Small, Marion Fuget, Bob Powell.

We would certainly welcome any suggestions and advice you might offer, also, if you could send us a book on Robert's Rules of Order...if you have any membership application blanks, we would appreciate about a hundred because we have many more potential members that haven't been contacted yet.

We will keep you posted as to our activities and are really going to try to turn out a good chapter.

Sincerely,
George E. Ray

The fact that George Ray requested one hundred "membership blanks" verified the growth of Quadalajara's spinal cord injured population from the handful of Pioneers who Maria Elena Cruz met nearly eight years earlier to a substantial community of people who shared common needs and experiences.

In a handwritten note dated May 10, 1964, titled, "Affiliation," National PVA Vice President Harold Stone wrote:

Dear George,

Please Pardon the note; I have been extra busy. Allow me to congratulate you on the fine job you have done. Soon the directors will be asked to vote for your affiliation as a PVA chapter. As a PVA chapter you will be entitled to send a delegate to the convention in Los Angeles at National expense—details later.

Will send Robert's Rules.

Sincerely,
Hal

On June 17, 1964, the Mexico Chapter, Paralyzed Veterans of America became a reality, and a new era was born. George Ray's vision had again brought results, much as his foresight and efforts had in enabling so many disabled individuals to realize a new life south of the border.

* * *

At the June 17 meeting, outgoing Mexico Chapter President Bill Bailey officially handed the gavel to the now nationally chartered Mexico Chapter, Paralyzed Veterans of America's first president, Charles "Joe" Miller. Joining Miller were Vice President Charles Ceska and Secretary/Treasurer George Ray, along with Board of Directors Bob Jackson, Stanley Prucnal, Ray Foland, Bill Bailey, Lee Schyler and Bob Beilsmith. (It was interesting to note that all three chapter officers had been nominated by former Alliance of Compassion Chairman George Small, who would remain in the background but continue to be an active member. Small also proposed "that all paralyzed persons not eligible for PVA membership be admitted as honorary members." George Ray seconded the motion and it was adopted.) Additionally, Ray was selected to represent the newly founded Mexico Chapter, Paralyzed Veterans of America at the National PVA's annual convention in Santa Monica, California from July 21 to July 29, 1964.

In the following months, the Mexico Chapter PVA continued to evolve and grow in numbers. The members decided to have different meeting places each month. The first was the Vienna Room Restaurant at the local bowling alley. The duties of secretary/treasurer were split, and Bob Barrett became the Mexico PVA's new treasurer with Ray remaining as chapter secretary. George Small, Bill Bailey, Ray Foland, and Larry Kegan were appointed to a social function fundraising committee. The committee decided on a BINGO party at the Jewish Community Club to raise funds for a Christmas party at the Hospicio Cabañas orphanage. A goal of 6,000 pesos was set.

At the January 18, 1965 Mexico Chapter PVA meeting, George Ray announced he had secured the facilities of a motel with "ample space for the Chapter BINGO games," which by now were a huge fundraising success. Ray also suggested that "a monthly bulletin be sent to all members and prospective members informing them of what has been accomplished and what we propose to accomplish." During that meeting, however, it was President Miller's detailed report on the children's Christmas party that was the highlight of this particular PVA meeting.

According to Miller, "It was a most moving and worthwhile occasion."

It was reported that, "The chapter collected 7,175 pesos and spent 7,172.50. Over four hundred orphaned and abandoned children received presents, candy, fruit, and nuts, and had a supper and entertainment. Without the contributions of the paralyzed veterans, these children would have had a very bleak Christmas."

* * *

From its infancy, PVA's Mexico Chapter had laid the groundwork for its primary source of revenue, outside of the generosity and compassion of its members, and had established helping Mexico's poorest children—especially at Christmastime—as one of its top priorities.

Former Alliance for Compassion chairman, George Small, passed away in 1966. From the August 1966 *Paraplegia News*: "Candy for three hundred youngsters, three big piñatas, and other party and fun materials were bought from a fund left by the late George Small for this purpose. Small, one of the first paraplegics to settle here and a leader in community projects that thus far have benefited more than three thousand poor children, died last month and left money to carry on similar child welfare work."

The Pioneers had laid the groundwork for those who would follow. Although uncertainty about this mysterious utopian city somewhere in Mexico remained, those who came to Quadalajara after the early-60s benefited from what the early wheelchair settlers had explored, endured, and conquered. Life in Quadalajara was still a unique experience for those who tried it, but it had been made all that much easier by those brave souls who first ventured into the unknown.

Chapter 14

Cold Weather and Cold Warriors

Eddie Lucier was injured while serving with the Army Airborne Division at Fort Campbell, Kentucky in 1961. The injury left Lucier a C5/C6 quadriplegic. After a medical discharge from the Army, the young man from Warwick, RI was transferred for further treatment at a VA rehabilitation center, close to home in West Roxbury, MA.

While there, Lucier's steadfast determination to rehabilitate his paralyzed body drew high praise from physical therapist Vinnie Anderson. Anderson would eventually publish a book on rehabilitating patients with spinal cord injuries. Eddie Lucier would be immortalized within its pages in photos illustrating how some quadriplegics can use certain devices and techniques to assist themselves when sitting up in bed, getting dressed, and transferring into a wheelchair.

With rehabilitation behind him and an uncertain future ahead of him, Lucier—as some of his hospital buddies already had—opted to check out a place in Mexico that promoted freedom and a new beginning for paraplegics and quadriplegics. After contracting with one of the West Roxbury hospital attendants to accompany him, Lucier was on his way to spend Christmas of 1963 at George Ray's Place in Quadalajara.

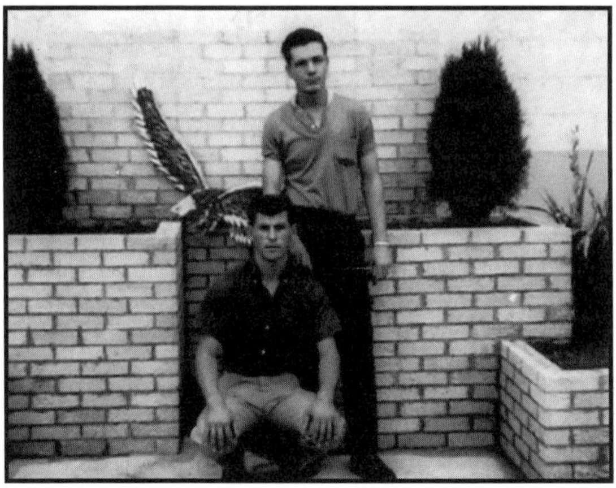

Eddie Lucier (front) with Army buddy at Fort Campbell, KY, circa 1960

Earlier that same month, a young man named Gabriel Chavez had been hired by George Ray, and trained to care for spinal cord injured residents at the popular gimp camp also referred to simply as *Cubilete*. Two adjoining houses on Avenida Cubilete in Colonia Chapalita had merged as one, thus converting George Ray's Place into a spacious eight bedroom residence for quadriplegic and paraplegic residents and visitors. Separate upstairs quarters housed attendants who worked the night shift.

Eddie Lucier was experiencing the carefree lifestyle that few places, if any at the time, offered, basking in the sunshine of this fascinating Mexican city far from the sleet, snow, and inaccessible buildings of Warwick, RI.

Little did Eddie and fellow newcomer Gabriel Chavez know how intertwined their lives would become.

* * *

Veracruz was the destination as three amigos from the West Roxbury VA, Claudio Bertoli, Billy Gilly, and Eddie Lucier, ventured out of their Quadalajara home to explore some of Mexico's famous tourist attractions. They left George Ray's Place in two convertibles. "*Claudio tenia un convertible y Billy Gilly tambien. Un Mustang,*"[42] recalled Gabriel Chavez, who was to accompany and assist Lucier on this junket. When asked if he was Lucier's regular attendant at the time, Gabriel replied, "*No, yo trabajaba para George Ray. Todos ayudaban a todos.*"[43]

"*Fuímos a Veracruz pero era tiempo de Carnaval y no tenian* rooms for nobody. *De alli fuímos a* Mexico City *y Acapulco,*"[44] recollected Gabriel Chavez, mixing Spanish and English.

Lucier was fortunate to have found this quad paradise only a few years post-injury. He was soon caught up in the momentum that would transform Quadalajara from its early wild era of *Tequila, Señoritas y Mariachis* to the more mature era of organized efforts helping fellow veterans, the local orphanage, and poor school children.

As these efforts grew, along with Quadalajara's gringo wheelchair population, Lucier found himself working with men such as

---

[42] Claudio had a convertible and Billy Gilly too. A Mustang.

[43] No, I worked for George Ray. Everyone helped everyone.

[44] We went to Veracruz, but it was Carnival time and there weren't rooms for nobody. From there we went to Mexico City and Acapulco.

George Ray, Bill Bailey, George Small, Joe Miller, Charles Ceska, and others in early 1964. All were among those who pledged their support for a possible chapter of the Paralyzed Veterans of America in Mexico. The idea and effort became a reality in June of that year.

The founding of the Mexico Chapter PVA further galvanized the growing community of American wheelers from across the United States. Men and women with diverse backgrounds and interests, residing at Bill Coe's, Larry Kegan's, and George Ray's Place were now meeting and greeting like never before. Lucier's role in all of this would soon evolve, just as the newly founded Mexico PVA Chapter had.

In 1966, after a time of living the "snowbird" way of life, spending his summer visiting family in Rhode Island (mother and father, six brothers, including twin brother David, and five sisters) and spending the rest of the year at George Ray's Place, Lucier and fellow New Englander Art Wheaton, as well as Bob Powell of Illinois, decided that it was time to get a place of their own. They now called Quadalajara home and the need to reside in an assisted living facility was no longer a necessity.

"*Despues de dos años es cuando Lalo dijó 'vamos a cambiarnos de aqui.' Es cuando se pusieron de acuerdo los tres, Don Roberto, Arthur Wheaton y Eddie y nos cambiamos a Vallarta San Jorge. Hidalgo 3333,*"[45] Gabriel recalled.

Although Lucier, accompanied by Gabriel Chavez, made annual trips to Rhode Island and side trips to the West Roxbury VA for medical checkups or just to shoot the bull with fellow hospitalized New Englanders, his role as social chairman for the Mexico PVA continued to emerge and expand.

Snowbird picnics became semi-annual events, send-offs in the spring or welcoming returning PVA members, friends, and visitors back home in time to escape the upcoming cold weather of their stateside hometowns in the fall.

From the February 1967 *El Sombrero News*, information on the semi-annual Snowbird Picnic by Lucier:

---

[45] After two years Lalo (short for Eduardo, Edward) said, "We are going to move out of here." That's when the three agreed, Don (a show of respect) Roberto, Arthur Wheaton, and Eddie, and we moved to Vallarta San Jorge. Hidalgo 3333.

Snowbird's Picnic

by Lucier

The trap is all set for the Snowbird Picnic Sunday Feb. 26, 12:00 noon at Granja Pavitos, Circunvalación #81 in Las Fuentes. This picnic was especially arranged for those flying down for the winter months. Anyone who attended the October picnic will verify the fact that Granja Pavitos is the perfect spot for a picnic and is very convenient for wheelchairs. It is a very generous gesture on the part of Col. Reggie Anderson and his lovely wife Collito to permit us to use their beautiful gardens and facilities for this occasion.

Fifty cases of cold canned Tecate and Bohemia will be on hand for the thirsty. You are also welcome to bring your own mixin's. There will be plenty of soft drinks. The bill of fare will consist of charcoal broiled hamburgers, with the big Tlaquepaque buns, Taeko's potato salad, and all the trimmins. Live music will start at 1:00 PM until who knows.

The National Vice-President Len Chrysler is trying to arrange his schedule so that he can attend the picnic. Len is a grand guy and will probably have a message of interest to all. He is also one of the foremost athletes in wheelchair sports.

There should be no transportation problem this time as a lot of members have volunteered to help those without cars to and from the picnic. See Jack Myrick and he will coordinate the transportation wherever needed.

Don't forget that someone is going to win a beautiful new Motorola television set. So, hope to see all of you, your friends, and guests SUNDAY Feb. 26.

From the March 1967 *El Sombrero News*, a report on the semi-annual Snowbird Picnic by Ray and Lucier:

Picnic

by Ray & Lucier

In my opinion and the opinion of several others with whom I've talked about our last picnic, it was one of the best to-date put on anywhere by anyone. I can't think of anything that could have been added to make it a greater success. The hamburgers were big, plentiful, and straight from the charcoal grill, Taeko's potato salad as usual was an experience in good eating, and the bread and butter pickles were like mother used to try to make. The 45 cases of beer consumed kept things moving along at a lively pace. The mariachis were on time and played loud and clear. We had a good wheelchair turn-out and a lot of distinguished guests. Among the distinguished guests we were fortunate in having with us were: National Vice-President of PVA Len Chrysler and his wife Cloey, President of the Instituto Cultural Frank Leakey and his wife Connie—who is a distinguished guest in her own right for the work and contributions she has made in getting a home started and operating for children who had no home, Veterans Affairs Officer from our local consulate George Hiraga, and Rev. Paul Hunter who we all know and know of by his contributions to the American and Mexican communities.

I think you would be safe in saying that the picnic was also a financial success as we showed a net profit of $3230 pesos. We could have possibly made a few centavos more except that the number one jefe of Circunvalación Sur #62 thought it would be a good idea to put on a bar-b-q across the street from us at the same time in order that we would not be swamped and have to turn anyone away. They must have run a little short as they sent over for hamburgers. We were only too happy to oblige as we had plenty.

Quadriplegics Lucier, Powell, and Wheaton continued to share their three bedroom home in Vallarta San Jorge for eight years. According to Gabriel, "*Vivian ocho años juntos. Luego Wheaton se casó, y Don Roberto fallació. Es cuando Lalo compró el lote y hizo una casa donde duró veinte años. En Jardines del Sur.*"[46]

Meanwhile, Mexico PVA workaholic Eddie Lucier welcomed fellow Mexico PVA workaholic Ray Clifford to his house on Hidalgo 3333, Vallarta San Jorge in 1972. Jimmy Lietz and attendant Miguel Lopez joined them a year later. Interestingly enough, both Gabriel Chavez and Miguel Lopez—who would later work for Jack Tumidajski—dedicated over thirty-five years to caring for quadriplegic veterans.

Eddie Lucier passed away in Quadalajara in 2001.

---

[46] They lived together for eight years. Then Wheaton got married and Don Roberto passed away. That's when Lalo bought the lot and built the house where he lived for twenty years. In South Gardens.

Charlie Newbold was 23 years old when an auto mishap left him a quadriplegic in October of 1961. "The accident happened in Spain," he explained. "I was actually stationed in France and should have returned stateside, but had my Army tour extended by three months when the Berlin Wall went up."

Newbold, one of the early "Cold Warriors," continued, "Since my tour had been extended and I was granted leave time, I decided to go to Spain." The ironic twist of fate changed the course of Charlie Newbold's life. He would spend part of that year at the St. Alban's Naval Hospital before being transferred to the Bronx VA Hospital in December.

"I was in the VA a long time. I just didn't know where I was gonna go or what I could do," recalled Newbold. "I was there in '61, all of '62, '63, and most of '64."

Asked about when he thought about checking out Quadalajara, Newbold replied, "My friend Joe Cicero is the one who really pushed us to go." Charlie Newbold was in the same situation as many. "I grew up in the Bronx. My mother lived in a three-story walk-up." Not exactly wheelchair friendly accommodations. "I'd never have gotten out on my own. We had guys living at the hospital for thirteen, fourteen, and even seventeen years. After a while, you just figured that was the way it was going to be."

On November 12, 1964, Charlie Newbold and hospital buddy Joe Cicero made their move to Quadalajara. "Because of some labor dispute or something, the plane landed at the Zapopan airfield and we came into the city on Avenida Vallarta. George Ray had sent a worker named Poncho to bring Cicero and me back to his place. One thing that impressed me was the big, wide boulevard with a median and the palm trees and bushes all around. I was very impressed with that. And then I got the culture shock. We're on this big avenue just cruising with no cars around, and then all of a sudden there's a guy on a burro.

"Anyway, when I got to George Ray's, it was evening. One of the first people I met was Larry Blinn," continued Newbold. "Since it was after dinner, Blinn and some of the others guys sent one of the aides out for roast chicken. They had a platter full of chicken and all I could say was, 'This place is heaven, look at the kind of food they serve you.'

It had been a long day for the latest arrivals from New York. "We had had to get up early at the hospital and my mother and step-father took Cicero and me to the airport, just the two of us. We didn't have any aides come with us. I remember before we went to bed just sitting at the dining room table in George Ray's Place. We talked and drank some beer. Another night they took us to the Jacaranda Bar, it was a popular place when I got there. Later, we went to Goldtooth's place, where you just sit in the car, drink beer, and the girls come out and sit in the car with you."

Charlie Newbold's initiation to Quadalajara-after-dark continued with an all-nighter in the city's infamous San Juan de Dios district.

"I had my aid tell the guy I wanted six to eight eggs. So we sat there and ate hard boiled eggs, and then wound up at the Mariachi Plaza."

On another occasion, Newbold got to try another popular street treat, "pulpo."

"My aid didn't know the name of it, but I found out the next day that I'd eaten octopus."

After spending time and familiarizing himself with Quadalajara, Charlie noted, "There seemed to be two camps: one comprised of guys from Long Beach, and the other of guys from Chicago." His statement tended to echo what Maria Elena Cruz had observed years earlier.

Newbold would eventually meet Pioneers Joe Miller and Bill Bailey, "who would come over to George Ray's Place every week to play pinochle." Bob Barrett lived right up the street. In February, George Ray, his wife, and Barrett accompanied Newbold to San Antonio to purchase a vehicle. George Ray's contact got Charlie a good deal on a car.

"All he wanted was a few bottles of liquor and a hundred cartons of Faro cigarettes, Mexico's cheapest. They only cost 40 centavos, or 8¢ U.S., and had only sixteen in a pack, at that time." The quad who grew up in the Bronx would later meet and become good friends with Minnesota quad Larry Kegan. Kegan ran a place in Las Fuentes, which was similar to George Ray's Place. Besides being known for operating one of Quadalajara's three main "gimp camps," the third being Bill Coe's also in Las Fuentes, Larry Kegan's claim to fame was knowing someone famous. He grew up with and was close friends with singer/songwriter Bob Dylan.

"They were friends since grade school," Newbold explained. "They were the only two Jewish boys in class." On a trip to visit and hang out with his paralyzed childhood friend in Quadalajara, Dylan accompanied Kegan to visit Newbold.

"I wasn't home when they stopped by," a somewhat

disappointed Newbold remarked years later. "My daughter is a big Bob Dylan fan. She's even read books about him. I didn't really get involved much. I sort of stayed by myself. I rented a place with Cicero for a while, but then got a place of my own. That's when I began to hang around with Bob Nemac, Manny Trujillo, and Kegan."

Charlie Newbold's Quadalajara experience began as uniquely as most and yet was familiar to many young quads who were on their own for the first time. Newbold would later twice marry Mexican women. He too would blend into the community, occasionally attend PVA meetings, and participate in charitable functions, including having his picture taken by a local newspaper at Hospicio Cabañas while he held one of the orphans.

* * *

JoAnn Raway first experienced Quadalajara in November 1964. "I went on a three week vacation to Las Fuentes with my sister Luella and our friend, Roselyn Mahowald." While Charlie Newbold and Bronx VA buddy Joe Cicero were discovering their newfound freedoms at George Ray's Place, the three women from Minnesota simultaneously vacationed in Las Fuentes. "Paul Patino and Larry Kegan ran the place," JoAnn recalled. That was where JoAnn initially met fellow Minnesotan Tom Kirch, along with Joe Darichuk and Señors Patino and Kegan. "We were ready to return home when we saw the living conditions at Las Fuentes—and the dining room. I can still remember the plastic plates with cigarette burns." Apparently, guys (especially those who escaped institutional living) tended to overlook such minor details.

JoAnn first heard about Quadalajara from Bob Peters, a fellow member of Minnesota's social club for the handicapped.

"He first went to Quadalajara in '63 or '64 and stayed for a few months." Larry Kegan, who was also from the Twin Cities area, "went to different local places, including the VA, telling people about the ideal climate and reasonable cost of living for winter visitors there." Asked about accommodations for disabled women, JoAnn Raway indicated that other women had visited Las Fuentes earlier. "I first met Eileen Van Albert in 1964. She was already established with her own home in Colonia Chapalita by then. There were two women from New York who also stayed there."

With all that Quadalajara had to offer, the three vacationing women from Minnesota wanted to make the most of their precious three week visit.

"When we first got there, we presented Kegan with a list of places in and around Quadalajara that we wished to visit."

Although Kegan's ads had mentioned local tourist attractions, the surprised landlord responded, "No one's ever done that to me before."

"He was so floored," added JoAnn.

The three visiting women got their wish. Larry Kegan proved to be a worthy host and tour guide. According to their hometown newspaper, "They got to see such sights as Jalisco's Lake Chapala with its resorts and fishing villages, the town of Tequila and the factory where the famous drink was distilled, Tlaquepaque with its popular Mariachi Plaza and glass and silver factories, bull fights at Entrada a la Plaza, the city's huge Mercado Libertad, and fiestas in mountain villages. Additionally, the women were impressed with Quadalajara's flower-filled parks and plazas, colonial architecture, palm trees, and fountains. Other points of interest included the Cathedral de Guadalajara, the seventeenth century Basílica de Zapopan, and the Hospicio Cabañas Orphanage which housed the famous paintings of Orozco." (José Clemente Orozco was one of the 20th Century's most famous painters. Known for his mural paintings, he decorated many public buildings both in Mexico and in the United States. His work frequently embraced the themes of the Mexican Revolution.)

JoAnn's secretarial job in cold country was still easily manageable, despite living with Spinal Muscular Atrophy (a type of Muscular Dystrophy, simply referred to as MD). It wasn't the climate, cost of living, or beauty of the city that caught JoAnn Raway's eye. It was the handsome skinny quad, Tom Kirch. JoAnn and Tom began a friendship that would continue by mail and occasional phone calls (calling the U.S. from Mexico and vice versa could easily set one's pocketbook back to the tune of a dollar per minute). Finally, they had a reunion of sorts in 1967. "Tom was in the Minneapolis VA from spring until November," JoAnn continued. "That's when things really heated up."

While JoAnn continued her work and long distance relationship with Tom Kirch, Roselyn Mahowald would return to Quadalajara with another friend, Mary Margaret Sommers, in 1965. "Roselyn passed away sometime later and Mary Margaret stayed for a few more years."

JoAnn Raway and Tom Kirch picked up their friendship-turned-romance by mail and occasional phone calls after Tom returned to Quadalajara, until 1970—decision time.

"I went down to Las Fuentes for ten days," JoAnn recalled.

"To deliver an ultimatum?" she was quizzed.

"We had a lot to talk about," JoAnn responded. "About quitting my job, applying for Social Security, which took six months, and getting the documents we needed to get married in Mexico."

JoAnn returned in early September 1971. "Tom wanted to get married that week. He had to check into the VA hospital in Long Beach in a week and wanted to get married before he left. We could take care of the legal stuff more easily that way." JoAnn Raway was visiting Tom at the Jardines Alcalde house he rented along with Jim Adkisson, Bill Kahler, and Ray Clifford, when Bill and Maria Elena Bailey stopped by.

"Tom asked Bailey if he could help make arrangements for our civil marriage before Tom left for Long Beach. Maria Elena said, 'How about tonight?' and went to find a judge to perform the ceremony. We all piled into one car and went to Bob and Teresa Beilsmith's house. They weren't expecting us."

Tom's roommates and friends soon followed them to the Beilsmith's home. "Maria Elena came back with a judge and we were married that night."

What began as a three week winter vacation to sunny Quadalajara in November 1964 would alter the course of JoAnn Raway's life. On September 12, 1971 Josephine "JoAnn" Raway from Hastings, Minnesota became JoAnn Kirch. The seven-year Quadalajara-to-Minnesota courtship with Tom Kirch of Kellogg, Minnesota culminated with the impromptu wedding at the home of Bob and Teresa Beilsmith. A church wedding would follow after Tom returned. On March 11, 1972 JoAnn and Tom Kirch were "officially" wed at Our Lady of Guadalupe Catholic Church in Colonia Chapalita.

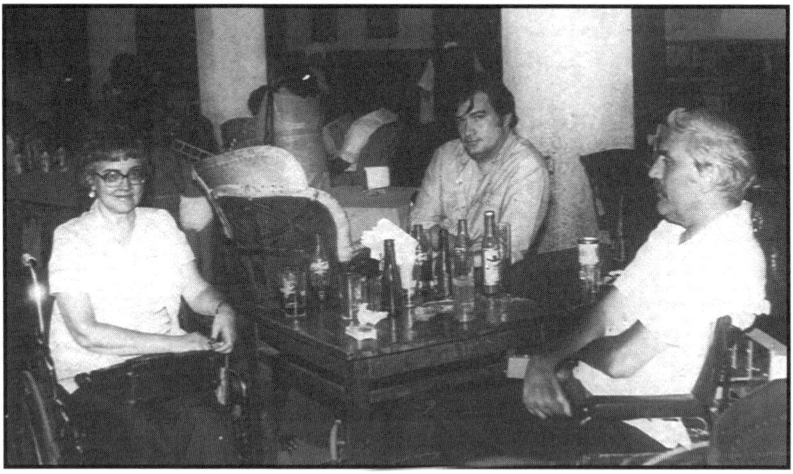

Jim Lietz flanked by JoAnn and Tom Kirch

Keith Ziegler was one of those few quadriplegics who went on to college after sustaining a spinal cord injury in 1960 at the age of twenty-one. Ziegler, another "Cold Warrior" who had earlier been stationed with the Air Force in Morocco, spent the next six months hospitalized in Denver before being transferred to the Long Beach VA. With the help of his parents, Keith returned to his now-modified and wheelchair accessible home in Colorado, and to an uncertain future in higher education. After three years, it became apparent that Ziegler's pursuit of a college English degree was becoming increasingly more difficult. His parents could only do so much, and full-time attendant care for a quadriplegic student on his own was beyond his financial means.

In 1965, Ziegler read an ad in the *Paraplegia News* about this place in Mexico that advertised:

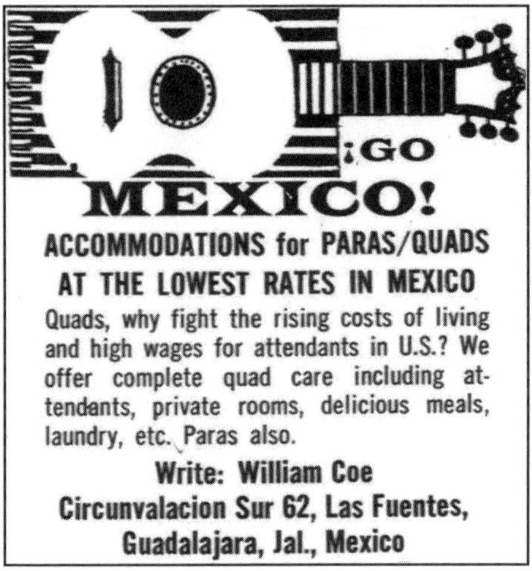
¡GO
MEXICO!
ACCOMMODATIONS for PARAS/QUADS
AT THE LOWEST RATES IN MEXICO
Quads, why fight the rising costs of living and high wages for attendants in U.S.? We offer complete quad care including attendants, private rooms, delicious meals, laundry, etc. Paras also.
Write: William Coe
Circunvalacion Sur 62, Las Fuentes,
Guadalajara, Jal., Mexico

A few months later, Keith and his parents were on their way to check out Bill Coe's. Asked what his first day was like in Quadalajara, Ziegler responded, "They were a bunch of drunks. The owner was drunk, his wife was drunk, and the room was all mildewed and wet. My parents didn't like it and went for a walk the next day and saw Kegan's Place and said, 'You're coming over here.' I had a nice room by myself. It was dry and comfortable. I knew Tom Kirch from Long Beach. Dave McDonald and Joe Darichuk, I'd seen before."

Unlike those quads staying at Kegan's who Keith already knew from Long Beach, the guys at Bill Coe's "were mostly paras with pressure sores who stayed in bed all day and shot their pistols at night. There was one guy named 'Cowboy' and another named Ben something-or-other. Bill Coe used to get drunk and curse at Kegan at night and fire his pistol."

"At Kegan?" Ziegler was asked.

"No, just in the air."

Might this be the "entertainment" mentioned in many "WHY MEXICO?" and "GO MEXICO" ads?

"The first time I went out was in Joe Darichuk's car," Ziegler recounted. "I met Frank Stocker, Chuck Devejanik, and this other redheaded para named Bob Enge. Just about everyone I met who didn't stay in one of the gimp camps had their own automobile. Even some of the guys who stayed at Kegan's had their own cars. Besides Darichuk, Steve Wilson had his own. Eddie Lucier had his own."

Asked about some of his more memorable experiences in Quadalajara in the mid-60s, Ziegler recalled the time, "I was with

George Ray and he pulled out his pistol and BLAM, shot a sparrow through Joe Miller's window."

"Didn't some of the guys belong to a shooting club in Quadalajara?" Keith was asked. Ziegler wasn't aware of it, but added, "Some of the guys used to shoot doves on the Tequila Highway."

On a more positive note, Ziegler was one of many wheelers invited to a graduation party at the Hospicio Cabañas orphanage. "It was soon after I got there," he added. Mexico PVA's unofficial chaplain and friend, Reverend Paul Hunter, did the inviting. The honoree was a very bright, paralyzed teen who had just graduated from *la preparatoria*, Mexico's equivalent to high school. Although the event wasn't Mexico PVA sponsored, a number of its members, including one of its newest, Keith Ziegler, attended and donated money toward the purchase of a wheelchair, bed, and help toward Arturo Hyer's college education.

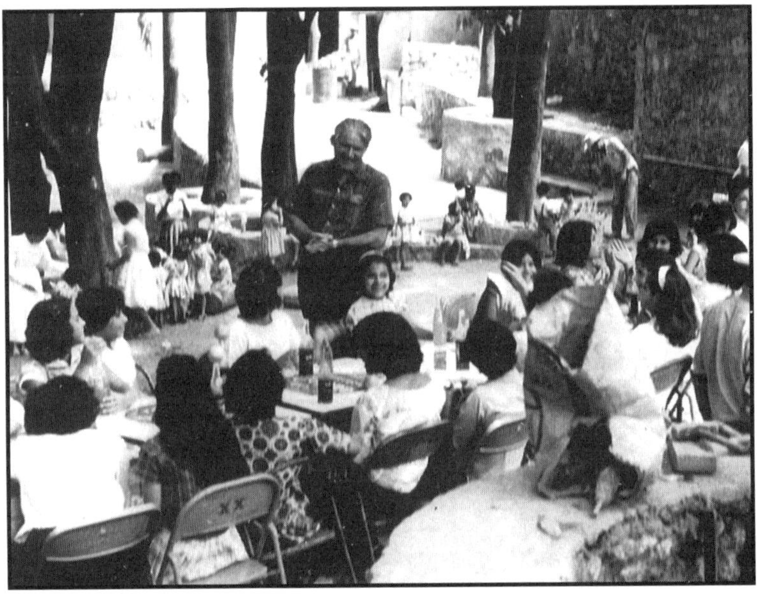

Reverend Paul Hunter at the Hospicio Cabañas Orphanage Quadalajara, 1964

The significance of Hyer's introduction to the Mexico PVA would have lasting implications. According to Ziegler, Hyer would go on to receive an engineering degree, a job in Santa Ana, California designing prosthetic equipment to better the lives of people with disabilities, and return home "to found a similar organization in Mexico."

La Asociación de Lisiados de Jalisco, A.C. (ALJAC), "would be formed around '72 or '73," according to Ziegler, with membership open to all of the state of Jalisco's disabled citizens.

Keith Ziegler returned stateside after about six months of getting to experience Quadalajara from rural Las Fuentes. He, too, would return with his own transportation and move out on his own to a different part of town.

He rented a house not far from George Ray's Place in Colonia Chapalita with fellow quad Jack Myrick. Myrick, like Ziegler, had attended college after his injury and discharge from the VA. Both became active in the Mexico Chapter PVA. But like many others living in Quadalajara, different interests and opportunities led them to take separate paths.

Keith Ziegler teamed with Steve Wilson and rented a farm in Ciudad Granja.

"We were going into the pig business," Ziegler mused. "We bought a bunch of baby pigs and Steve was the one who was going take care of them. It didn't turn out to be a profitable venture," Keith added. "We got lazy, he had trouble with the aides, and the pigs all died. I ended up in the Granja with a farm of my own that had ducks, geese, turkeys, and goats. I was raised a country boy," Keith sang.

"Didn't your wife's family live in La Granja?" he was queried. "Might that have had something to do with your moving out and staying in La Granja?"

Ziegler slyly replied, "That too. . ."

Keith Ziegler married Josefina Arana in 1968 and soon the couple was raising a family of their own. Ironically, years earlier, Josefina and her sister Olivia worked on the fifth floor of one of Quadalajara's taller buildings. They would look down at a convertible parked outside of the building. It was lunchtime, and the driver would pull up outside the building to talk to his girlfriend. She was the daughter of the owner of one of the businesses located there. He was Jerry Fesenmyer, another of Mexico PVA's members.

"I thought he was so handsome," remembered Josefina. The thought that she someday would marry one of these American wheelers never crossed her mind.

"Did the fact that he used a wheelchair cause you to view him any differently?" she was asked.

"No, I just thought he was like anyone else."

But Josefina wasn't the only one to find an earlier attraction. "I was at a party in La Granja. We were talking and drinking and I noticed this girl," Keith recalled. "So I started making eyes at her." The uninterested señorita was Olivia Arana, Josefina's sister. "She went home and told Josefina about me."

* * *

Jerry Fesenmyer took his first trip to Quadalajara in 1965. Fesenmyer was neither a "Cold Warrior" nor someone trying to escape the cold weather, although no stranger to cold weather, having grown up in Iowa. Jerry was a World War II veteran who had been shot during combat in Okinawa in May 1945. "I couldn't tell you what day I was shot, I was out before I hit the ground," he confided. "I woke up lying in a hole in the ground. They built a hospital, of sorts, over the hole I fell into. It was the second or third week in May. I was later transferred to Corona Naval Hospital. There were forty-two of us with spinal cord injuries on two wards. Nobody knew nothing about nothing." Indeed, most people with spinal cord injuries prior to World War II died within a year or two. Fortunately for Fesenmyer his paralysis was at L1 (first Lumbar vertebrae), and the medical community was now responding to the growing need for a better understanding of spinal cord injury.

A couple of years of hospitalization left the para from Iowa unprepared for what to expect. "You couldn't go anywhere. You couldn't find a place to live. Hell, nothing was fixed for wheelchairs."

After bouncing around different hospitals, from Southern California to Chicago, Fesenmyer wound up at the Birmingham VA in Van Nuys, CA. Upon his discharge the good shape para managed to survive—and thrive—post SCI. "I was married three times," he confided. "I had a number of jobs, mostly in electronics. I remembered being hospitalized in Hawaii before they brought me to Corona. After my third divorce I figured it would be a good time to quit my job and go lie on the beach!"

Fesenmyer, now a twenty year spinal cord injured paraplegic, had already outlived most other SCI injured men from his war. Asked how he first heard of Quadalajara, Fesenmyer responded, "I had been living in Honolulu, Hawaii when my friend Jerry Baker first mentioned it. He had gone there before and liked it." Baker had indeed, moving his family there a couple of years earlier. Fesenmyer decided to see for himself.

Twenty years after being wounded on the battlefield, Fesenmyer found a unique place where he could pursue his passions—women and staying active—in a Mexican city he never knew existed.

"I never stayed at a gimp camp," Fesenmyer continued, "I visited Baker three or four times before I decided to stay, although George Ray's Place was practically across the road from Baker's house. I did meet Lee Shyler, who I knew from the Long Beach VA Hospital, and later met Chuck Derevjanik, Krekler—the wild bunch. When I returned to Quadalajara I rented a house of my own in Colonia Independencia close to where Shyler lived."

Shyler, a high-level quad, according to Fesenmyer, "liked to go downtown at night to some of the bad places." Maybe Fesenmyer was accustomed to living in a different paradise where everything was pristine and upscale, but nonetheless, would accompany his more severely disabled friend on excursions into Quadalajara-after-dark. "Some guys married girls who they met in cantinas and bars. Most turned out to be good wives." Fesenmyer was not the first to mention that a few residents of Quadalajara actually did meet their future wives in the most unlikely of places.

Although Fesenmyer made frequent trips back to Hawaii, Quadalajara became his new home. The active para, not one for hanging around with groups (he once declined a nomination to fill the vacancy created by George Ray's resignation as Mexico PVA president at the November 1967 membership meeting), enjoyed driving his Cadillac convertible around town, to the ocean, to meet señoritas, or wherever else he pleased. The freedom and accessibility that Mexico's second largest city provided was just what the doctor ordered—or would have—if only he knew Jerry Fesenmyer and what those like him needed to thrive on and survive.

Chapter 15

Paradise Central: The PVA Clubhouse

By the mid-1960s, Quadalajara's growing wheelchair population included folks from all across North America and beyond. The mostly veteran, mostly male, and mostly quads had heard of the city from patients in VA hospitals and members of their local PVA chapters, or had read of it from the *Paraplegia News* and other periodicals. Eddie Lucier from Rhode Island, Tom Kirch from Minnesota, Bill Christensen from South Dakota, Jack Myrick from Louisianna, Joe Anderson from Nebraska, Domingo Santos from Puerto Rico, Joe Candalaria from Colorado, Joe Cella from Pennsylvania, Barney Vigil from Wyoming, Herb Miller from Florida, Joe Darichuk from Michigan, Jack Lastor from Texas, and Pat Fitzgerald from Massachusetts, all joined and blended into the "community" with the Pioneers from Long Beach and Chicago. This was a "colony" which spread from East to West, North to South, and to the lakeside towns of Chapala, Ajijic, San Antonio, San Juan Cosola, and Jocotepec.

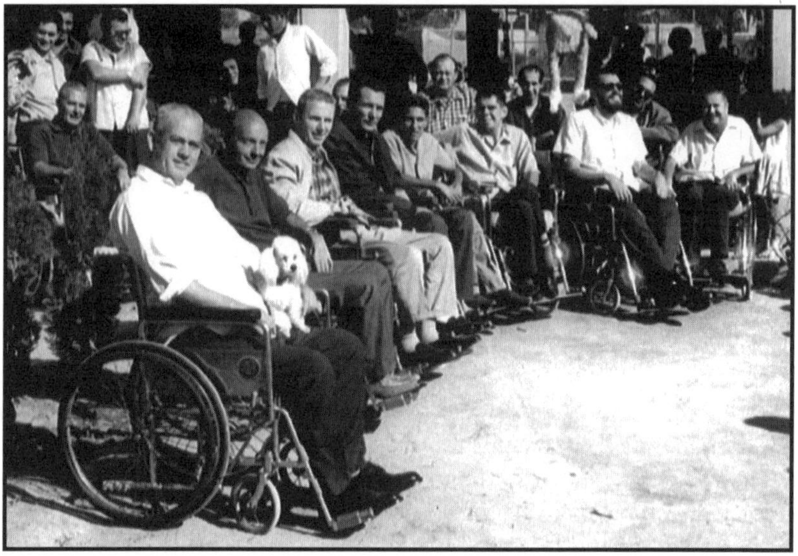

Ed Creegan (in back), Joe Miller with chapter mascot Peppy, Roger Allen, Sam Frazier, Jack Myrick, Joe Cicero, George Ray (in back), Bart Corbett, Doc Foland (in back), unidentified man (with glasses), Bob Peters (in back), and Lee Schyler (left to right)
Annual Christmas Posada, Quadalajara, 1966

As the veteran population grew, so did the Mexico PVA and its membership. Parties and picnics were a way of raising funds and rewarding members with social events that served to expand friendships and unite this diverse group who shared so much. The *Paraplegia News* reported on this expansion in both February and October of 1966:

Membership grows

Rev. Hunter said, "When I came here three years ago, there were only about 40 paraplegics in this area, and they were just looking for a way to integrate into the American community. Today there are more than twice that number, and they have become an influential and important segment of the American community. In fact, no American effort in Guadalajara is going to get off the ground without the paraplegics' support."

Guadalajara sets membership goal

The Guadalajara, Mexico, chapter has set their membership goal for 1966-67 at 100 members. The decision was made at a dinner meeting in August.

The chapter hopes to encourage membership in the chapter at their picnic this month which will feature a roast pig "Mexican style." Also at the picnic a hi-fi, donated by former president Joe E. Miller, will be raffled. The Club is planning to find a permanent home for the chapter.

The idea of a Mexico Chapter bulletin, as raised earlier by George Ray, became a reality when the membership voted to purchase a mimeograph machine. *Spokes 'n Wheels* would lose out to *El Sombrero News* as the name of the official newsletter of the Mexico Chapter PVA. Kenny Van Albert would become the first *El Sombrero News* editor. Kenny's wife Eileen, herself a wheelchair-user and affiliate PVA member, would assist her husband with the tasks of typing and assembling the articles for the monthly chapter bulletin. Eileen Van Albert would continue helping the Mexico Chapter produce an interesting and informative newsletter years after her husband passed on.

In one of the earliest editions of *El Sombrero News*, dated December 1966, Mexico PVA President George Ray wrote: "We are doing everything we know how to make this bulletin helpful, interesting, and entertaining. If anyone has a talent or an interest in helping us to attain these goals please come forward as we can use your help. We would like to run any kind of want ads each month, free of charge that might help anyone locate a house, an attendant, buy something, sell something, or render any type of service. If you have anything of this nature let one of the chapter officers know about it and it will be published."

By this time, George Ray had moved out of George Ray's Place and settled on the northern outskirts of Quadalajara in the farming community of Ciudad Granja. "George Ray was the first one to live there," according to Keith Ziegler. Although Ray continued to rents rooms to residents and visitors, he would marry his Japanese-born girlfriend, Taeko, and live out his final years in "La Granja."

Many of Mexico PVA's functions were now run from the American Legion Hall in Las Fuentes. Early in 1967 some of the members came up with the idea of buying or building their own Clubhouse. A location in Colonia Independencia was looked into, but due to scarce funding nothing materialized.

Shortly thereafter, according to Keith Ziegler, "George Ray found this property in La Granja that he thought was a good deal. He's the one who brought it up. He was the driving force behind it." Since George Ray was the driving force behind most of what took place in Quadalajara from day one, it was no surprise that the majority of the members backed his idea. But there were those who had doubts. Where was the money going to come from? Why Ciudad Granja, which was a long drive for many members who lived across town in Colonia Independencia, or the many who lived in Las Fuentes?

The members decided to float bonds with a 10% annual interest rate. Most bonds were purchased by the Mexico PVA members themselves, some for the interest alone, while others showed support by "putting their *dinero* where their *boca* was." Additional fund raising within their own Clubhouse, combined with savings on rental fees to other organizations for chapter functions, enabled the members to cut down on prior monthly expenses.

PVA Clubhouse a "First"

From Quadalajara's weekly newspaper, the *Colony Reporter*, dated July 29, 1967:

> The men of the Mexico Chapter of the Paralyzed Veterans of America (PVA) are not content to sit around.
>
> Rather the hundred or so members, all of whom have suffered injuries or diseases of the spinal cord, have done what almost every other group in Guadalajara said they themselves would do first: they bought a Clubhouse.
>
> After three years of planning, the PVA purchased a fully accessible building with six rooms and two baths in the Ciudad Granja. The Clubhouse is situated on over one-half acre of land with rooms utilized for offices, storage space, and game area. There will also be an exceptionally large room suitable for meetings and bingo. The group intends to have a ramped swimming pool that can be used by all.
>
> The only chapter of PVA on foreign soil, the group began to form in 1957 when a few "rebels" came to Guadalajara to "find new auras," since they "had nobody and nowhere to go," according to George Ray, president of the chapter.
>
> The men came down to investigate the warmer

climate, find cheap help, and perhaps marry. According to Ray over 90% are disabled veterans with 75% having been injured while in service. After they are hurt, too many problems are created and what home life existed before, usually then fails, he said.

When the first men arrived in Guadalajara it was "almost like opening the frontier," according to Ray. Many Guadalajarians agree with this statement although they have said the men lived like it was the Wild West. The group began to acquire a bad reputation as many people claimed the men came down for marijuana and cheap liquor.

Members of the group admit that this is how things were but also state it was because the men here had responsibilities only to themselves. However, as more men came from the States, commercial houses were established (where the men could live and receive help) and in 1963, the chapter of the PVA was formed.

According to Ray, "In those days a few people thought it would be a good idea to have a PVA chapter in Mexico but didn't know exactly why. Since those days, they have found out why and have been progressively going forward to fulfill the high ideals and aims of the National Organization."

The group, which numbers upwards of two hundred in the winter months, has advanced to a solvent organization with a net worth of over 30,000 pesos. The group has a service program, a special fund for anyone in financial distress and has held annual Christmas parties for over one thousand children.

Money for the Clubhouse was raised by issuing bonds in denominations of 500 pesos and upwards. The chapter has pledged itself to pay 10% annually on these bonds.

(The chapter was actually founded in 1964 and chartered by National PVA on June 17, 1964.)

From the Mexico Chapter, Paralyzed Veterans of America Annual Report for the year 1967–68:

We reached a total of seventy-five members, including dual members.

The biggest progress of the year for the Mexico Chapter has to be its acquisition of its Clubhouse. By having it we have been able to greatly increase the service to our members in many ways. It gives us a central location to have our offices, to store spare medicines and prosthetic appliances; a place to hold all types of social and fundraising events. It is a place members of our chapter, visitors from other chapters, or any other Americans that are in the area, can go to get something to eat or drink at a reasonable price, play a game of checkers or cards, borrow books from the library, check the bulletin board for information about available aides or houses to rent, or if they want, just visit. Before we took this step, there was doubt among some of our member as to whether this venture could even be a success or not. But in the seven months since the Clubhouse was opened I think that most of those doubts have been dispelled. With the more than 40,000 peso profit that the Clubhouse has shown, we have been able to easily pay the interest on the bonds that we sold to buy the property and still have money left over to make additions and improvements.

Respectfully submitted,
Raymond R. Foland
Chapter Director
Mexico Chapter

With the Mexico PVA chapter functioning as both a viable veterans service organization and a source of charitable community programs, it would be safe to say that the addition of the new PVA Clubhouse only served to confirm that the Pioneers had done their job—and done it well—for all who would follow in the path they had cleared.

Shortly thereafter, George Ray would lose his battle with lung cancer. He joined many of his followers who lived their final days and were laid to rest in Quadalajara. *Paraplegia News*, April 1970:

Mexico PVA founder dies

George E. Ray, a founder and past president of the Mexico PVA, was buried with full military honors in Guadalajara last month.

Mr. Ray died on February 28, after several months of illness. At the time of his death, he was a member of the chapter's board of directors.

Ray "Doc" Foland, a tireless worker and all-around good guy, wife Maria, and son Arturo, would soon return to the U.S. for a new life in Garden Grove, California. He was honored not only by his fellow Mexico chapter PVA members, but also by the *Paraplegia News* in September 1969:

Mexico honors Foland

Mexico PVA president Keith A. Ziegler presented a silver plaque to retiring chapter director Raymond R. (Doc) Foland during summer ceremonies at the chapter's Clubhouse in Ciudad Granja.

South-of-the-border PVA members honored Foland for his long efforts on behalf of the organization. A charter member, he had also served as chapter secretary and director. Foland, according to the chapter bulletin, gained his nickname because of his "midnight black sombrero" and consequent resemblance to a legendary character of the Old West.

Foland, who returns to the United States after 10 years residence in Guadalajara, will make his home in Garden Grove, Calif., with his wife, Maria and son, Arturo.

The following letter was read at the August 7th membership meeting and published in the August 1969 edition of *El Sombrero News*:

Dear Members,

I would like to take this opportunity to thank everyone connected with the Mexico PVA for the plaque that was awarded to me recently and for the kind words that went along with it. Although I think the honor was more than I deserved, I am very proud of it and it will always be one of my prized possessions.

The individual thanks that I have received from individual members and the self-satisfaction of trying to do something constructive would have been enough for me. I also remember that all of the time I was working for the Mexico PVA there were some very dedicated persons serving as President and other officers who were working right along with me. Also, if another dedicated person had not had the idea and done a lot of hard work to begin our chapter, none of what we have accomplished would have been possible.

There is no doubt that Maria and myself are going to miss Mexico, the PVA Clubhouse, and all the friends that we left. We hope to return to live in Mexico again some day and when we do, I hope that we will be associated with the chapter for more than the five years that we were this time. In the meantime, nuestra casa es su casa, so come by and see us if you are in the area, or at least write to us and let us know what is happening there. Good luck to all of you and to the Mexico Chapter PVA in future years.

Yours truly,
Raymond R. (Doc) Foland

Part Five

The End of an Era

Chapter 16

Gambling With the Gringos

After two and a half years of living in the house at Monte Olimpo 1046, Colonia Independencia, it was time to move on. I'd miss my Compadres Bailey and my newly adopted Mexican family, but the youthful gypsy blood running through my veins told me it was time. The Mexican peso had been devalued and my landlady wanted to be paid in dollars. "*¿Para usted le da lo mismo, no?*"[47] she asked. Well, yes and no. I was paying about $200 per month, and the devaluation would now bring my peso rental equivalency down closer to $100. Saving close to $100 per month would allow me to boost Alberto's wages and help find the most attractive, friendly, and competent housekeeper (in that order) that a few extra pesos would afford. Truth be told, it wasn't merely how Hilda had asked for dollars, or how much more I could afford to budget, but it was the perfect excuse to check out greener pastures.

It was back to familiar turf for me. Joe Anderson welcomed me back with open arms—the most reliable house sitter in Quadalajara—complete with a full time attendant for those nights when a guy just had to go out on the town. We agreed it would be temporary, but I knew Anderson would love nothing better than if I spent the summer there while he made his usual six-month sojourn to Omaha.

Alberto had been working for me for over three years, ever since I had had to let Sergio go, and he was as comfortable as anyone at Joe's place. That was just the problem. Alberto had started to view our working relationship as a sort of partnership. This was a common problem when either the gringo employer treated his Mexican helper as more of a friend than employee, or when human nature would tend to make the employee feel irreplaceable and entitled to make decisions, insignificant as they may be.

The first sign of any problem between Alberto and myself started just before I left Monte Olimpo and moved back to Joe's house. Some of the college kids, mostly from rich families in the state of Sinaloa and attending school in Quadalajara, befriended me while I sat in front of the house drinking one or two (or three) cervezas. Once one

[47] Because it's the same for you, isn't it?

of the male students stopped by to chat with the wheelchair-bound gringo from across the street, the ice had been broken. Chuy was outgoing and enjoyed complimenting me on my Spanish-speaking abilities, while getting a kick out of the fact that I couldn't roll my R's. He finally let up on me after I butchered the name Raul. I had to explain to them that we Newinglandas never bothered pronouncing R's in our own language, except for emphasis in the word "idear." It was way too late to start now.

After Chuy came his sidekick Manuel, whose signature look was one of trying to make himself resemble John Lennon as closely as possible. He seemed to pull it off, because every time I saw him I thought of the round-rimmed member of The Beatles. Manuel rarely stopped by on his own—merely waved—unless with Chuy. Even then, he rarely spoke.

Soledad, or Sol, was next. Sol had long blonde hair and was as friendly as Chuy, and much more appealing to this gringo's eyes. Unlike the Sinaloans, Sol was middle class from Ciudad Guzman, not far from Quadalajara. She would never fail to ask, "*¿Quieres un refresco, Jack?*"[48] whenever I was enjoying the mid-day sunshine of this fabulous city and she was on her daily soda run to the corner grocery store.

Other students renting rooms in *la casa de asistencia* were less friendly than these. Some Mexican families would rent to out-of-town students as one after another of their children would leave the nest and make available a rentable room. In fact, the gorgeous twin sisters who rounded out the across-the-street student population never even shot a glance my way, although I certainly noticed them.

Whenever any of the students dropped by for a visit with me, Alberto would get huffy. He couldn't stand these rich kids who didn't work and looked right past him as though he were a piece of furniture or completely invisible. Being from the poor socio-economic class of the Mexican society, there was no love lost for rich Mexicans who too often flaunted their wealthy status and birthright of being far superior to the uneducated, poorer class of Mexico's citizens.

I resented Alberto's overt disapproval of my college friends. This was my life, and I enjoyed experiencing another aspect of Mexican culture—interacting with people from the privileged class. This was my first contact with any Mexicans above the middle class level, and I would make friends with anyone I chose.

---

[48] Would you like a soda, Jack?

The transition back to Anderson's went smoothly, although I did have to sell, store, and give away many pieces of furniture and household items I had collected since Vinnie and I had first purchased Jack Lastor's stuff. My having made so many friends in four years made the task of moving relatively easy.

Problems with my helper only got worse when fellow poker player and dealer, Fred Baker, moved back stateside. I first met Baker at Bill and Gil's house. Since most of the regular players were quadriplegic with limited hand use, Fred and a couple of the poker playing paras would take turns dealing cards for those unable to deal their turn. Baker was one of the better players in the game. An able-bodied retired man in his forties, he was constantly harassed because of rumors that he was either hiding out from the mob or in the witness protection program. It didn't help that he arrived in Quadalajara in an auto that, according to Quadalajara folklore of the time, had both snow tires and Florida license plates. Bill would refer to him as Bacarelli. It was Bill's house and Bill's game. Fred would seem agitated and tuck his head down and in like a nervous turtle. One PVAer from Florida claimed he knew of Fred, and that his actual last name was Bagleoni. Whatever the case, Baker/Bacarelli/Bagleoni was not only a good poker player, but an excellent gambler. He intimidated almost everyone except Gerry Maurer. Maurer, a para from Indiana, was the other main dealer, both at Bill's and at the Big Game. Bluffing was a skill Baker had mastered, not only on his own part, but being able to read whenever another player was trying to "buy" a pot while not having the best hand. Fred was the intimidator, and usually one of the evening's big winners.

With Fred gone, someone suggested we "drag" the pot to pay some of the helpers to deal on a shift basis. Although some of the attendants, including Alberto, dealt cards and helped their employer's already, the "professional" dealer idea had its downside, especially for those of us with helpers who had worked for years helping quads play anything from Gin Rummy to Red Dog. You name the card game and someone had played it at some point in Quadalajara. Card games were a big part of life for gringos living in paradise. With no jobs, idle time, and often extra pocket money, gambling was a bigger part of the Quadalajara experience than drinking or carousing cantinas for available women.

After a few weeks, Alberto was making almost as much from his poker dealing gig and some healthy tips from appreciative lucky winners, than he was as my attendant. The effect of his dealing for three or fours hours, sometimes more, was a tired attendant who just wanted to do a minimal job of helping me to bed and then crashing in front of the TV set. I had developed a few blisters on my heels from sleeping all night on my back—not a good idea. Left unattended to, as they now were, the possibility of the blisters becoming pressure sores/bedsores had become reality.

As I lay in bed one night after a marathon poker game and getting some sarcastic comments from my helper-turned-dealer while assisting me to bed, I contemplated making one of the biggest decisions of my four year stay in Quadalajara. I had no choice but to reclaim control over my life. After getting out of bed, showering, and dressing, I informed Alberto—much to his surprise—I had decided to fire him.

Needless to say, Alberto was shocked and caught off guard. I wasn't certain of Mexican labor laws, but had heard that a fired employee was entitled to three month's wages. *"Toma los centavos* (meaning real money, not coins) *que tengo en el cajón y lleva la televisión,*"[49] I instructed him. The money that I kept hidden in a drawer, combined with the thirteen-inch TV, would come close to three months wages. Alberto gathered his belongings, took the money and TV, and left with wounded pride. Maybe he needed a break from me as well?

What I needed now, and the sooner the better, was another attendant. I called Tom Kirch.

Tom was always there if you needed anything, and I sure needed something.

Within an hour or so, I was in the back of Tom's van headed to where Javier lived. Javier, who formerly worked for my Gin Rummy and poker-playing pal Leo Bourdosis, was currently unemployed and had made a few stops around Quadalajara inquiring about work. He would be a good fit as a helper: experienced and someone with whom I had a good rapport, the only problem being that Javier didn't drive.

All it took was one phone call and a quick drive out to one of Quadalajara's suburbs, and I again had an attendant. As a matter of fact, Javier's younger brother Martin was also looking for work. Although Martin had little experience, we agreed that the brothers would split the week, details to be worked out later. Apparently, Javier

---

[49] Take the money that I have in the drawer, and take the television.

was not interested in the usual six-day workweek, his stated reason for leaving his job with Leo. He wanted more time to spend with his new novia.

There were many advantages for a quad living in Mexico's second largest city. With so many members of this strange fraternity having similar needs, opportunities were always waiting for someone to claim them.

The phone rang while I was still in bed. Javier, who hadn't even finished his third day helping me yet, answered.

"*Es Jaime Lietz. ¿Puede hablar con el?*"[50] my new attendant asked.

"*Sí, traiga el teléfono para acá,*"[51] I replied, as I wondered what Jimmy wanted so early in the morning. Having a residential phone in 1977 was much more common than when I had first arrived in Quadalajara, and Jack-of-all-trades Sofia had long since figured out that splicing ordinary electrical cord to the usually too short cord supplied by Telefonos de Mexico enabled many a quad to have a phone cord that could be dragged anywhere in the house. It was well worth it, as long as someone was willing to reel it back in, in somewhat of an orderly fashion.

Sofia was now "working for" and dating Jimmy. It was a good arrangement for both, as Sofia was able to come and go daily and spend more time with her kids, while Jimmy had his full-time attendant, Miguel, to help him prowl around the city after dark. Sofia trusted Jimmy, or tolerated his womanizing up to a certain extent.

"Jack," he began, "there's a house up the street from me for rent. It's fairly accessible, has the same floor plan as mine, but it's two stories. The rent is only slightly higher than mine. The landlord stopped by and asked if I knew of any Americans who might be interested. He's afraid to rent to a Mexican family with a bunch of kids." The idea was intriguing. Jimmy lived on the other side of Circunvalación, the main boulevard that divided Jardines Alcalde, and only about a dozen streets north of Joe's house.

"Let me think about it, Jim, I'll stop by as soon as I get up."

Having been to Lietz's house a few times, I had a fairly good idea of what the house would look like. Oftentimes, houses built adjacent to one another in newer colonias, had identical floor-plans, except that adjacent houses were reversed. Kitchen walls would be

---

[50] It's Jimmy Lietz, can you talk to him?

[51] Yeah, bring the phone over here.

back-to-back, for example, as would master bedrooms, etc. Looking up at the second floor was an odd sight for a wheelchair user. The only part that caught my attention was the balcony. I suddenly had an idea. Since I had two helpers splitting the week, I'd have Javier and Martin each work four days. One brother would work Sunday through Wednesday, the other Wednesday through Saturday. This way I could utilize and justify my two-story house by having the brothers carry me upstairs, wheelchair and all. I could invite friends, or dine alone, on my novelty balcony. Spaghetti and red wine immediately came to mind. I imagined how unique this would be, eating and sipping wine—beer would work just as well—while overlooking Jardines Alcalde's north side.

I agreed to the rental price and began the moving process immediately, rounding up stored furniture and settling into the house five doors up Gaspar Bolaños from where Jimmy lived.

My new arrangement lasted all of one week, as brothers Javier and Martin, objected to both having to work on the same day. I relented, and we set up an alternating two-three-two schedule so that neither brother would have to work more than three consecutive days, and each would have every other weekend off. Was I already forgetting what I had just learned from the experience with Alberto making decisions for me, or was I merely being practical and fair? Time would tell.

My friendship with Jimmy was more of the love/hate variety. Lietz was extremely moody and, unfortunately, like a number of combat-injured veterans from the war in Southeast Asia, would self-medicate with alcohol to make the pain and memories go away. I could handle the drinking aspect more easily than those days when Jimmy was in one of his moods. There were days when I felt uncomfortable around him, as if he resented me for whatever reason. Most days though, Jimmy Lietz was just like the rest of us enjoying life south of the border, happy and carefree, looking for someone to visit and hang around with—be it card playing, drinking, girl watching, girl chasing, or simply shooting the breeze on a sunny afternoon or pleasant evening.

In five years living in Quadalajara, I'd moved into Colonia Independencia with Vinnie Nash, to Jardines Alcalde at Joe Anderson's house, back to Colonia Independencia on Bill Bailey's street, back to Alcalde and Joe's, and finally to my own two-story bachelor pad in Jardines Alcalde. A definite pattern was developing.

I quickly came to like living on the North side of Jardines Alcalde. Although Joe's house was within pushing distance of two other quads, Bob Nemac and "Captain" Ben Borish—not to mention former friend, Quadalajara resident, and PVA President Jack Black—the North side was home to seven other houses, rented or owned by fellow gringos. A few quads of scarce financial resources rented rooms in the neighborhood and managed to have active social lives and contacts, without the benefit of owning automobiles. Someone was always congregating at Helen's, Jimmy's, Jerry's, Buddy's, Herb's, Chico's, or my place. I was glad I had also decided to take a break from the rigors of over-involvement with the Mexico PVA. My new neighborhood was the perfect place to start over.

I'd met all my new neighbors already while visiting mutual friends, working at the PVA, or enjoying Clubhouse functions. The only exception was Harry Wilson, a.k.a. "Chico." Chico Wilson was anything but small, as his name implied. He was a muscle-bound para with biceps that would make many a gym rat envious. Lietz explained that Chico had lived in Quadalajara for about one year, but mostly kept to himself, except for when it came to courting Helen Dunn's former helper and his now-fiancée, Rosa.

"He had been tagged with the nickname "Chico," explained Lietz, "because there had been another para named Harry, also a Black American, who used to live in Jardines Alcalde and who supposedly was bigger."

Chapter 17

Wedding Bells

October 1977. I was beginning my sixth year in Quadalajara. I had already seen, done, and accomplished more than I could have ever imagined at any time during rehab or while living at home. Poker king, Fred Baker, had stated it best a couple of years earlier, "Jack, you've found your niche."

One evening, Jimmy pushed himself up from his house.

"Let's go over to Chico's," he suggested. "He's a really nice guy and he wouldn't mind company. He's an interesting guy to talk to." I was the new kid on the block and Chico was sort of new to the whole Quadalajara social circle.

"I don't know, Jim."

"Come on," Lietz insisted. "He'd enjoy the chance to meet you. He's heard of you."

Hesitantly, I followed Jimmy down the driveway ramp, onto Gaspar Bolaños, around the corner, and down Calle Bruno Moreno to a ramped house exactly one street north of where Jimmy and I lived. One of the advantages to living in this neighborhood was more independence. If you were able to push a block or two, there was no need to bring along an attendant. Everyone's helper was willing to assist. They understood this was a good way to get a break for a few hours to relax, watch TV, or flirt with some of the neighborhood maids. Next time they might be tabbed to assist another attendant's employer, but it was well worth the trade off.

Once we arrived, I noticed Chico's car was blocking the driveway to his ramped entrance. Before I said anything, Jimmy yelled out, "Rosa!" A dark complexioned Mexican girl came out from the kitchen and greeted Jimmy while helping each of us around the car and up the slight driveway incline of the house next door.

This was the Quadalajara that Vinnie Nash had told me about years earlier at West Roxbury.

Chico was sitting at the dining room table with his massive arms crossed in front of his chest. As with many houses in Quadalajara, the living room and dining room were indistinguishable. Usually quite spacious, with a doorway leading to the adjacent kitchen, it was perfect for large families and entertaining guests. Chico's warm smile proved to be an accurate indicator of the personality inside the muscle-bound body of this gentle giant with the wide mustache and '70s-style Afro.

After Jimmy formally introduced us and we had a few minutes of chit-chat, I noticed a light skinned Mexican girl peering out from one of the rooms behind Chico. It was the room where Rosa had disappeared to earlier. Lietz had noticed also and called, "*¡Cuca, ven para acá!*"[52]

The somewhat shy and reluctant girl emerged from the room with Rosa standing behind her.

"*Este es mi amigo, Jack,*" Jimmy informed the blushing girl, as the on-looking Rosa giggled. "*El no tiene novia.*"[53] I wasn't sure who was blushing more as Jimmy introduced Maria de Refugio (Cuca) to the newest gringo on the block. After the awkward introduction, the girls left and returned to the room just behind Chico. I could hear them talking and giggling as Chico himself got a kick out of what had just transpired.

I learned that Cuca was Rosa's cousin, and that she was new to Quadalajara. The attractive nineteen-year-old had just arrived from a town named San Juan Capistrano. She planned to take some classes while in the city, English among them.

A three-way game of Gin Rummy was suggested as the main event of this icebreaking visit. Chico remained where he was when we arrived, facing the entrance, while Jimmy sat to my left. From my vantage point, I was able to look right at the doorway where the curious girl would periodically sneak a peek and smile nervously every time I caught her. Trying to concentrate on the card game while being unable to resist the urge to look up and catch another glimpse of Cuca was too demanding. I preferred the latter.

As Jimmy teased me about Cuca, Chico just grinned. He seemed to enjoy the entertainment provided by Jimmy's mischievous matchmaking over the small game of chance. It was an interesting night.

On my way out the door, Chico told me, "If you want to ask Cuca out it's okay with me. She's just staying here helping Rosa."

One thing there was definitely no shortage of in Quadalajara was attractive señoritas. Unfortunately, Javier had also noticed the "new" girl. "*Me la voy a _____,*"[54] I overheard him vulgarly tell one of

---

[52] Cuca, come here!

[53] This is my friend, Jack. He doesn't have a girlfriend.

[54] I'm gonna _______ her.

the other attendants. Apparently, having a new girlfriend took a back seat to a possible meaningless conquest in this macho Mexican culture.

I started driving again since neither of my attendants did. Even though I'd never gotten up the confidence of applying for a driver's license after being shot down at the Providence, RI drivers' license department. I had gotten hand controls installed in both my old blue Plymouth Satellite and my maroon Cordoba. I finally felt comfortable driving in Quadalajara, as long as I picked streets that were easy to negotiate and didn't seem to be traffic nightmares.

My apprehension about driving in Quadalajara stemmed from an incident that took place a few years earlier. Jerry Andrews requested that Alberto and I follow him home from the Clubhouse after a night of poker playing. Jerry, an almost independent quad, was temporarily without a helper. Since it wasn't unusual for the Big Game to break up after 1:00 a.m., we comrades of the poker wars followed a sort of buddy system where we looked after one another—even if the recipient of the good deed had been the main culprit responsible for lightening your wallet by a couple hundred dollars. After all, it was only money.

I must have consumed an adult beverage or two, because that would be the only way I would have felt comfortable enough to get behind the wheel at that time. Alberto hopped into Jerry's car instead of riding shotgun with his *patrón* (employer). He must have known something I hadn't yet realized. As I tried to keep up with my poker playing pal, friend, and neighbor, I suddenly felt uneasy. Jerry had taken Quadalajara's *Periferico* (the circular highway that ran around the outskirts of the ever-expanding city) and the lights of his Chrysler New Yorker were getting smaller as I fell further behind them.

I was now driving about as fast as I had ever driven my Cordoba, when I came to a slight canyon incline. My speed quickly picked up even more. Seeing the steep canyon drop-off out of the corner of my right eye caused me to drift to the left. I attempted to correct the problem, but it only got worse as I overcorrected. Suddenly, stone cold fear set in as my heart rate went through the roof. I attempted to remain calm. *Relax, Jack*, I told myself, trying not to panic. Fortunately, my performance adrenaline kicked in and I was able to extricate myself from my nightmare as I slowed down just in time. "Local Quadriplegic Dies in Mexico after Auto Plunges into Canyon—Mexican Authorities Investigating" was not the headline I would have wanted my family and friends to see on the front page of the *Pawtucket Times*.

I decided to invite Cuca to accompany me that Sunday to

dinner at Bill and Maria Elena Bailey's. My reason was two-fold: to keep her away from my helper, and to gratify my own curiosity from our little sneak-a-peek meeting a few nights earlier. The thought of Javier taking Cuca's innocence infuriated me. That wasn't going to happen to "my girl."

Sunday would be perfect. Martin would be helping me, and the Bailey's, namely Maria Elena, were planning on cooking a turkey dinner. Bill had long since taught his wife of twenty years to prepare American-style food. Maria Elena was an excellent cook.

Cuca readily accepted my invite. I had a feeling that both Jimmy Lietz *and* Chico were playing Cupid. We arrived at the Bailey's around 2:00 p.m., and were soon seated at the large dining room table. To my surprise, Cuca hardly touched the turkey dinner.

After dinner, Cuca volunteered to help with the cleanup and dishes, but that was a no-no at the Bailey home. Lucy, Bill's daughter, and a few of the female family members took care of that. Guests were treated as guests, no matter what socio-economic class they belonged to.

The table wasn't even cleared yet when Bill suggested we play cards, but not before first lighting his signature cigar. He always said, *"Después de un buen taco, un buen tabaco."*[55]

Cuca wasn't interested in the penny ante poker game either. The fact that she had no clue as to what was going on might have had something to do with that. I also knew that Cuca was nervous around so many people she didn't know—that seemed to be the reason she had just pushed her fork through her mashed potatoes and barely tasted the turkey. I later learned that American-style cooking was as foreign to my date as Mexican food still was to me. I should have known, but the meal was the last thing on my mind. After watching me play a few hands, she went over to the living room sofa where the non-participants were watching TV. I felt uncomfortable playing poker with friends while Cuca was sitting there on the living room sofa with practically no conversation going on. *Jack, you're blowing this date big time,* I thought to myself. The only saving aspect of the afternoon was that whenever I glanced over my shoulder, Cuca seemed to be looking my way.

After a few hours of visiting my Quadalajara family, we departed for home. I took the roads less traveled and passed a vacant lot, one where there was a soccer field adjacent to a park. It was the

---

[55] After a good taco, a good tobacco.

long way home, but convenient for this unlicensed gringo driver. After dropping Martin off at my house, I drove past Chico's street and headed back toward the now-empty and darkened field. As I did so, Cuca slid over next to me. Maybe she was as attracted to me as I was to her. At any rate, we'd hardly had time to talk on our date, but talking definitely wasn't the only thing on my mind.

I pulled off the road and drove to a secluded area at the far end of the soccer field. Within seconds, Cuca and I had skipped the chit-chat and exchanged our first kiss.

The secluded area beamed with just enough moonlight to make this romantic night all the more special for Quadalajara's newest novios. Kissing the girl who had caught my eye merely days before was magical, and I knew right away that this would not be a one or two date fling. The girl from San Juan Capistrano and the gringo from Pawtucket had found instant chemistry.

My first night alone with Cuca in my arms took an unexpected twist. The moon was not the only object beaming light upon us. We opened our eyes to find two Mexican policemen, one with a flashlight in hand.

I rolled down the window to the question, "*¡Espero que ustedes no estén haciendo cosas inmorales aquí!*"[56] Although run-ins with Mexican law enforcement officials could be intimidating (everyone from the border guard *aduana* to the *transito* traffic cop were experts at supplementing their income by shaking down whomever they could), I attempted to remain calm and impress my novia with quick thinking.

"*Estamos como a cien metros de la avenida. ¿Qué les parace si les doy un peso por cada metro?*"[57] I was surprised by their quick response, like an unsuspecting tourist offering full price without bargaining with a vendor at *el mercado*. From my wallet to their hands—the easiest 100 pesos they'd probably made thus far on this soccer field gig.

We were left with the admonishment, "*No quiero verlos aquí, y no hacen cosas inmorales.*"[58]

Cuca just laughed, "*¡100 pesos! ¿No más?*" she jested. Was that all she was worth to me?

It was late enough to get my date-turned-girlfriend home. I

---

[56] I hope you aren't doing indecent things here!

[57] We're about one hundred meters from the avenue. How about if I give you one peso for each meter?

[58] I don't want to see you here, and don't do immoral things.

didn't want "Mr. Muscles" giving me any flack for keeping his future in-law out past whatever curfew he deemed appropriate. I gave Cuca a goodnight kiss at the end of this strange date. "*Te llamo mañana,*"[59] I told her. I dropped her off in front of Chico's house and waited for her to go inside. She waved goodnight and disappeared from view. As I drove home, I was sure Rosa would be grilling her cousin for all the juicy details of our first date.

* * *

Love can motivate a man like nothing else. I began driving to Chico's house on a nightly basis. Cuca and I would sit in my car in front of the house alternating between talking and fogging up the windows, mostly the latter, on Quadalajara's cool fall nights. I fell more deeply in love with the girl ten years younger than me with each kiss we shared. An hour or two would be like a minute in time. I thought I had loved other girlfriends, but the feelings that overtook me while kissing, talking to, or merely thinking about my novia from San Juan Capistrano, were like nothing I had experienced with any of the girls I'd dated before.

I decided to apply for a Mexican driver's license, something I would never have contemplated before. What is that mystical power women possess that can make a lackadaisical man suddenly want to conquer the world? A Mexican driver's license wasn't exactly Napoleanic, but it was a harbinger of things to come.

Javier jogged up a few flights of stairs inquiring about how his patron could obtain a driver's license. He soon returned with a uniformed official. The surprised transito cop stared at the gringo sitting in the wheelchair asking in Spanish for a road test. After thinking about it for a moment, he pointed to the upper parking level and said, "*Usted, vaya para allá y espererme un minuto.*"[60]

The skeptical man looked at my hand controls, looked again at me, and exited my maroon Cordoba.

"*Pongalo en reversa,*" he instructed as I backed out of the parking space high above the ground below. "*Metalo otra vez,*" was his next command. "*Està bien,*"[61] he spoke as he walked toward the office.

That was easy enough, I thought to myself as I waited for the

---

[59] I'll call you tomorrow.

[60] You go over there and wait a minute.

[61] Put it in reverse. Put it back. That's fine.

official to return. When he did, the nervous look on his face signaled something was just not right.

"*Usted tiene que demostrame que puede manejarlo.*"[62] I suppose his supervisor wasn't satisfied with the brief demonstration I had just provided.

"*Tienes que dar una vuelta al rededor del edificio y regresar para acá.*"[63] The jittery traffic cop wasn't exactly thrilled that he would have to accompany me onto the street that circles the Transito building itself and then return to the upper level of the parking garage. He quickly buckled his seat belt as I followed his instructions. Once out onto Calle Circunvalación, I came to a slow crawl as I approached the traffic sign, Ceda El Paso, checking for traffic at the yield sign. "*Muy bien*,"[64] the relieved Transito official sighed.

After the test, I had my picture taken and was the proud owner of a State of Jalisco Driver's License.

The decision to take a year off from the work I'd been doing with the Mexico PVA, coupled with the move to my new house in Jardines Alcalde, was paying unexpected dividends. The working arrangement with brothers Javier and Martin was again functioning smoothly, until I hired a young housekeeper named Edith. When I asked Edith to fill out an impromptu job application, I was surprised that she couldn't spell her own name correctly. "Ediht," she wrote. She had an extremely sweet innocence about her that made me feel responsible for her welfare.

My main problem was keeping Javier from taking advantage of the somewhat naïve, uneducated girl. It didn't take long for him to try to corner and persuade her to help him with something upstairs. As I rolled out onto the back patio looking for him one afternoon, I overheard part of a conversation from the top of the stairs where Edith was sweeping.

"*Hay viene El Señor Jack*,"[65] she cautioned him. At least my main attendant had set his hormonal sights on someone other than Cuca, but his act was beginning to wear on me. I let Edith know that she didn't have to put up with any harassment from either of my helpers. Then I put Javier on notice that my new housekeeper was not there for entertainment purposes.

---

[62] You have to show me that you can drive.
[63] You have to go around the building and return here.
[64] Very well.
[65] Here comes Mr. Jack.

Unfortunately, Edith wasn't the first maid to incorrectly assume that if she rejected the advances of the boss' main helper, her job might be in jeopardy. Between some of their gringo employers and the male drivers and attendants who helped them, being an attractive domestic servant in this macho culture meant putting up with sexual harassment from both directions (long before the term became a common phrase).

The difference in the flirting/harassment that went on in Quadalajara's version of the "battle of the sexes" was striking. Many of the paras and quads who had rolled the dice and ventured to Quadalajara in search of a better life married Mexican women, often the very señoritas or *madres solteras* (single mothers) whom they initially hired as domestic helpers. Other naïve young women weren't as fortunate, having only a love child to show for their brief affair with a long-gone former driver or attendant.

A number of American/Mexican unions were of the kind Reverend Hunter had told me of years earlier. An American para or quad, now unable to father a child, would marry a Mexican single mom. He thought it to be a win-win situation, an instant wife and family for someone who, only years before, was hopelessly trapped in an institutional environment. It also gave security and a father for the child of the young Mexican woman. Other couples unable to have children would adopt, while some of the guys, depending on their disability or damage to their spinal cord, were able to father a child.

Reverend Hunter's words would remain with me, but had the reverse effect. Subconsciously, maybe, I was determined to meet and marry someone who loved me for who I was, not for security or financial reasons.

My romance with Cuca was becoming routine and predictable. Almost every night we'd park in front of Chico's house, talk, and make out. On the nights when Cuca and Sofia went to English classes, I'd spend more time hanging out with Jimmy and the neighborhood crowd or make an appearance at the poker game. Chico had broken off his engagement with Rosa, and Cuca was now officially working for him. He'd hinted to me that I was monopolizing her evening hours. Was Chico now jealous of me dating Cuca?

I wanted to spend more time with my girl. We had talked about everything imaginable, as much as two people could between kissing, including the possibility of marriage and adopting children. I suggested she move in with me. We had been dating for two months. Cuca rejected the idea.

I respected the fact that my Mexican novia had sound moral convictions. If two months of dating wasn't sufficient, then my initial thoughts that Cuca was a virtuous señorita had been happily vindicated—frustrating as that could be.

My parents had married relatively late in life. Pop was thirty-four and Mom was twenty-nine on their June 3, 1946 wedding day. World War II had interrupted their courtship for a few years. Coupled with the fact that I chose Matthew as my confirmation name, after my only bachelor uncle, I wasn't sure if I wanted to wait until I was older to get married, or if I too wished to remain a "confirmed bachelor," as one of my early girlfriends had predicted.

* * *

Christmas 1977. I decided that the idea of marrying older in life suited me better than a lifetime membership in the bachelor's club. I was in love with the kind of girl who I would proudly bring home to meet Mom. I was also approaching my milestone "Big 3-0" birthday.

Cuca and I spent *La Noche Buena* (Christmas Eve) at the home of Bill and Maria Elena Bailey. The Bailey's were always entertaining family and friends, especially at Thanksgiving and Christmas. This was my third year as an honorary member of their extended family, and I was pleased they accepted Cuca as my novia. Maria Elena was very picky of the young Mexican women who dated some of the remaining bachelor residents of Quadalajara, and the fact that she seemed to like the girlfriend of her "*Muchachito*,"[66] as she had dubbed me when I first became a regular visitor in their home, further validated my choice.

New Year's Eve was spent at the PVA's annual celebration *Del Año Nuevo* at the Clubhouse. Four years earlier, I brought in the New Year seated with a different girlfriend at almost the same table. Maria and I had received compliments on what a "cute couple" we made. Little did the maker of those compliments realize that that would be the last appearance together Maria and I would make. Little did *I* realize my soon-to-be-ex-girlfriend was expecting a child.

Much had transpired in four years. I was no longer the new guy in Quadalajara. I had grown up all over again in my post-injury life: learned to be independent, wined, dined, and gambled with the best of them, and was now ready to take the next step.

Asking Cuca to marry me on New Year's Eve was a romantic

---

[66] Dear boy.

notion indeed, but I'd decided to wait a few weeks. I didn't need a hundred or more witnesses to celebrate our announcement. I knew the answer would be "yes," but I preferred it to be at the appropriate time and in the appropriate place—in front of Chico's house. Where else?

My Tolman High School Class of '66 ring would serve as our official engagement ring. I had always carried it on the key chain with my car keys. I had removed it earlier in the day.

I pulled up in front of Chico's house, parking in the same place that annoyed his busybody neighbor who feared I might do damage to the sidewalk bushes that served to shield Cuca and I from view. Cuca was perched on the sofa peeking out the curtains, reminiscent of our seemingly long ago game of peek-and-catch peeking, waiting for the now-familiar '75 maroon Cordoba that carried her gringo novio.

After our first embrace and kiss, I took the ring from my shirt pocket and said the words guys dreaded saying and women longed to hear, "*Cuca, te quiero mucho. ¿Te casarías conmigo?*"[67]

A tentative March 18 date was chosen for our upcoming nuptials, less than two weeks before my thirtieth birthday. Cuca and I had only known and dated each other for three months—three short months to pick a life's companion. I questioned myself: was I rushing things just because I wanted to be married before my thirtieth birthday? I was in love with Cuca and she with me I was certain, but were we actually "in love" as a couple? Maybe she was so taken with the idea of marrying a gringo that her judgment had been clouded.

Though these questions plagued me at first, that indescribable feeling I had for Maria de Refugio from *San Juan Capistrano* was unmistakable—I was in love and ready to prove it.

Our first separation was coming in February, as Cuca was planning a trip back home to visit family, and to tell her mother the news. Word had already spread from Quadalajara to San Juan that one of their pretty señoritas would be marrying an American. The only thing Cuca's visit would do was confirm what was already the talk of the town.

Two weeks, which felt like two months, was akin to emotional torture. I missed talking to, holding, and kissing my girl from the moment she boarded the bus to San Juan Capistrano. Counting the days until her return was like counting the days on my short-timer's calendar in Vietnam. I don't know which two week period dragged on longer: my last two in Nam or my first two absent from my future bride.

[67] Cuca, I love you very much. Will you marry me?

I was so excited talking to Cuca on the phone the day after her late night arrival back to Quadalajara. There would be no waiting until sundown for this long awaited trip around the corner and down the block. I had missed Cuca so much that I couldn't hold back my enthusiasm to see her as soon as possible.

A vehicle was blocking the street in front of Chico's house. I parked directly across the street as my novia was waiting for our first reunion. Cuca was practically inside the Cordoba before I had finished parking it. Our embrace was like something from an old movie or romance novel, at least for me. As we temporarily let go of one another to talk face-to-face after an eternal two week period of time, I noticed she was crying. Were they tears of joy or was something wrong?

"*Te estrané mucho*," I told her. She remained silent as I asked, "*¿No me extrañaste?*"[68] Tears began to flow more freely as Cuca removed my high school ring and placed it on the front seat as she slid away from me and closer to the passenger door.

"*Mi Mamá no quiere que me case contigo. No quiere porque dice que me vas a llevar a Los Estados Unidos. Te estrané, Jack, pero también estrané a mi prima Rosa y mi sobrino Jose. Y si voy contigo allá, voy a extrañar a mi Mama y a mis hermanos.*"[69]

That being said, the love of my life and girl who held the key to my future happiness ran across the street and out of my life…

---

[68] I missed you so much! Didn't you miss me?

[69] My mother doesn't want me to marry you. She doesn't because she says you are going to take me to the United States. I missed you, Jack, but I also missed my cousin Rosa and my nephew Jose. And if I go with you, I'll miss my mother and my brother and sisters.

Chapter 18

Life Goes On: The Deadly Saltillo Highway

I had been dumped before. My first girlfriend, Maureen, had broken up with me, gotten back together with me so she would have someone to take her to her prom, and then left me again just a few weeks before my own high school prom. My first romantic hurt could never be outdone. I was so doubly devastated that I thought it impossible to be emotionally hurt any worse than my first taste of broken-heartedness. I was wrong.

I wandered through the next few months like an emotional zombie. I couldn't think about anything or anyone but Cuca. I would occasionally see Cuca on her way to or from the store, or when my Cordoba couldn't resist the temptation to drive down Calle Bruno Moreno and past Chico's house, as if on autopilot. But the most painful sighting happened one innocent Sunday afternoon. I was driving home from Bill and Maria Elena's when, upon turning the corner onto my street, I spotted my former fiancée walking hand in hand with one of Herb Miller's attendants. My heart just sank.

I realized the only thing that could possibly keep me from thinking about the girl who had torn my heart out, was to find another love interest—and quickly. I knew Catalina still had a crush on me. One of the attendants had previously questioned why I chose Cuca over the sexy young waitress at the PVA Clubhouse. I knew that Catalina was jealous of Cuca, and although the eighteen-year-old Catalina and I had only fooled around in the past, she was a sure thing. I would resume my mischievous rendezvous with Catalina, while searching for a second or third girl to fool around with. My new dating philosophy was going to be just like my pre-Cuca dating habit—*puras amigas y amantes*.[70] No more commitments or falling in love for this hurting gringo; falling in like and lust was all any señorita or young single mom could expect. I would never allow myself to experience that horrible gut-wrenching feeling again.

I began to hang around with my quad neighbors again. I'd join

[70] Only friends and lovers.

the afternoon and evening bull sessions, have a few beers, and enjoy the afternoon sunshine and cool Quadalajara nights.

I also became a regular at the PVA meetings again. The time away had rejuvenated me to the extent that I considered becoming actively involved in the chapter once again. Jimmy and I started to spend more time visiting and talking. He was contemplating running for Mexico PVA president in the upcoming June election, and having already served in the role of chapter secretary three times (as well as one brief stint filling in as vice president), I knew I'd be welcomed back in whatever capacity I chose.

I decided on vice president, and when the ballots were tabulated, the Mexico PVA, for the first time, had the infusion of younger, newer blood, in the form of two Vietnam veterans holding down the top chapter positions.

As chapter vice president, I inherited the job of membership officer, or bill collector for those lazy members and those part-time "snowbirds" that spent six to nine months in Quadalajara and the balance of the year stateside. I also reclaimed the role as editor of *El Sombrero News* from an overworked Keith Ziegler. Editor was more of a misnomer, as publisher would have been a more accurate title for the time-consuming duties of gathering info, typing, writing articles, and getting one of our active paras, Ray Clifford, Frank Stoppiello, or Jerry Maurer, to crank out the finished product on the chapter's old mimeograph machine. As difficult as it was to get the newsletter to chapter members on time every month, I enjoyed the challenge and it reinforced my confidence as a former numbers-cruncher turned would-be wordsmith.

* * *

I would go through a few attendants over the coming months. Javier was next to leave.

"*Quiero un aumento de 500 pesos al mes*," he casually informed me one morning. "*Me voy a bañar y quiero su respuesta cuando salga.*"[71] The last thing any attendant or helper could get away with by me was an ultimatum. Rafael had made that mistake a few years earlier. Javier's ultimatum, if he was serious about an additional 500 pesos or walking out, would find only one end result. At least

---

[71] I want a 500 peso monthly raise. I'm going to take a shower and I want your answer when I'm done.

Martin was scheduled to come in within the hour, so I would still have one helper. The thought of being left alone with no helper, as had happened months before with Alberto, had never entered my mind.

Javier finished his shower and dressed for home. The cocky attitude was even more blatant, as my soon-to-be-ex-helper demanded, "*¿Me vas a dar un aumento o no?*"[72] Either Javier didn't know me as well as he thought, or he merely wanted a quick out.

"No," was my answer as he calmly walked out the door.

"*Adios*," was his response.

I wasn't at all disappointed in losing Javier. The young man who worked for my poker and Gin Rummy playing friend, Leo Bourdosis, had gone from a friendly easy going attendant for Leo to a sexual predator and macho pain in the butt for me.

But what happened next was totally unexpected: Martin showed up, learned that his brother had just walked out, and did the same.

"*Si Javier no va a trabajar aquí, yo tampoco*."[73] Martin was now following in the footsteps, literally, of his big brother. Flashbacks of being stranded at Anderson's house when I let Alberto go popped back into my head. This time I called Jimmy. Tom Kirch had solved my last temporary problem, but Jimmy was only a few houses away. I knew I could count on Jimmy's attendant Miguel, or Sofia, to fill in until help arrived.

Help arrived in the form of a wide mustached stocky attendant named Rodolfo, or Rudy, as he preferred. Rudy had previously worked with a few quads in town whose names were unfamiliar to me. His elder brother, David, actually showed up for the interview, but wasn't interested. David was well known for having worked for some of Quadalajara's early Pioneers, so I felt comfortable giving Rudy the job.

The fact that Rudy had previously traveled stateside with other quadriplegic residents of Quadalajara was a plus. He had a passport, and I had a June wedding to attend. My baby sister Debbie, now twenty-one, was marrying the love of her life, her first and only boyfriend, Chuck. (My oldest sister, Diane, had also married her first and only boyfriend. Diane had married Alan when she was eighteen, right after his discharge from the Navy.) With an experienced driver, I could travel back to Rhode Island as I'd already done a few times with Alberto.

---

[72] Are you going to give me a raise or not?

[73] If Javier isn't going to work here, neither am I.

As things worked out, Rudy was much more comfortable behind the steering wheel than I. Since Cuca was no longer in the picture, driving wasn't as important now. I'd be free to venture outside of the Jardines Alcalde neighborhood and roam Quadalajara wherever and whenever I wanted. Javier and Martin, as luck would have it, had done me an unexpected favor.

I crossed paths with Cuca a number of times. She was always walking with or talking to one of the neighborhood attendants. Each incident would bring a mixture of emotions from jealousy to anger. I never realized how much of a flirt my former fiancée was. I'd never given her the chance to show that side of her personality, or to experience dating Mexican males from outside her hometown. I had spotted her so early on in her stay in Quadalajara with Chico that she hadn't had the opportunity. Even though I had dated and fooled around with Catalina and whoever else was interested, my feelings for Cuca would gnaw at my gut just thinking about her with another guy. How long would this go on?

I made plans for my stateside trip from Quadalajara to Pawtucket. A May 4, 1978 departure date would give me ample time to travel, settle in at home, visit with family and friends, and attend my baby sister's wedding. Debbie had planned her wedding to coincide with that of Mom and Pop, who were married on June 3, 1946.

Rudy was eager to visit his family the day before the scheduled trip. I relented, although warned ahead of time that it was not a good idea to give your driver the day off before a long trip. As had been the case previously with other "understanding" patrones, my driver showed up in the morning, sleep deprived and slightly hung over. Stuff like that happened whenever large families gathered for special occasions. Beer, tequila, family and festivities were part of the tradition in the colorful Mexican culture.

As Rudy and I began our journey north, I noticed that my maroon Cordoba had taken a familiar route, around the corner and down Calle Bruno Moreno. Stopping by Chico's house was not on my travel agenda. The Cordoba seemingly parked itself in its favorite spot as Rudy jumped out to talk to a waiting señorita from San Juan Capistrano. I could barely see them from behind the bushes, but I had no trouble recognizing the female voice. Cuca ended the brief exchange with the word, "*grosero.*"[74] What had he told her to solicit such a response? My mind wandered to the gutter. Had he told her he'd bring

[74] That's rude.

her back a vibrator from the States? I was already infuriated by Rudy's side trip. The fact that my former fiancée never bothered to say hello or goodbye to me further compounded my emotional state.

As we restarted our journey from that point, an eerie feeling came over me. This was not going to be a pleasant trip back home for Debbie's wedding.

* * *

After having made our way from Quadalajara, through the winding mountain barancas, we arrived safely outside the picturesque city of Zacatecas. After a brief rest at the roadside Pemex (Petrolios de Mexico) gas station, we were once again headed north toward the U.S./Mexican border town of Laredo—620 miles from Quadalajara.

The Saltillo Highway, a stretch of relatively straight two-way traffic between the cities of Zacatecas and Saltillo, gave one an opportunity to open it up and make up for the seemingly lost time spent in endless lines of vehicles waiting their chance to pass slow moving truck traffic between Quadalajara and Zacatecas. Unfortunately, this is exactly what most travelers did. The false sense of security traveling on a quality straight highway, albeit sparsely sprinkled with two-way traffic, would find drivers often pushing their vehicles oftentimes over eighty miles per hour.

I had cautioned Rudy to slow down once already since we left the *gasolinera* some thirty miles behind us. As I felt the Cordoba again start to pick up speed, I leaned over to check the instrument panel, as well as our speedometer.

BANG! A loud explosion from underneath the hood shook the vehicle now traveling eighty-five miles per hour. Rudy instantly hit the brakes. A moment in time that lasted mere seconds, while at the same time feeling as if it were taking place in eternal slow motion, had me praying, "Oh God, oh God."

The Cordoba skidded off the highway on an angle and rolled down an embankment of some fifteen to twenty feet. Our speed allowed the vehicle to descend almost parallel to the highway, avoiding a steep drop-off from the roadway above. I couldn't tell whether the Cordoba rolled one and a half or two and a half times, but it finally came to a stop amidst a cloud of dust kicked up from the dirt road that cushioned our fall. The death-defying ordeal left me totally disoriented.

The twenty to thirty seconds that flew by in an instant of fear and confusion immediately confirmed two things—I did believe in God and I was still alive.

As I attempted to regain my bearings, it became apparent that I was upside down. My knees were just above my face. The sensation of being upside down was strange to this quad, nine years post injury. I hadn't been upside down since I was a child doing kid things at the local playground. The motor and air-conditioning were still running. I was alone in the flipped over vehicle, basically still in the passenger's seat, yet with my head resting on the car top roof, now beneath me. Broken crumbs from the chocolate chip cookies JoAnn Kirch had baked for my trip home laid next to me on the inside roof of my maroon Cordoba.

A voice cried out, "Are you okay, Mr. Jack?" It was Rudy.

He turned off the ignition. A small group of ranch workers from across the highway had made their way to the accident scene to lend assistance. The dashboard clock read 5:05 p.m. I could hear them talking with Rudy.

My vehicle had come to rest against some kind of old dirt and fence barrier. The trunk was difficult to access.

"*Rudy, pon mis cojines de la silla en la tierra y sacame de aquí*,"[75] I instructed. Soon, Rudy and a couple of the ranchers slid me out of the vehicle and placed me on my back atop the cushions I used while sitting in my wheelchair. Getting my trusty Everest and Jennings wheelchair out of the trunk could wait for a while.

I lay comfortably on the ground "enjoying" the late afternoon sunshine while contemplating what had just transpired. The "explosion" I thought I heard from the car motor was that of a blown tire. After helping Rudy extract my wheelchair from the trunk, the ranchers returned to their work across the highway, leaving behind a girl about sixteen or seventeen years old. We talked for more than an hour.

"*Pensé que usted se había muerto*," the girl remarked. "*Murió un hombre más o menos de su edad aquí la semana pasada*."[76] Knowing that another American about my age had lost his life under similar circumstances merely a week before made me feel uneasy, while at the same time quite fortunate and thankful. My self-appointed guardian angel remained by my side while Mexican truckers stopped to ask Rudy if we needed assistance. Not one American bothered to stop.

---

[75] Rudy, put the cushions from my wheelchair on the ground and get me out of here.

[76] I thought you were dead. Last week, a man about your age died here.

With Mexican law being as backward as it was most American drivers knew that stopping for an accident, even if not at fault, could have negative consequences.

With a little assistance, Rudy finally lifted me into my chair. I had no apparent broken bones or injuries, except one. The knuckle on my left middle finger had a scratch resulting in a momentary trickle of blood.

Once I was in my chair, my angel bid farewell. I wanted to give her something for staying by me. Scattered on the ground were a number of hand carved wooden animals I'd purchased in Manzanillo as token gifts for family and friends. I told her to take them. Why hadn't I given her a few pesos? It was too late. My angel had disappeared as darkness was setting in.

With the sunset came the cold night air as Rudy and I waited for help to arrive—help that should have been there hours before.

A patrol car came slowly toward us with lights flashing. It was approximately 9:00 p.m. It had been four hours since the blown tire had nearly killed us some thirty miles outside of Zacatecas.

Even an experienced helper like Rudy had trouble squeezing me into the front seat of the patrol car. The police official had to move a rifle that was resting against the passenger seat, and the radio and other modern Mexican technology seemed to occupy the area where my long legs belonged. Additionally, our rescuer wasn't exactly thrilled to drive some forty-two kilometers from his office in Zacatecas to bring us back to face charges. More paperwork? Charges for what? We had sent word back with a number of truckers that we'd been in an accident. Why had it taken his sorry ass so long to at least check on our welfare?

Once back at the police station, I learned what the charges were: *Daños a la carretera*[77]...only in Mexico.

Cold, hungry, tired and a bit shaken from the ordeal, we waited around for the nice policeman to finish his paperwork while shooting us intimidating glances now and again. It was after 11:00 p.m. when I finally instructed Rudy, "*Preguntale cuanto quiere por los daños del accidente.*"[78]

Without viewing the accident scene in daylight, or even saying exactly what damage my precious, former mint condition Cordoba had supposedly caused "his" highway, "*Ochenta dolares*," was the answer.

---

[77] Damage to the highway.

[78] Ask how much he wants for the damage caused by the accident.

Though I was annoyed, it was worth $80 just to get out of the strange room and away from Mr. Policeman.

"*Rudy, busca un carro de sitio que nos lleve a la casa.*"[79] All I wanted was for Rudy to return with a taxi willing to make a midnight run back to Quadalajara. Another five or six hours of nighttime driving would be required to get back home and finally get some rest in my own bed. It would be worth it.

* * *

Less than a week after returning to Quadalajara via taxi, and having to explain to my friends how one starts out on a journey with their own automobile yet returns at sunrise the following day in a taxi from Zacatecas, Rudy and I parted ways.

The night Rudy left had begun routinely. Jimmy offered me, his transportationally challenged friend and neighbor, a ride to the Club. While Jimmy and I played in the Big Game, Rudy and Miguel mingled with fellow attendants and BINGO players in the hall. Something to eat or drink from the kitchen was simply tacked on to the boss' bar and restaurant tab. On this night, Miguel helped pad Jimmy's bar tab with one or two drinks more than his body could handle. Although Miguel insisted on driving Jimmy's car home from the Club, his inability to walk upright was sufficient reason to transfer the keys to Rudy for the ride home. Feeling as though his manhood was in question, Miguel balked at the idea of turning over the keys to another driver. By the time Rudy had helped transfer me from my chair to Lietz's car, Jimmy fired Miguel, just as he had on more than one occasion over the nine years Miguel had worked for him.

Once home, Jimmy and I remained outside of his house as we talked in his carport. I offered Rudy's services to help Jimmy get to bed, but he opted for a beer instead. I soon joined my neighbor as he contemplated his next move. A beer or two did wonders for keeping this quad warm on those cold Quadalajara nights when *Te de Manzanilla* wasn't available or strong enough to warm the body's temperature.

It was well after 2:00 a.m. when Rudy decided to mouth off.

"*Jimmy no debe de correr a Miguel por eso,*"[80] he chimed in.

"*Dame las llaves y vete también,*"[81] I responded. It was the

[79] Rudy, look for a taxi that will take us home.

[80] Jimmy shouldn't have fired Miguel for that.

perfect opportunity to rid myself of this punk. His attitude had been getting worse leading up to our ill-fated trip to Rhode Island. Maybe that was why I had that eerie feeling in my gut when we first departed Quadalajara. I consciously or subconsciously blamed Rudy for the accident on the Saltillo Highway days earlier. I didn't want him around any longer.

Déjà vu all over again, first, Alberto, then the tandem of Javier and Martin, and now Rodolfo (or Rudy or whatever he cared to call himself, as long as he did it out of my sight and mind). I lost four attendants in one year. If only Mom could see her vulnerable quadriplegic son sitting alone—well, not quite alone—in this foreign land, with a Tecate to keep him warm and fellow quad Jimmy Lietz to keep him company. Mom would either think I was crazy, brave, or, for whom I'd become, an independent man capable of making his own decisions and taking care of himself.

After another hour or so of talking, Jimmy went inside to wait for Sofia's morning arrival. I pushed up the sidewalk and up the ramp into my house. I'd wait until sunrise to call Bob Nemac's home. Bob had passed away a couple of years earlier, and his widow's sister Maria would surely be available to help me back to bed.

Within hours, sandy-haired Ramon Perez was at my door. Ramon, who had a fairly good reputation around town after working for Steve Woosley for a few years, was one of those experienced attendants who seemed to be floating around Quadalajara looking for work. Throughout my stay in Quadalajara, I found it to be quite common to run across experienced personal care attendants who had lost their jobs either when a fellow quad moved back stateside or passed away. Some attendants looked to return to work helping disabled gringos after testing seemingly greener pastures, only to return to what they knew best and the security of the American dollar.

* * *

Most "snowbirds" returned to Quadalajara every fall, and the ranks of Mexico PVA membership would rise accordingly. My goal as membership officer was to sign on seventy members. Membership in the Mexico PVA had stagnated to the high sixties for a couple of years. I was determined to increase our previous year's number of sixty-seven. About half of our memberships were "Life Members," meaning

---

[81] Give me the keys and get out of here too.

they opted, as I had in 1974, to pay one lump sum for a lifetime membership. Life membership gave the chapter a solid base upon which to build our numbers. Members didn't have to be concerned with being hounded annually by aggressive goal oriented membership officers attempting to meet their self-imposed quotas.

It was on one of the early October game nights in 1978 that I first felt a cold clamminess around my neck and shoulders. The warmth from the heat of our Clubhouse's artificial fireplace was most welcome. I had experienced a number of urinary tract infections throughout my time as a quad, but those always seemed to start with the chills and subsequent high fever. I had been a "guest" in the Hospital Mexico-Americano on a couple of occasions dating back to 1973, but this was different. I experienced the same sensation the next night at Jimmy's house. Again, I got as close to Lietz's space heater as possible.

The insurance company, inappropriately named Progreso, which I always referred to as "Regreso," still refused to fork over even one peso for my Cordoba. Instead, a quick visit to the auto body shop, where I was repeatedly assured it would be "*Listo en una semana más*,"[82] revealed that my vehicle was merely being used for spare parts. How dare they tell me it was being worked on and would be ready in another week, when in fact, it was being cannibalized for a small part here and a small part there. Got to take the bad with the good, I supposed.

Having returned with Ramon by plane after Debbie's wedding made it easier to leave the country, sort of legally, in the same manner. I wasted little time and flew directly back to Rhode Island and on into the West Roxbury VA Hospital.

Ironically, my friend Richard Jaros had made the same trek as me, arriving at the admission's office of the VA facility less than one hour before me. Two quadriplegics with Polish last names arriving from Quadalajara back-to-back with similar complaints of feeling cold and sweating—what were the odds?

What happened next was totally unexpected. I was told I needed a procedure called TUR (Transurethral resection), and that I had a number of micro-organisms growing in my urinary tract. My bladder neck was sliced and diced before I knew what exactly was taking place. Richard joked that they had attempted to prep him for my surgery, getting the two Polish quads from Quadalajara confused. I didn't believe Richard was fabricating his story. Everything happened so fast.

---

[82] Ready in just one more week.

Once out of surgery and placed into the recovery unit, one of the nurses wisecracked, "If you had arrived a month sooner, they were running a special on penile implants." I'd heard of that procedure, but had managed to enjoy an active sex life in Quadalajara without it. Little did I know what to expect post-TUR surgery. Maybe I should have taken ill a month sooner...

* * *

After spending Thanksgiving of 1978 in a four patient room which included my former educational therapist Harold Stone (the very person who represented National PVA's efforts to help establish a chapter in Mexico), I was discharged home for Christmas. Ramon was already going nuts being cooped up in my parent's home, only getting out on family trips to visit me at the hospital. Ramon's limited command of the English language compounded his homesickness.

Mom expected me to spend Christmas with the family. Everyone did. But after being an in-patient for several weeks in the VA hospital, I too was eager to go "home."

After an acquaintance drove my slightly twisted Cordoba from the junk yard in Quadalajara to Indiana in an unsuccessful attempt to sell it, I knew it was time for a new vehicle. I settled on my third vehicle since my injury, all purchased from Smokey Cerrone's Chrysler/Plymouth dealership. First was my '71 blue Plymouth Satellite, and next was my precious '75 maroon Cordoba. Now, however, the pickings were slim. They had a '79 beige Cordoba and a green car that sort of looked like a Cordoba. I settled on the beige Cordoba and, within a week—much to my family's disappointment—Ramon and I headed south to escape any inclement December weather. Interstate 95 would get us out of the worst states weather-wise, but also placed this less than worldly highway navigator into uncharted territory.

Driving through Atlanta during late rush hour traffic and the darkness that welcomed us, only affirmed my lack of navigational experience, although I had spent time at Fort Gordon, near Augusta, GA, and had initially received orders to report to Fort Benning, GA before my Pentagon visit. I never did get to visit Atlanta and hadn't realized how large the city was.

Once we passed Atlanta, Ramon's and my nerves seemed to settle down as familiar territory drew closer. We would be entering Mexico in another couple of days. The remainder of our December return trip to Quadalajara was routine. Until, *BAM!*

Shattered glass covered my upper body and lap. What felt like a cannonball hitting the windshield was actually a large rock hurled through the darkness from between the tires of a passing truck that impacted directly in front of my face. The rock left a small hole in the now sunken shatterproof windshield surrounded by almost glassless lining and long cracks that stretched to the driver's side. My brand new beige Cordoba was now permanently scarred. We were within meters of kilometer marker forty-two on the Saltillo Highway, where my maroon Cordoba met its fate some seven months earlier. The irony of what had just transpired didn't hit me until my heartbeat returned to normal. If windshields were still made of glass alone, I would have lost my head—literally—on a cold December night in '78 on the Saltillo Highway.

Chapter 19

A Taste of the Real Mexico?

Friday, February 19, 1971. The increasing popularity of BINGO and game nights since the purchase of the PVA Clubhouse a few years earlier had not gone unnoticed. On this particular night, five or six municipal Zapopan police, armed with rifles and accompanied by photographers, entered the "Casino PVA." Members were soon detained in the front room, but not before a few incriminating photos were taken.

According to Pioneer Bob Beilsmith, "We were in the front room playing pinochle when they came in." Beilsmith, Bill Bailey, Jack Black, and Doyle Holt had their card game interrupted. "They piled poker chips in front of us and took some pictures," Beilsmith remembered.

Members' wives, attendants, and able-bodied people present were rounded up and forced to endure a ride "downtown."

"They came into the other room in the back where we were playing poker and told us not to move, to leave everything there," recalled Teresa Beilsmith. "I think it was 11:00 p.m. They treated us like criminals. There were two of them. Both police had rifles pointed at us. They saw the poker chips on the table and got all excited. They thought it was a lot of money. They thought it was a clandestine thing. Maria Elena was there, some of the helpers, Eduardo who worked for Bob, Eddie Lucier, and Gabriel were there, and I think Taeko was there too. They took us in a truck that was like an ambulance, but it had bars on the windows," she continued. "They left the men in the front room and two police stayed outside so they wouldn't escape."

While Teresa Beilsmith recalled that night some thirty-three years prior, she couldn't stop laughing. "It was so funny that night!" It may have seemed funny to her years later, but I couldn't believe it was as funny that Friday BINGO night many years earlier.

"They took my brother with us. He wasn't doing anything but watching the cars parked outside. He was singing as they drove us to Zapopan. My sister-in-law went out the back of their house next to the club to tell Keith Ziegler."

Members present were left to fend for themselves. Tom Kirch, who suffered from pressure sores from time-to-time if he sat too many hours in his E&J, was helped on to the couch by paraplegics Holt and Clifford. The paras present suddenly had new responsibilities—they became the emergency attendants for their quadriplegic friends who might need help while their wives and personal care attendants were being detained. But for how long?

Ziegler, who lived close to the PVA Clubhouse in Ciudad Granja, was soon contacting U.S. Consulate officials. "The U.S. officials contacted the Zapopan cops and told them what was going on," Keith continued. "The Zapopan police were looking for money, that's all."

Indeed, recounted Bill Christensen who left the Clubhouse with family and guests an hour or two earlier, "They were there one afternoon less than a week before wanting something like 5,000 pesos a piece. That was about $400, a lot of money back then. Bill Bailey spoke with them first, but wasn't getting anywhere. I was elected to try next because my Spanish was better than most of the other member's. They mentioned drugs and prostitution. I explained to them that we helped the local community, especially at Christmas time, and had good relations with our neighbors."

When asked if he remembered anything about photos taken the night of the Clubhouse "bust" or anything that appeared in the local newspapers, Christensen responded, "Oh yeah, I think an article came out in *El Informador*, but I'm not sure about the pictures." Christensen recalled, "After I told them about our good reputation there, one of them said, 'It only takes one bad story to wipe out ten good deeds.'"

According to Teresa Beilsmith, "The police took us to some place like an office. They didn't take us to jail. The judge was questioning everyone. He wanted information we didn't have. He asked about drugs. They were stupid questions because we didn't know about that. About three in the morning, Consul General Wilkinson showed up. He was so mad. He said, 'Let these people go.' Oh no, he didn't ask them please. He said, 'For what reason are these people here when the other men in wheelchairs are alone without their helpers? This is not work. These people didn't do anything wrong. You take these people back right now.' By the time we got home it was four in the morning."

"There was a fiesta to raise money for the kids the next day," remembered Teresa Beilsmith. "We all finally went home to get some sleep."

"Did many of you make it to the fiesta?" she was asked.

"A lot of people showed up for the party. We had all the invitations and everything ready for the next day."

The situation was finally resolved when it was agreed upon by all parties involved that the Mexico PVA would take out a renewable gaming license, but not before a number of members' photos made the front page of the local newspaper. "Casino PVA" had been "busted" for running an illegal gambling operation. While the trumped-up story accompanied by the bogus photos was not 100% journalistically accurate, the BINGO and high stakes "Big Game" would continue for many years.

* * *

Monday, January 28, 1980. "*¿Quién es Jack?*"[83] inquired the tall, fair-complexioned man with wavy brown hair wearing a long tan coat. The intimidating man moved as would someone of authority. I was seated with my back to the wall opposite the front room fireplace, in the process of raking in multicolored poker chips won on the very first hand I had played. A second man, wearing a short brown jacket with a noticeable bulge on his right hip, positioned himself by the game room doorway. It was approximately 10:30 p.m. The apparent ring leader and point man handed me an official looking document written in Spanish, as Joe Anderson and others asked me who they were. A sense of extreme nervousness overwhelmed me as I attempted to read the paper while being peppered by questions, initially from my friends, and now from the interrogating official. "*Departamento de la Defensa Nacional*" was stamped at the top of the bogus document. I had sufficient experience with cutting and pasting articles for Mexico PVA's *El Sombrero News* to realize that the supposedly official document was nothing more than an amateur attempt at legitimacy. The "official" seal had been cut and pasted. I had never heard of "*Departamento de la Defensa Nacional*." The paper listed my name (spelled incorrectly) in the first sentence, followed by a number of charges, including drug possession and distribution, prostitution, gambling, pornography, and more. There was also mention of me going to Mexico City to face charges. The misspelling indicated someone had set us up, as all official chapter correspondence with my name on it looked nothing like the hatchet job now being done on my Polish surname. As chapter president (having taken office on June 14, 1979), I was now the alleged ringleader of this notorious band of dangerous quadriplegics who had settled in this fair city to rain evil of all sorts

[83] Which one of you is Jack?

upon the populace.

I wasn't given time to read the complete document. The extreme nervousness had long since turned to a feeling of fear unlike any, save for a few isolated incidences that I experienced while on duty in Vietnam.

By this time, the second man had moved into the game room, and another man took his place at the doorway. The third man was the most menacing in appearance. He was a short and heavily built ranchero type with a large droopy mustache, wearing a multicolored sarape, and brandishing what members later described to be a .30 caliber carbine complete with banana clip. The second man, who looked familiar and spoke English fairly well, had begun the process of taking possession of poker chips, cards, and eventually the wallets of my confounded fellow gamblers.

I was taken from the game room as the interrogation began in earnest in the hallway leading to the Mexico PVA chapter office next door. As I opened my mouth to answer, I was literally speechless; no words in either Spanish or English passed my lips for a long moment. Asked for my wallet, which I never carried in Quadalajara, the intimidator readily settled for approximately $200 worth of pesos that were in my shirt pocket.

Once inside the chapter office, the man questioned me about some of the listed charges, specifically gambling and pornography. The high stakes poker game was the worst kept secret in Quadalajara. Everyone knew about it, and any Clubhouse visitor could readily see playing cards with stacks of poker chips on the game room poker table. It was a wonder the game hadn't been "raided" since 1971.

The desk of the official chapter office was open. Macario, Gil Turetsky's helper (who I later learned was rifle-butted when he bravely asked if these men had a right to be doing what they were), had borrowed the key to the desk so that he could retrieve the phone lock key for Gil to make a local call. The phone lock was kept to prevent people from making expensive long distance calls. With the desk open, another item, namely a book titled *Sexual Options for Paraplegics and Quadriplegics* that was also kept locked in the chapter desk, was visible. The book conveniently opened to an apparently often-viewed page depicting an aroused male quad engaged in an intimate sexual act with his able-bodied female partner. "*¡Pornografia!*" declared my interrogator. Could things get worse?

For the first time, the threat to take me to Mexico City was articulated. I was totally paralyzed with fear. The situation was getting worse, as I was pushed back into the Clubhouse game room where the "innocent" Monday night poker game had originated. Ray Clifford and Chuck Hawkins were the only players still engaged in battle across the chessboard when our visitors arrived. Monday night was Chess Club night and a convenient excuse for the diehard poker players to take full advantage of the game room and open kitchen facilities. Poker players outnumber Chess Club members by about 2:1. Some of the members and guests participated in both, as I did. I had just finished a game of chess when Bill Bailey and Bob Brassfield left around 10:00 p.m., opening up two seats in the first-come-first-served game of chance.

Within minutes, personal care attendants Javier and Ramon, were relieved of their valuables and told to join us. Teresa, our Clubhouse kitchen cook, and her waitress daughter Patti, were next. Once inside, the English speaker started questioning certain members. When he attempted to search the bag John Rogers carried on the back of his E&J, the slightly inebriated fellow quad voiced his displeasure. My buddy, the interrogator, quickly took charge and rifled through John's bag. Once he got past the stuff on top, he came across Roger's personal bottle of hot salsa and a suspicious looking bottle of pills. "*¡Drogas!*" exclaimed the interrogator. Indeed, the main intimidator had found Cevelin—vitamin C tablets that were supposed to make the urine more acidic and reduce the chance of urinary tract infections.

When the realization of how ridiculous he looked set in, both John and I were ordered back into the Mexico PVA office. More harassing questions followed, but the limited Spanish speaker and fuzzy thinking poker player was useless to Mr. Interrogator. Back into the game room went John, but the point man, up until now, continued past the doorway while physically leading me into the front room. Chess boards still sat unattended to as pawns, knights, bishops, rooks, king, and queen were frozen in time awaiting further orders from their absent human field generals.

The English speaking man was holding the keys to my '79 Cordoba. The threat of facing charges in Mexico City was repeated. I was now as scared as any time in my life.

"*El Comandante quiere hablar contigo*,"[84] declared the interrogator. El Comandante? Wasn't the interrogator the leader of this gang of three? The rifle toting sarape wearer was guarding the main Clubhouse door. Could he be El Comandante?

---

[84] The commander wants to speak with you.

"*Dale una propina al Comandante*,"[85] the interrogator suggested.

"*No puedo*," I responded. "*Usted tomó todo mi dinero*,"[86] I added, surprising myself. It must have been an instinctive reaction. Where did I get off giving this man a semi-sarcastic response under these circumstances?

A medium height, graying man wearing a blue jacket appeared from nowhere.

"*¿Tiene cocaína aquí?*"[87] El Comandante questioned. I had heard the word before, but wasn't aware of this narcotic and wouldn't recognize it if I saw it.

"No," was all I said.

"*Prometes que tu no vas a seguir esta operación ilegal,*"[88] (referring to the drugs, prostitution, gambling and pornography).

"*Si Señor*," I assured him, showing as much respect as my being could summon.

"*Te voy a dar otra oportunidad*,"[89] the fifty-something-year-old man announced.

"*Gracias*," was all I could say.

El Comandante and the English speaking man, who had entered the poker room approximately one hour before, walked out the front door. The interrogator motioned to the sarape wearing, rifle-toting "ranchero," and he now physically pushed me back into the game room, semi-automatic on his right arm and my wheelchair handle gripped tightly in his left hand.

Once inside, the intimidating interrogator ordered, "*No salgan de este cuarto hasta que yo les de permiso*."[90]

Nine quads, one para, three attendants, and two kitchen employees sat around dazed, but able to freely speak for the first time since the hour long ordeal began. After about ten minutes, long-armed Joe Anderson used his functional right hand to slide open the double doors opposite of the main game room entrance.

One by one we filed out into the Clubhouse front room. All confiscated wallets lay empty on the long meeting room table, all

---

[85] Give the commander a tip.
[86] I can't, you took all my money.
[87] Do you have cocaine here?
[88] Promise that you will not continue this illegal operation?
[89] I'm going to give you another chance.
[90] Don't leave the room until I say so.

except Paul Saine's, which I theorized might have been taken for identity theft purposes since it was close to the Spanish surname Sainz. Somehow, Joe Cella, an incompletely injured quad able to stand and take a few steps, had stood up and flipped his wallet from the poker table while sitting back down on top of it unnoticed.

I requested that all members, guests, and employees present a list of the valuables which our recent visitors had taken. Inventory revealed the following:

Total cash (pesos)	3,000
Total cash (dollars)	700
Camera (approximate dollar value)	85
Silver Coins (approximate peso value)	3,500
Traveler's Checks (dollars)	300
Check made out to "Cash" (pesos)	2,800

A total of over $3,000 U.S. dollars

Ironically, non-poker playing Ray Clifford, who had come for Chess Club and was waiting for the Clubhouse kitchen to close, was hit the hardest. Clifford, who didn't trust leaving his valuables at home and who had recently returned from the States, lost cash in both dollars and pesos, two troy ounces of silver, Mexican 100 peso collector's coins, and his camera. A good guy helping fellow members on Chess Club night, as well as one of Mexico PVA's most tireless workers, Ray Clifford lost between $700–$800 worth of money and property that night.

While some of the tired and stunned members left for home, Ray and I, along with a few others, stayed at the Clubhouse to call local PVAer, Keith Ziegler, and attempt to reach the U.S. Consulate. It was useless, as the intruders had disabled the phone by removing the inner voice and hearing devices.

With the lifting of fear at what had just transpired, I suddenly remembered that the English speaking man looked familiar to me. It was from a car search that had been going on in Quadalajara for a couple of weeks. A number of members had been stopped in a similar fashion, some more than once. It happened to Ramon and I as we were returning from Eddie Lucier's house across town: a pickup pulled up about fifty yards in front of us. About a dozen armed men dressed in street clothes had jumped from the back of the pickup and stopped all vehicles coming from either direction. A few of them approached and searched my Cordoba, first the glove compartment and then the trunk. As soon as Ramon opened it, revealing my E&J wheelchair loaded there, the men waved us through. One of the men was the same man who had just robbed us. I was absolutely sure of that. He was the leader of that vehicle search team, and spoke English.

Plain clothed men stopping and searching vehicles were commonplace in Mexico. Maybe these auxiliary authorities were on loan from Mexico City? No Second Amendment right to bare arms nor Fourth Amendment right to protect against illegal search and seizure was necessary in Mexico. How else could a corrupt political system control millions of citizens, leaving most poverty stricken for decades?

Those of us present agreed we should pay the U.S. Consulate an early next day visit. We would contact as many of the victimized members and helpers as possible for a hastily arranged meeting with U.S. Consul General J. Donald Blevins, as soon as I was able to call and set up the meeting.

Consul General Blevins and I met to discuss the events of the previous night. About six to eight of the members present during the robbery were able to attend the mid-morning briefing. Mr. Blevins had already contacted the Mexican authorities who assured him every effort would be made to find the Clubhouse robbers. He was also told that local authorities knew nothing of the raid.

My one-on-one briefing with the consul general ran long, leaving a few members (who busted their backsides to get to the Consulate early) a bit disgruntled for not having had an opportunity to vent their frustrations with Mr. Blevins personally. Still, most returned the next day to go through a few rather large binders containing mug shots.

After tediously searching hundreds of photos from these binders, few of those present were able to identify anyone, except for Patti and me. Both our Clubhouse waitress and I identified the interrogator and the rifle toting "ranchero" from the binders. Other members had suspicions about some of the men in the photos they viewed, including one person who labeled the interrogator as a "possible" suspect.

The investigation was officially on. Mexican law enforcement, to calm any apprehension, assured us through the U.S. Consulate that any suspects apprehended would be viewed by us via a two-way mirror.

Ramon and I had mutually agreed to terminate our working relationship at the end of January. I had hired Juan, a former local police officer and brother of an attendant who had worked for Richard Jaros, Bill Christensen, and myself a few years earlier. Juan, like his brother Kiko, had work experience that pre-dated my arrival in Quadalajara, and spoke nearly flawless English. Rounding out my team of new helpers were housekeeper/cook, Marta, and recently hired weekend helper and medical student Luz del Carmen (Lucy). I customarily gave my driver/attendant the day off every Wednesday, as well as alternating Sundays. Marta had most weekends free, as Lucy would help out Saturdays and some Sundays. I was quite satisfied with my team of helpers. Things were finally beginning to fall into place again.

There had been a recent number of residential robberies that predated the Clubhouse incident. In one instance, PVA member Domingo Santos was visited by some three men who knew he kept a substantial amount of cash in a briefcase. Before leaving with Domingo's money and valuables, one of the men referred to another as "El Comandante."

Two other robberies appeared to have been the handiwork of young amateurs. In one robbery, after an unsuccessful attempt to break into the vacant Jardines Alcalde home of Herb Miller, the young men walked up a few blocks to the home of Helen Dunn. Helen, who had muscular dystrophy, was one of the Quadalajara community's kindest souls. Helen rented rooms in her Gaspar Bolaños four-bedroom home to those with the least financial support. But the unwelcome strangers were anything but kind. A pistol was brandished by one of the three or four men. Money and valuables were taken, including bottles of perfume. The two personal care attendants present were tied up on beds in different rooms. Upon leaving the scene of their cowardly robbery of three of Quadalajara's poorest and most severely disabled residents, one of the young men shouted obscenities about Americans. He then fired a shot, which grazed totally paralyzed Sandy Welborn's shoulder and lodged in the back of Sandy's caregiver, Sr. Gil Chavez.

Rumors floated around Quadalajara that one of these young punks had worked briefly for PVA member Richard Jaros. It was with that pretext that these lowlifes entered Helen's home on an otherwise quiet Sunday afternoon in quad paradise. Herb's good fortune of not being home that day proved to be Helen's nightmare.

The meeting with Consul General Blevins brought results to the "investigation" of the string of robberies perpetrated against U.S. citizens. I was contacted by Mexican officials through the U.S. Consulate, and told that I was to meet the point man of their effort, an undercover Mexican detective. My instructions were a bit unconventional. I was to meet this unnamed man on the street adjacent to the Consulate building at 3:00 p.m. All I was told was that he would be driving a green Volkswagen. (Ironically and tragically, undercover DEA officer Kiki Camarena was kidnapped, repeatedly tortured, and finally murdered just a few years later in a story that made international news. He was abducted from his vehicle just around the corner from where Juan and I waited to meet Mr. X.)

My contact showed up fashionably late, but still in accordance to some unwritten Mexican law that says "Three o'clock can mean 3:15, 3:30, 3:45, sometimes never, as long as the other person is on time." The door to the green Volkswagen, which parked directly behind my Cordoba, finally opened to reveal Mr. X. My contact came in the form of a short Mexican man in full disguise. Actually, the man was disguised as himself, a middle-aged Mexican of strikingly Asian decent.

My new amigo was a pleasant man who had obviously been briefed on the Clubhouse robbery. After filling him in on the missing details and discussing the residential robberies, Mr. X and I exchanged contact info. I rarely heard from him again, and his "investigation" bore no fruit.

Juan and I immediately broke into *Starsky and Hutch* mode. I was determined that the robbers couldn't get away with what they did, while Juan felt right at home with being the wheelman of this impromptu team of self-appointed detectives. Together, we tracked down every lead from a fellow PVAer's house to an orphanage on the far outskirts of Quadalajara. Baltizar and another young Mexican, who called himself Steve, were first on our list of possible suspects. I doubt it even occurred to me that I was a quadriplegic and that Juan was a former city cop without a weapon.

It was on a Wednesday night in mid-February when I heard a number of men laughing and joking as they approached the front door. I took advantage of not having a driver on these nights to work on *El Sombrero News* and other PVA business. Marta would help me to bed, get medications and water, and stay the night. This had been standard procedure for all of my housekeepers for most of the past five or six years.

Marta nervously answered the door as I stared through the curtains at the silhouettes of the previously laughing men. Typing at the dining room table afforded me a glimpse of my visitors before they officially rang the doorbell.

"*Policia*," was the answer to Marta's inquiry as to who was at the door. Marta felt somewhat relieved, but recent memories still haunted me. The two police officers, who just moments before had been joking around outside with other men, entered the house with two possible "suspects."

As the two policemen entered with the two suspects, an eerie feeling came over me—the formerly jovial group of four was now divided into two "good guys" and two "bad guys."

After introducing himself, one of the cops asked, "*¿Son los que le robaron a usted y a sus compañeros?*"[91] The face-to-face approach took me off guard as a wave of apprehension ran through my body from head to toe.

"*Puede el caminar desde allá hasta donde estoy y preguntarme '¿Quien es Jack?*'"[92] I requested of the man who looked like the one who "interrogated" me. As he complied, I noticed that this man did not appear to be quite as tall.

The suspect walked without purpose toward me and sheepishly asked, "*¿Quien es Jack?*" It definitely was not an instant replay of what would remain tattooed to my brain for years to come. Nevertheless, I thought this might be him.

"*No estoy seguro*,"[93] I honestly responded to the policeman's earlier question. The ranchero suspect sat quietly on the sofa. Without the semi-automatic and colorful sarape, he looked like any stocky Mexican, with or without the mustache.

"*¿Puede usted hacer contacto con algunos de sus compañeros para que vengan aquí ahora?*"[94] I had recently moved back to Colonia Independencia, close to Quadalajara's soccer stadium, to this cold and damp house that had one thing going for it: a telephone. None of those present during the Clubhouse robbery lived remotely nearby. I thought about Tom Kirch. He was probably already in bed at this hour, but his attendant Javier might be able to help.

An extremely nervous and reluctant Javier was sent over by taxi. In what had to be record time, Javier walked through the doorway, briefly glanced at the two suspects, and mumbled a quick, "*No son*,"[95] before being formally requested to identify the two men.

---

[91] Are these the men who robbed you and your friends?
[92] Can he walk over here and ask me 'Which one of you is Jack?'
[93] I'm not sure.
[94] Can you contact any of your friends for them to come here now?
[95] That's not them.

With that, Javier left and the "good guys" informed me that the suspects would be held overnight for any interested member or employee who cared to take a look through the police station's two-way mirror in the morning. *Thanks a lot*, I thought to myself

Word traveled fast within the Quadalajara community. Bill Bailey's driver, Jose, showed up shortly after with instructions for him to take Marta and me for security purposes to Bailey's house overnight. Tom must have called Bill, who determined that this quad and his female helper would be no match for any other suspects who now knew exactly where I lived. It was a heck of a night for Hutch to be off…

I readily accepted the invite, and soon found myself being put to bed in Bailey's guest room. There was a separate bed for my now-nervous housekeeper, Marta, who watched over me like a mother bird over a recently hatched offspring. Marta conveniently lived within walking distance of Juan's house. I sent her home early in the morning with instructions to stop by his house and tell Juan to get to Bailey's house as early as possible.

My trusty wheelman arrived earlier than I thought possible. Within an hour we were driven back to my place and transferred to the Cordoba. Ironically, Bailey's house was within a mile or so from the police station, but I needed to go clear across town to see if I could find Patti. Luckily, Juan and I arrived while both mother and daughter were still in their Ciudad Granja home. Teresa and Patti accompanied us back to Colonia Independencia and our destination. Juan had to park my Cordoba about twenty or thirty yards from the station, just off the main street of Calzada Independencia. I sent Juan inside with our Clubhouse cook and her daughter. I wished to find out if the building was relatively accessible, so I could accompany them. Juan returned with a message that I need not go through the hassle of getting out of the vehicle and going inside.

Shortly, Teresa and Patti returned. I was fairly certain that the interrogator was one of the suspects brought to my house the night before. Surely, Patti could confirm that.

"*No son*," Patti assured me, knowing how my adrenaline was pumping. But something didn't feel right. Why did the authorities discourage my participation? And when Patti told me, "*No se parecen a ninguno de los que robaron el club*,"[96] my suspicion grew. What if the police had pulled the bait-and-switch routine, and had two ordinary stand-ins replace the two who were unexpectedly brought to my house

---

[96] They don't look like any of the men who robbed the Club.

the night before? How would anyone know? Outside of appearing shorter and being purposefully soft-spoken, Patti would have had to at least say one of the suspects looked like the interrogator.

The more I thought about it, the more upset I became with myself for not taking charge of the situation and insisting to go inside the viewing room with the two kitchen employees—how dumb.

Weeks went by before my suspicions were confirmed.

After it was all behind us, Javier confided in me, "*Sí, fueron los que robaron el club*."[97]

"*¿Porqué no me dijiste antes?*"[98] I lectured Tom's attendant.

"*Mire, Jack, yo vivo aquí. Tengo familia.*"[99] Javier had a point. By identifying the bad guys, quite possibly Mexico City police officials themselves, how could he live in this city fearing for his and his family's welfare?

Time had passed. I felt vindicated for my efforts and suspicions. What might have been the end result if we had identified these men? How much danger had I placed others in simply to prove my point? How much was principle worth?

Memories of that night would remain with me for years. Questions. Who did set us up? Were they actually Mexico City police officials? Why did they feel so comfortable spending an hour hassling us when they could have robbed us and been out of there within minutes? Who could it have been?

We finally did receive some consolation, as the authorities arrested at least one of the young men who had allegedly robbed Helen's home and shot Sandy and his attendant.

The Mexico PVA membership voted unanimously to pay outstanding hospital bills for Sr. Gil Chavez. Sandy dictated to Helen a warm note of gratitude to the Mexico Chapter, which I had the pleasure of reading at the next PVA meeting. Sandy Welborn soon returned to New Jersey and an awaiting nursing home. He passed away shortly thereafter.

---

[97] Yes, they were the men who robbed the club.

[98] Why didn't you tell me before?

[99] Look, Jack, I live here. I have family.

Chapter 20

Adios Mexico: The Northern Migration

Like many of my Quadalajara friends, I considered the possibility of moving back to the States. The Clubhouse robbery had taken a toll on me, but other factors came into play. I had settled into this sorry excuse for a house because of the scarcity of accessible houses for rent. The influx of people to the city, the emergence of a "middle class" in Mexico, the rise of the cost-of-living, and several other factors made one weigh the pros and cons of continuing to live in Quadalajara. Excluding the cost of attendant care, living in the "good ol' U. S. of A." would be comparable to living in Quadalajara—but with many advantages. It would be neat to have central heat and air-conditioning, to be able to take a shower without first having a helper fire up the hot water boiler, to eat American food in America, and to transition back into the mainstream of American society.

The main sticking point for most of us was attendant care. A number of Quadalajara residents had married local women. Many were single moms. Those quads who had already left Quadalajara were, for the most part, married to Mexican women who served as their caregivers as well. A few of my single friends: Charlie Gilliam, Eddie Lucier, and Jimmy Lietz had already built or were building homes in Tucson, AZ. Phoenix, Tucson, San Diego, Florida, New Mexico, southern Texas, and one's old hometown were the destinations of choice for most stateside returnees.

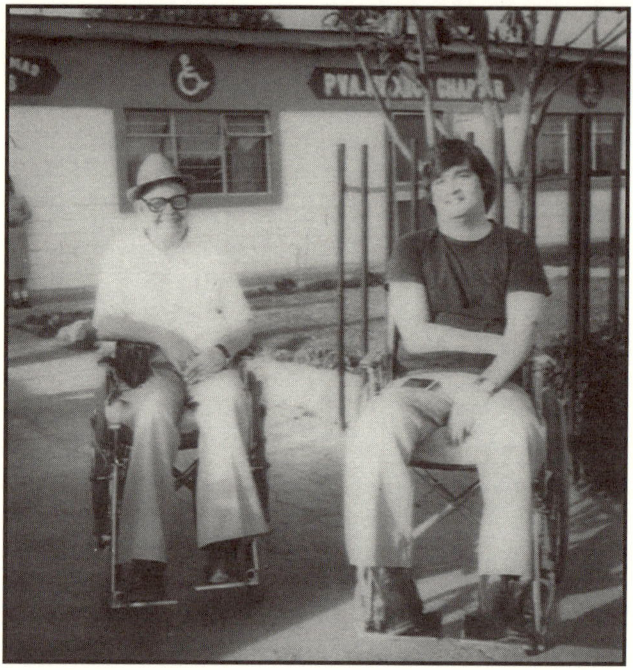

Charlie Gilliam (left) and Jimmy Lietz in front of Mexico PVA Clubhouse

Another motivating factor for some of us were VA forms requesting information on when and if we intended to use our one-time grant for purchasing a VA approved wheelchair accessible home: one year, two to five years, etc.? This benefit had grown to $40,000 by 1980. Rumors that the seemingly constant questionnaires were a harbinger signaling the end to this housing benefit prompted many of us to consider the stateside option sooner, rather than later.

As I looked back over my years spent living in this quad paradise, I couldn't help but reflect on just how I'd matured from the scared kid who'd spent the first three and a half years of his post-injury life in hospitals, rehab, and as a virtual shut-in, to president of one of the Paralyzed Veterans of America's thirty-three chapters. When poker king Fred Baker had told me years earlier that I'd found my niche here in Quadalajara, I never could have imagined sitting at the head of the PVA meeting table calling the meetings to order. It was a definite power trip, but remembering that PVA was a veteran's service organization, and all the hard work involved in it, brought everything into perspective.

My Monday morning ritual of contacting Mrs. Lillian Cartlidge at the Hospital Mexico-Americano to check on hospitalized Mexico PVA members, and to Vice Consul Joe Delaney in charge of Social Security and veteran's benefits at the U.S. Consulate, made clear I was an important member of Quadalajara's American community. Having befriended Vice Consul John Bennett at a veteran's gathering months earlier had led to what was probably the first parking space dedicated to the handicapped in the country of Mexico. Quadalajara's English language *Colony Reporter* September 29, 1979:

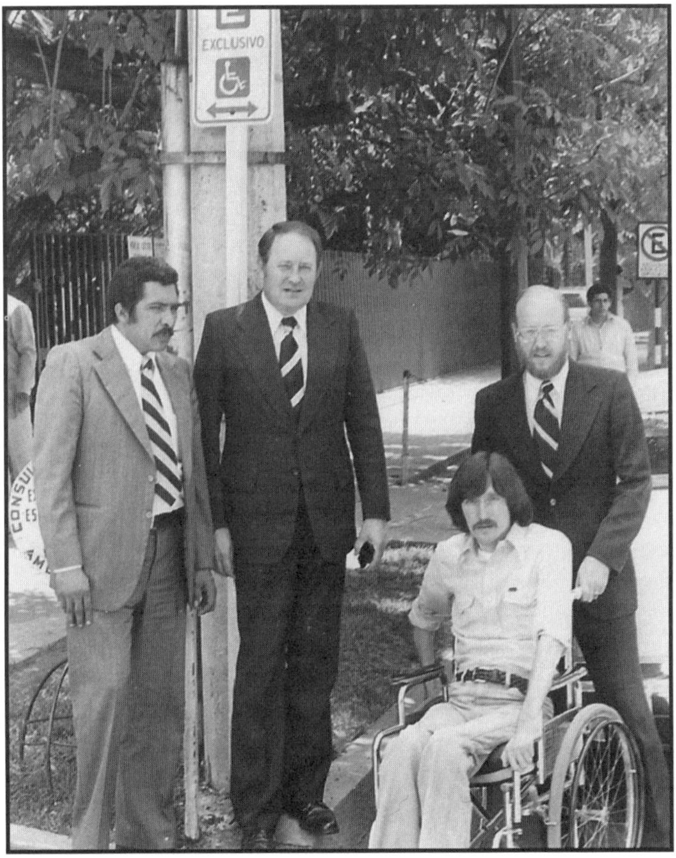

Transito Chief Lic. Jose Antonio Martinez Ramos, Consul General J. Donald Blevins, Vice Consul John Bennett, and Mexico Chapter PVA President Jack Tumidajski dedicate handicapped parking space outside the United States Consulate

A write-up in the *El Sombrero News*, September 1979, expresses Mexico Chapter PVA's gratitude:

> AMERICAN CONSULATE DESIGNATES RESERVED PARKING SPACE FOR THE HANDICAPPED -Editor-
>
> Operating in a foreign country, as our chapter does, Architectual Barrier and Advocacy programs are all but non-existant. But with the help and understanding of Consul General J. Donald Blevins and Vice Consul John Bennett along with special permission granted by Lic. Martinez Ramos, Chief of Transito for the State of Jalisco, the American Consulate is designating a reserved parking space for the handicapped on the street Lopez Cortilla (just in front of visa section of consulate building). The curb has been painted and the signs have been put up - both in English and Spanish - indicating that this parking space shall be reserved for the handicapped.
>
> I would like to express my sincere gratitude to Consul General Blevins for donating Consulate parking space, to Lic. Martinez Ramos for granting Transito authority and for getting one of the signs done up in Spanish, to Mayor Glenn Jarstaat (of Bremerton, WA) for furnishing the signs, and a special "thank you" to Vice Consul John Bennett for his time and effort in seeing this project through.

Interviews with *Rolling* Stone, Quadalajara's English language newspaper *The Colony Reporter*, and the publication that served Quadalajara's Mexican disabled community, ALJAC's *Superación*, only added to my heightened sense of importance.

The *Colony Reporter* interview came on the heels of the string of robberies. *Superación* was looking for my input on recent changes in U.S. law beneficial to the disabled. The interview with *Rolling Stone* was based on the reporter's erroneous assumption, fueled by a member of PVA's Eastern Chapter, that there was a group of disgruntled expatriates living in Mexico as some sort of turn-your-back on the United States protest. It was interesting, but no story here.

Compliments from other chapters on the new improved *El Sombrero News* were flattering, as were others from National PVA and local officials, but the satisfaction of working my butt off and seeing results, even though often taken for granted, made my tenure as Mexico PVA president a rewarding experience.

* * *

Vice Consul Delaney contacted me one day inquiring about a Jim M. His family in New York hadn't heard from or about him for a year or two. Apparently, his benefit checks were being cashed on a monthly basis, but where was he?

"I've heard of him," I informed the Vice Consul, "but I've never met or spoken to him. His name remains on the Mexico PVA membership roster because he signed on to be a Life Member some years earlier."

"If you can ask around or find out anything about him, please give me a call," Mr. Delaney requested.

Although I had never met Jim M., a number of my friends spoke of him from time to time. He was a quad from the New York area who seemed to have vanished just after his marriage to a young Mexican señorita. I had seen the name on membership lists during my tenure as membership officer, and as *El Sombrero News* editor. Rumor was that as soon as Jim had married the girl, the mother (who supposedly coaxed her daughter into this scheme), took control of all of Jim's benefits, including his VA compensation check. Once married to the veteran with service connected disability benefits, this girl (and her mom) were assured a lifetime of goodies, compliments of U.S. taxpayers. Whether or not he was pent up in a second floor house somewhere in Quadalajara living on sandwiches and water fed to him by a *chamaca* (a young Mexican girl too young to yet work as a housekeeper), while his "mother-in-law" and "wife" lived off of his monthly benefit checks, remained a rumor.

Suddenly, Calle Bruno Moreno popped into my head. Why not? It was the street that Chico lived on, and the street my formerly mint conditioned maroon Cordoba drove down many times to take me to hugs-and-kisses rendezvous with my ex-fiancée Cuca. I looked at the membership list for the street number.

A quick drive by that address confirmed that the listed house on Calle Bruno Moreno was indeed a two-story building. Whether the rest of the rumors were true or not still had to be confirmed.

Juan casually asked a passing neighbor, "*¿Cómo està el Americano Jim?*"[100]

"*Oh, El Señor Jim està en el hospital,*"[101] replied the neighbor. Bingo; potentially bad luck for Jim M., but a lead worth following up on.

Mrs. Cartlidge remembered Jim, but he wasn't a patient at the Hospital Mexico-Americano. Might mom and wife have taken him to some lesser-known hospital where Americans admitted for treatment flew under the radar screen, away from contact with the Quadalajara U.S. Consulate?

We finally tracked Jim M. down in a small hospital unknown

---

[100] How's Jim, the American?

[101] Oh, Mr. Jim is in the hospital.

to me. Upon entering the room, I found myself looking at an emaciated American quad who I doubt weighed 100 pounds. He seemed appreciative of the visit. I never brought up anything about family in New York or anything that came via the rumor-mill, but from what I observed, most or all of what I'd heard might just be true.

Based on what I'd learned, Vice Consul Delaney paid Mexico PVA member Jim M. a hospital visit. He called soon after to inform me of his findings. Apparently and sadly, what had heretofore been merely rumor was now mostly confirmed to be accurate. Jim M. was indeed being used mainly for his benefits and monthly compensation check.

I was surprised at what came next: "As long as the recipient of the benefits is coherent and accepting of his life situation, nothing can be done about it." That would probably be all the news Jim M.'s "real" New York family would learn.

Mr. Delaney, whose job it was to verify such situations, went on to inform me that many times a deceased Social Security recipient's relative would assume his identity to keep the U.S. taxpayer money flowing. It wasn't that uncommon, and often difficult to track down.

With the children's Christmas parties, our New Year's Eve party, and our annual Spring Fiesta now behind us, the next event of note was the June membership meeting. The membership meeting included a changing of the guard—handing over the reins as chapter officers to our successors. I decided that after the change was made and I was no longer chapter president, I would take an extensive stateside trip with Juan that would include driving back to Rhode Island for my family's Independence Day reunion, driving cross-country to visit friends in Arizona, and making a long overdue Las Vegas visit.

* * *

July was spent visiting family and friends, as I had the good fortune of doing most summers. Driving from Quadalajara to Rhode Island was arduous enough, but taking care of a quadriplegic as well made the five-day, 3,000-mile trip (in the days of the fifty-five miles per hour speed limit) all that more demanding for whoever my driver was.

Juan didn't seem to mind, except for my miscalculation of the driving distance between Ohio and Rhode Island, which necessitated back-to-back seven hundred plus mile driving days. The faithful father of five fit in well with family and friends, making my Rhode Island visit as enjoyable as any in recent memory. But the desert southwest was calling, and soon we were back on the road. Destination: Tucson, Arizona.

Zigzagging diagonally through Mew Mexico, we drove through the town of Roswell, made famous by the 1947 UFO incident. Or was it a hoax? Either way, we didn't see any little green men, so we pushed on to Tucson and the home of Charlie Gilliam. Charlie, and attendant Timateo, made Juan and I feel at home in the hillside hacienda, which doubled as a sanctuary for quail and other small birds and desert creatures.

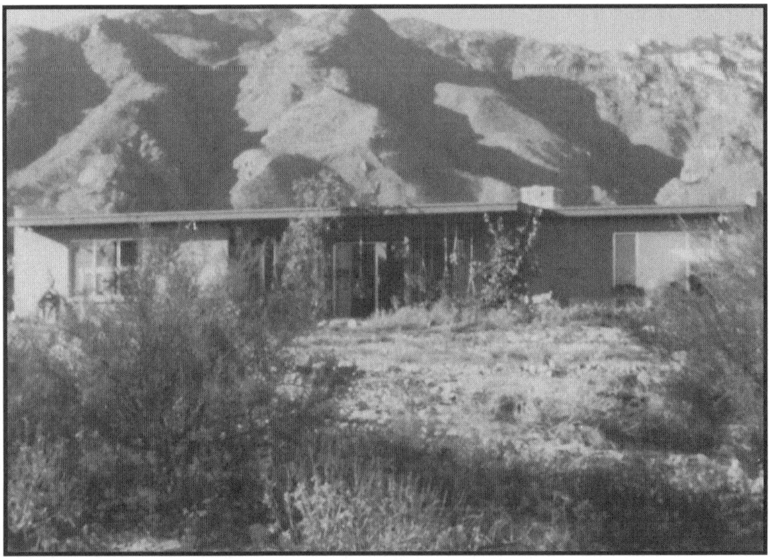

Charlie Gilliam's home in Tucson 1980

After a couple of days visiting with the jolly bald-headed man, who had introduced me to the *Colony Reporter* and my first Quadalajara house eight years earlier, it was on up the road to Scottsdale.

Bill Christensen and I had known one another since my first stay at Joe Anderson's house. Chris, as he was known in Quadalajara, had been the big brother I never had. He and Lorena had moved from Sioux Falls, South Dakota to Scottsdale a couple of years earlier. Along the way, Bill and Lorena Christensen had taken on legal guardianship of two of Lorena's youngest sisters, Aurora and Norma, who, along with their ever-growing daughter Anna, rounded out the Christensen household.

What Chris made up for in the big brother category, was counterbalanced by his lousy directions—or was that my lousy sense of following them? Whatever the case, Juan and I soon found ourselves about as far away from Scottsdale as one could get and still be in the greater metro Phoenix area. The unusually "cool" ninety-four degree August day, coupled with my auto air-conditioning failing, gave me the false impression that I could take the summertime Phoenix heat.

While visiting Chris and family, we were invited to the home of Jack and Imelda Myrick. Jack and Imelda owned a home in Quadalajara up the street from Joe Anderson's house and, along with Bob and Teresa Beilsmith, the visit made for a mini reunion of sorts. While the women continued to socialize, Chris, Jack, Bob, and I made our way to a small game table, where, to no one's surprise, a card game broke out.

The game, mixed with a few beers and drinks, lasted past midnight. I came away with over $100 in winnings—mostly from Myrick's wallet—and as we were leaving, made the stupid comment to Jack, "You couldn't have been a more gracious host if you had served steak and eggs for breakfast!" In response to this comment Myrick shot me a disapproving glance.

From Scottsdale, Juan and I headed to Sin City. This was my first trip by car, and my first visit since my hastily shortened stay in 1972 with Big Earl. Chris suggested I check out a small casino on Tropicana Boulevard called the Treasury.

My adrenaline was already pumping, and upon entering the casino itself, I felt like I was at home in this adult Disneyland. The two gorgeous blonde KENO girls made a normally hormonal All-American quad temporarily forget there was such a place as Quadalajara. The allure of the poker table was too much to ignore, and I was soon checkin' 'n raisin' with anyone who wanted a piece of this slightly tipsy and curious stranger from south of the border.

Juan came down from the room and mentioned something about the buffet.

"What time is it, about eleven?" I asked.

"It's 2:30," was all I heard my hungry and slightly annoyed helper say. One trip though the buffet line and my helper soon forgot the time of day. A few hands of blackjack, followed by an extended morning nap, and we were back to breakfast and KENO—and the two extremely attractive KENO runners who would collect a couple of dollars in exchange for a new game card and a pretty smile.

Poker and blackjack. Blackjack and poker. In a couple of days, my bank account had grown to over $800 in profit. That would more than double the amount I lost at the roulette wheel of the Imperial Palace in '72. Unfortunately, a couple more days of gambling at the Treasury had inverted my plus $800 to a minus $500. Damn black jack. I should have stuck to poker.

I decided to get some fresh air—literally—and found myself cruising Las Vegas Boulevard after dark. Four days and nights punctuated with a few hours of sleep here and there, which ran together in the clockless casino, made me forget there was a whole other world out there. There were girls everywhere. A sexy little blonde in a miniskirt caught my attention. Tempting, but another gentleman suitor noticed her before I had, and she accepted a ride from the kind stranger. It was as if each street pole had its own decorative ornament below. I saw a cowgirl holding up one light pole, but the effects of the beer were beginning to wear off and I decided not to ask her if she was a "real cowgirl."

I still had time to play a few hands of black jack. Maybe if I bet more and caught some cards, I could recoup my losses. Another red beer (beer mixed with tomato juice) and I was increasing my wagers. Funny thing about Las Vegas—when and if you got ahead of the casino, you tended to stay just long enough to do what I had. After losing your winnings, it was phase two—getting them back. After that failed, it was phase three—getting back what you lost in phase two. And then there was reality—if you were lucky enough to accept it—realizing that the once handsome $800 surplus had now grown to an ugly $800 deficit. Defeat. But it was fun while it lasted. Wasn't it? Like most, I'd be back.

Too much of a "good" thing in Sin City had caught up with us. Juan, the family man, was eager to see his wife and children again. My overindulgence had taken more of a toll on my driver/attendant than on my wallet. I hadn't actually realized it until he helped me to bed after night four, about the time the sun was rising.

By the time we got to the traffic signals on Phoenix's Grand Avenue, the old business route through Phoenix, I noticed that Juan would attempt to rest his eyes, or maybe time the lights for a quick minute nap. Whatever the case, I wasn't about to say anything to my now-grumpy driver. I'd sneak a glance each time to assure he was awake. We still had over one hundred miles ahead of us to our final stop, back to Charlie Gilliam's house before returning to Mexico.

Arriving at Charlie's around bedtime, or later, Juan quickly helped me to bed.

"Goodnight," I made the mistake of telling Juan.

"What!"

I repeated my, "Goodnight," to Juan. He turned away and said nothing.

It's amazing what a good night's sleep can do for a sleep deprived driver. After a quick breakfast and farewell visit with Charlie and Timateo, Juan repacked the necessary items he had unloaded the previous night and, after a final "thanks for everything," we were on our way to the border crossing at El Paso, Texas: Ciudad Juarez.

Once past the U.S./Mexico border, and after the usual shakedown by the Mexican checkpoint Aduana, it was on to our final destination: Quadalajara. Driving from noon to midnight, as had been my habit since I brought down my '71 Plymouth Satellite years before, had its drawbacks. First off, *never* drive in Mexico after dark. This was stressed repeatedly by the Mexican Auto Insurance company's travel manual. The many horses and cows that grazed the grass close to the highway often wandered onto the road itself. Sudden death awaited any poor animal that happened to be in the wrong place at the wrong time, and animals weren't the only ones in danger, as many tragically found out.

Considering I was the victim of an auto "mistake" myself didn't alter my driving schedule. Somehow, ironically, I had reverted back to the "it won't happen to me" mentality.

With the darkness came rain, and miserable driving conditions, but we pushed on. There was no place to stop and no turning back. Juan would pick out a vehicle to follow, and maintain the same speed for as long as possible before focusing on his next "leader." I had felt comfortable with Juan's driving ability from day one.

Back "home" I had sold or stored with friends my furniture, appliances, paintings, and everything I'd accumulated over my eight years in Quadalajara. The plan was for Juan's brother, Kiko, to spell Juan for two weeks while I stayed at Bob Nemac's old house, now being rented by my closest friends, Tom and JoAnn Kirch. From there it would be back to Anderson's house, one block north.

It was the redundant "déjà vu all over again," as I once again became Joe's official housesitter. Tom and I would visit daily. Outside of poker games and PVA stuff, where I would fill-in wherever and whenever needed, we spent time talking about viable post-Quadalajara options. Tom and I each were considering relocating to the Phoenix area. Attendant care, once again, was a major issue. Tom's situation was compounded by limited financial resources and JoAnn's disability, as well.

Vietnam combat veteran Bob Flowers was also looking at the Arizona option. Bob was a para who didn't require a personal care attendant. Bob, wife Angela, and toddler son Robert, might be Scottsdale bound. They had also made a swing through Arizona, and Bob was impressed with "How clean Scottsdale was."

Jimmy Lietz had already purchased land and was having his 702 home built in Tucson in 1979. (702 VA regulation specifying accessibility, door width, number of exits, etc...) Only a broken leg, suffered on a night of drinking and not noticing a small indoor step at a friend's house, kept Jimmy in Quadalajara until 1980. Eddie Lucier followed Jimmy to Tucson, purchasing land close to his good friend a year later. Buddy Pinnsonault and his wife Teresa had already left for New Mexico. Richard Jaros, who formerly owned a home in Tucson before returning to Quadalajara, was headed to San Diego with his wife and their young son Robert. My other single friends, besides the Tucson twins—Lietz and Lucier—were looking elsewhere as well. Mexico PVA workaholic Ray Clifford had purchased a home for his parents in El Paso. Ray soon moved to his southwest Texas home when his father, and fellow PVA member, passed away. The faithful friend was every bit the faithful son, moving to spend more time with his widowed mother in El Paso.

How times had changed. The Northern Migration had rocked the very foundation of Quadalajara. Mexico PVA membership dwindled, and finding members willing to become active in the chapter was next to impossible. Some residents felt a sense of betrayal, ignoring the obvious changes that were taking place around them while expecting everything in Quadalajara to continue as it had for over two decades.

January 1981. I decided to call Bill Christensen.

"Can you check around and find out if there are any 702s available in the Phoenix area?" I inquired of my big brother. After the experience I'd had with the addition to my parent's home ten years before, I had long since made up my mind to purchase, when ready, an existing house—no more surprises or disappointments.

The phone rang early on Saturday morning. It was Chris.

"Jack, there are two available 702s here. One I think you'll like has a pool and another near the mountain foothills. I'm not sure if you'd like it, but both are reasonably priced. They'll be closing soon on the house with the pool, would you be able to come up here soon? I can put down a small non-refundable deposit, and I know they'll wait a few days so you can take a look at it," reported my friend and big brother.

"Let me see how soon I can make it," I told Chris. "I'll check Juan's papers and call back."

I sent Juan home as soon as I got up. "Let me know if your documents are up-to-date," I instructed. With everything set, Juan and I departed Quadalajara for Phoenix.

This would be my first trip on the Nogales Highway, one that would take us from Quadalajara to Mazatlan to Guaymus and on to the border crossing of Nogales, Mexico/Nogales, Arizona. It was a journey of over 1,200 miles. I had avoided the Nogales Highway when Juan and I had returned from my extended stateside trip, opting for the El Paso/Ciudad Juarez crossing. Despite whatever horror stories I had heard about the Nogales Highway, it couldn't be any worse than our return trip months earlier.

With stops in the ocean-side city of Mazatlan, and the Bay of Cortez town of Guymus to rest and sleep, I wished I'd taken this highway earlier. Unfortunately, I was a point A to point B kind of guy who didn't have time to stop and smell the roses; in this case, enjoy what thousands of tourists paid real money to go out of their way to do.

It was evening of day three when Juan and I reached the Nogales border. I went inside with Juan, and waited as he stood in line for his U.S. visa permission to be approved. Usually, the immigration service was understanding and approved visa stays of up to six months. I didn't need that long. I had no problem with Juan's previous visa request.

I saw my driver attempting to explain something to the immigration official. Frustration filled the air. I pushed over toward him in time to hear the official exclaim, "*¿Qué quiere?*"[102] as if annoyed by Juan's persistence.

"I'd like to speak to your supervisor," I expressed. We were motioned off to the side where a kindly looking man approached us. For whatever reason, U.S. immigration officials of Mexican decent, or at least Hispanic themselves, were tougher to get assistance from than regular gringos were. Surely, his Anglo boss could straighten this out.

After glancing at Juan's passport, the not-so-understanding supervisor handed the passport back to my attendant saying, "His visa has expired." I looked, for the first time, at Juan's documents.

"Can't you give him a few weeks permission to accompany me

---

[102] What do you want?

to Phoenix? I'm supposed to look at a house for sale and need to be there as soon as possible," I explained.

"Only in emergency cases," he informed me.

"But this is like an emergency to me. I have to be there and have already placed a non-refundable deposit," I pleaded.

"That doesn't qualify as an emergency," he insisted, standing his ground.

"What am I supposed to do? You're telling me we can't cross into Arizona," I continued. "We drove here all the way from Quadalajara."

"Can't help you," he went on, "There's a U.S. Consulate in Hermosillo."

"But it's nighttime and there's no convenient place I can stay here in Nogales," I exclaimed.

"Don't you drive at night in Quadalajara?" he shot back.

Frustrated and tired, we drove through the darkness from the Nogales border back to the city of Hermosillo. Arriving tired and late, I sought out the U.S. Consulate building, and proceeded to find the closest suitable lodging for, hopefully, an early morning Consulate visit.

The official I initially spoke to was skeptical. "You want a tourist visa for your attendant?" he questioned

"It's commonplace in Quadalajara," I explained, "There's a large population of disabled wheelchair-bound residents there, and the Consulate routinely allows us visas for our attendants to drive us to the States."

He looked over his shoulder and another official came to speak with me. After explaining again the procedures adopted years earlier by the U.S. Consulate in Quadalajara, I added, "You can contact Vice Consul John Bennett, Vice Consul Joe Delany, or Vice Consul Williams who works in the visa section. I'm sure any one of them will vouch for me and explain our situation in Quadalajara." It paid to know people with influence. Heck, I had influence, didn't I?

The first official returned within minutes. "You can wait in the next room. The visa should be ready in about thirty minutes." I guess I did have influence…

We were back on the road and sailed through Nogales, this time without a problem. Juan was approved for six months, which might come in handy in case everything went well for me.

As we left Mexico and entered the United States, I was sure I would return to Quadalajara in the future. I was excited to be beginning a new chapter in my life, but unprepared for just how much I would miss Quadalajara.

I would have the opportunity to return to Quadalajara in 1982, 1986, 1987, 1988, 1989, and 1992. Each return to my former home-away-from-home showed changes. The '82 trip was brief, but many old friends still resided there and many more returned to visit. The Mexico Chapter, Paralyzed Veterans of America officially folded due to lack of membership in 1983. After a brief, but hectic visit in '86, the following years found fewer and fewer old friends still living in Quadalajara. Some eventually moved back to the States, while most who had stayed beyond the great Northern Migration fell victim to Father Time. We affectionately referred to this as going to "the big poker game in the sky."

I remember being invited to Herb Miller's house for dinner in 1986. A number of old friends were there. The topic of current residents of Quadalajara came up. Within the small group of us we counted about thirty-three. The following year Herb was gone, and through an ironic twist of fate, I rented Herb's old house for about five months while his estate was in probate.

It was during this lengthy visit that Cuca and I began dating again. I heard through the grapevine that Cuca's husband had abandoned her in the early-80s while she was expecting their second child. I paid her a surprise visit during my brief 1986 stay.

Maria de Refugio from San Juan Capistrano was living with her sister Alicia, who was married to my friend and "almost" *concuño,* (brothers-in-law by virtue of marrying sisters) Barney Vigil. Barney and Alicia had built a house in the Lake Chapala community of San Antonio, and had taken Cuca and her now three- and four-year-old boys into their home. Our reunion proved that we still had the magic and the chemistry we once shared. We kept in touch by mail until my return in 1987.

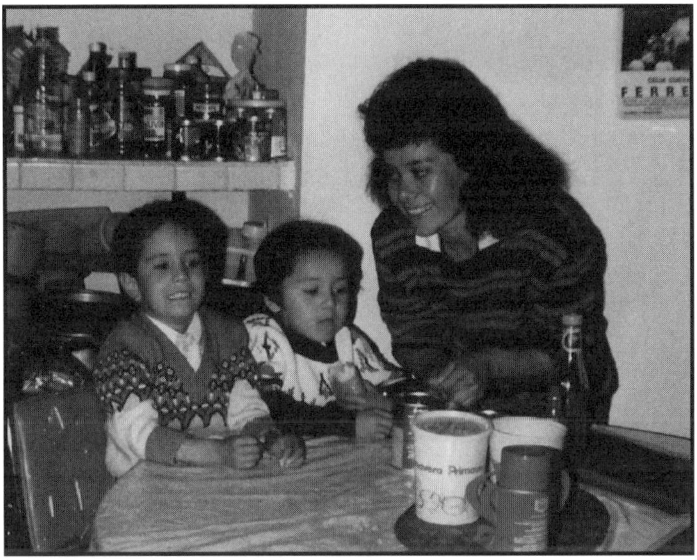

Alex, Willie, and Cuca 1987

It was impossible not to like Willie and Alex, and Cuca and I were once again discussing the possibility of a future together. Frequent trips to the Chapala community to spend time with my former fiancée and her two sons had me thinking about what Reverend Hunter had mentioned to me so many years ago. I remember on two occasions going to bed and thinking—this was it. I would do what so many of my friends and former Quadalajara resident had done. I would marry Cuca and have what was missing in my life—a wife and two adorable sons.

I guess some things in life are not meant to be. Although my señorita from San Juan Capistrano and I would continue to correspond for a few more years, our on- and off-again plans for the future eventually fizzled.

I considered selling my Arizona home with the pool in both 1989 and 1991, and returning to what once was the place that forever changed so many of our lives. I never did. Memories were all that remained: memories of getting a second chance in life, memories of those who touched our lives, memories of a unique place in a unique time—Quadalajara.

This was not the Guadalajara, Mexico (or "Villa Dulce") as depicted in Oliver Stone's movie Born on the Fourth of July. The only portrayal of Mexican women in Stone's movie was unfortunately that of whores and prostitutes. This is a demeaning misrepresentation of the fabulous señoras and señoritas of our neighbors to the south.

Ron Kovic's experiences during the short time he spent in Mexico, as detailed in his autobiography by the same title, differ greatly from that of most who visited or resided there. Although many of us who spent time in one of the "gimp camps" did explore the seedy side of this wondrous city, not everyone spent the majority of their time inebriated in cantinas or whorehouses. Most of us explored all aspects of the city, including its rich history, culture, and wonderful people.

I only regret that I, or someone knowledgeable of this unique time in history, had neither the voice nor the fortitude to set the record straight earlier.

Chapter 21

A Final Tribute

The earliest Explorers and Pioneers of this quad paradise, which began with few unknown explorers and followed by a trickle of brave souls who first stayed with George Ray, Joe Miller, and Bill Macleary, gave way to a steady stream of newcomers who rented rooms at Bill Coe's, Larry Kegan's, and George Ray's Place. By the late-60s, the population had grown to over two hundred residents and visitors. Villa del Sol, Casa de Vida Nueva, and Sun Haven—better known as Mrs. Cartlidge's Place—were some of the options for visitors and group living in the late-60s and early-70s. A May 1968 article in the *Paraplegia News* advertises these options:

> **New housing unit planned in Mexico**
>
> A new housing facility designed for wheelchair living is now under construction in Las Fuentes, a suburb of Guadalajara, Mexico, according to a report from that city.
>
> The new facility being built by Dr. A. D. Williams of Guadalajara reportedly will consist of a series of bungalows with a planned total capacity of 20 guests. A large community dining room and recreation room and patio are also planned.
>
> Necessary services, aides, chauffeur, and medical attention will be provided, according to the Guadalajara report.
>
> Persons seeking additional information may write: Dr. A. D. Williams, 856 Pedro Moreno, Guadalajara, Jalisco, Mexico.
>
> Other establishments in Mexico offering accommodations to wheelchair residents are those operated by PVA members William Coe and Lawrence Kegan, both in Las Fuentes, and George Ray in Chapalita.
>
> The 75-member Mexico Chapter PVA has its chapter clubhouse in the nearby suburb of Ciudad Granja.

A July 1968 *PN* advertisement:

> *Announcing*
>
> **VILLA del SOL**
>
> (A DESIGN FOR GOOD LIVING)
>
> Brand new — a medically supervised non-institutional paraplegic residential center providing cheerful, gracious, wheelchair living.
>
> Villa del Sol offers the privacy of apartment living to quads and paras of both sexes... informal atmosphere magnificent climate... trained attendants enjoyable recreational program.
>
> **TOTAL CARE**
>
> The most advanced, imaginative facility of its kind now in Latin America.
>
> For full information write to:
>
> **A. D. Williams, M.D., Director, Villa del Sol • San Antonio 45 Las Fuentes — Guadalajara, Jalisco, Mexico**

Quadalajara was in its heyday. A new breed of younger men could be seen at the increasingly popular Villa del Sol. Vietnam veterans—"Cold Warriors" who had served their country in an uncertain war against communism in Southeast Asia—were now finding their way to this interesting and inviting city in the heart of Mexico. Richard Jaros, Jimmy Lietz, Ray Clifford, and Frank Stoppiello among them.

Throughout the 1970s, the newest of the newcomers would hear old-timers talk about how great Quadalajara *had* been. But Quadalajara was still a fascinating and fantastic place for those who managed to find their way south of the border in the early-70s. The era of tequila, señoritas, and mariachis may have calmed down some, but how could Quadalajara have been that much better a decade earlier?

By the early-70s, a substantial number of those residing in Quadalajara had married Mexican women. Many, including Ray Foland, Bob Beilsmith, Steve Wilson, Jack Myrick, Bob Harmon, Richard Jaros, Bernie Munoz, Bill Christensen, and countless others, had returned to live in the U.S. with their Mexican wives and families. Others would follow.

The trickle of early settlers in the 1950s, that became a steady stream of newcomers by the mid-60s, would be reduced again to a slow trickle by the late-70s. Gimp camps dried up just as had the steady stream of newcomers, with the fitting exception of *Cubilete,* formerly George Ray's Place.

The Mexico Chapter PVA's Clubhouse remained the center of gravity for the Quadalajara community. Members and non-members, wheelers and walkies, would congregate there for twice weekly BINGO and game nights, monthly membership and Board of Directors meetings, Spring and Fall Fiestas, New Year's Eve parties, awards banquets, and other social functions. But with declining membership and loss of key chapter "workers" (mostly due to the great "Northern Migration"), the handwriting was clearly visible on the proverbial wall. Despite the hard work and dedication of men like Keith Ziegler, Ray Clifford, and Eddie Lucier—who combined to hold every chapter office of the Mexico PVA practically year-in and year-out since the late-60s—the chapter workload had become a Herculean task, and the PVA Clubhouse an albatross.

From Keith Ziegler's President's Message in the July 1982 *El Sombrero News*:

> *Fiscal year 1981-1982 has come to an end and I find that Mexico PVA has begun its fall. I do take partial responsibility for our decline, but no organization can be run by one man. Because of having to do many jobs, some quarterly reports have not been sent out. This report is to let you members who have not been to our meetings or have not been in touch know what has happened during the past year. I apologize for not keeping you completely informed during the past year.*
>
> *I would like to bring to all members' attention that during this past year we have lost six active members. These members have chosen to go back to the States for various reasons. Two of these members have been past presidents and*

two have been our treasurers. One has helped in the treasurer capacity when the treasurer wasn't here, one was our El Sombrero news editor, and one was a vice-president and Clubhouse chairman. These men were workers in our organization and we have missed them during the past year. Now we need replacements. If you members who live here in Guadalajara want a Mexico PVA Chapter you are going to have to come and help. We need your assistance in order to keep going on.

National PVA, at its 1983 annual Board of Directors meeting in Portland, Oregon, finally pulled the plug on its chapter in Mexico. According to Ziegler, "National called Ray Clifford and myself into a room and informed us they were no longer able to maintain a PVA chapter on foreign soil." Ironically, former Alliance for Compassion and early Quadalajara resident Ernie Chavez, who went on to serve National PVA as its service director for many years, was one of those who informed Mexico PVA President Ziegler and Director Clifford.

The unique time in history that began in the mid-50s in the Mexican city of Guadalajara would last for close to three decades. The Quadalajara era basically ended when the Mexico Chapter, Paralyzed Veterans of America folded. Although a number of residents continued to live there, while others visited frequently or infrequently, it was time to remove the letter "Q" and re-insert the letter "G." Quadalajara—the utopia that once was—was gone, and gone forever.

From the April 1984 *Quadalajara Review*:

Mexico Chapter To Be Dissolved

The Mexico Chapter of the Paralyzed Veterans of America is being dissolved after twenty years of service to veterans in the Guadalajara area. Chapter Director Raymond J. Clifford made the announcement when contacted at his home in El Paso, Texas. "Dwindling membership," was cited as the prime reason.

Clifford reported, "Chapter members voted fourteen to three to dissolve the group rather than to become a sub-chapter of one of five PVA chapters located in the southwestern United States." Members are being given a choice of affiliation with another PVA chapter or member-at-large status.

The Mexico PVA Clubhouse, which served as a focal

point for chapter functions and social gatherings, is up for sale.

According to Clifford, "The members voted to donate all chapter monies to PVA's Technology and Research Foundation (TRF) and building fund."

The final distribution, according to Ziegler was that, "$5,000 be donated to the Asociación de Lisiados de Jalisco, AC (ALJAC), $5,000 to the National PVA Building Fund, and the balance to the Paralyzed Veterans of America's Spinal Cord Research Program. The donation to ALJAC was in pesos. It was money that we had in our operational fund, along with what we collected from the sale of chapter and Clubhouse property. A bunch of us, including Ray Clifford, Eddie Lucier, Frank Stoppiello, myself and a few other members and wives went to one of their meetings. We donated roughly $5,000. They were extremely appreciative, and thanked us for the donation and help that we had given them over the years. Mario (Avila, who was ALJAC's president and most active member throughout the 1970s and into the 1980s) and I continued to write one another for a number of years."

In 1987, four years after the Mexico Chapter PVA held its final meeting, the Clubhouse sale was finalized and the funds distributed.

In a May 13, 1987 letter to National PVA, Keith Ziegler wrote:

Enclosed is a check for $5,000 which the past membership of the Mexico PVA voted to have sent to the National Office to be donated to the PVA Capitol Campaign Fund. We would like for our chapter to be remembered with our name engraved on a brick or whatever you do to remember those who donate such an amount for the PVA Building.

Your office will be receiving the remainder of our funds shortly which have been earmarked for spinal cord injury research.

From a May 22, 1987 letter to Ziegler from National PVA:

Dear Keith,

On behalf of National PVA, I would like to express our gratitude to you and the other former members of the Mexico

Chapter for your $5000 contribution to the PVA Building Fund. Your decision to donate these funds to the PVA Building is an important expression of confidence and support for the work being accomplished by your national organization and it is deeply appreciated by the officers and staff.

As a lasting symbol of your support and tribute to the past membership of the Mexico Chapter, a recognition plate will be appropriately engraved and placed on a brick in the front lobby of the PVA Building. In this way, the Mexico Chapter will be remembered by everyone who visits the PVA Building.

Once again, thank you for your support and please convey our appreciation to the other former members of the Mexico Chapter.

Sincerely,
R. Jack Powell
Executive Director

On August 18, 1987, in a letter to National PVA, Ziegler wrote:

Enclosed is a check for $21,393.58 which we, the members of the Mexico Chapter of the Paralyzed Veterans of America, have chosen to donate to the Spinal Cord Research Foundation of the Paralyzed Veterans of America. This is being done at the request of all the members of the ex-Mexico PVA.

Zieglar was graciously thanked by Linda K. Coughtry, Director of Development, in an August 28, 1987 letter from the National PVA:

It was a pleasure talking with you earlier in the week, and again, thank you for the check of $21,393.58 from the members of the former Mexico PVA chapter.

From our discussion and your correspondence, I understand that it is the intent of the Mexico chapter members to dictate this contribution to spinal cord injury and disease research. As you and I discussed, the PVA Board of Directors passed an important resolution regarding PVA's future activities in SCI research (copy enclosed). The resolution *provides the permission for PVA to enter in a co-venture arrangement with Yale University over the next five (5) years. The project, consisting of a physical building and SCI scientific research, will be called the Yale/PVA Center for Neuroscience and Regeneration Research. This extraordinary partnership will in large part be due to the $1.5 million commitment PVA has made to the Center over the next five years.*

I have enclosed a brief fact sheet about the project and a profile on the individual who will be heading the Center, Dr. Stephen Waxman. We are currently in the contractual negotiation stage with Yale and expect to have the arrangement formalized over the next month.

You may also be interested to know that 21 of PVA's 31 chapters have pledged a total of $450,000 over the next five (5) years towards fulfillment of PVA's $1.5 million pledge. Therefore, it seemed only natural that the members of the Mexico chapter would like to join with this effort.

* * *

In a September 2, 1987 follow-up letter to National PVA, Zieglar concluded:

It has always been the wish of the founders and members of the Mexico PVA that any monies which are left in our treasury, if and when the chapter should fold, would be used for spinal cord research. So I think that this would be an appropriate memorial for all who were part of the Mexico Chapter.

Many quads, paras, and other wheelers rolled around this unique city during this unique period in history. Unfortunately, just as the Quadalajara era will never be duplicated, forgotten others will remain unknown—many of them the original Explorers and Pioneers of an almost forgotten moment in time. Maybe one was a long lost family member or acquaintance? This tribute goes out to them as well.

Jimmy Adkisson—An extremely thin quad from Texas, Adkisson was the victim of an accidental shooting while in his teens. Although he was totally paralyzed from the neck down, Adkisson took on a number of endeavors; from PVA Clubhouse concessionaire to insurance salesman and investment counselor. He was an excellent chess player (see Appendix B, pages 333-334).

Roger Allen—Roger was from Indiana and the Hines VA Hospital. He stayed at Kegan's Place and was elected to Mexico Chapter's Board of Directors in May 1967.

Tommie Anagnostis—Anagnostis was a "snowbird" who resided at Patino's Place in the early-70s, formerly Hacienda Las Fuentes or more commonly referred to as Kegan's Place until the late-60s.

Joe Anderson—The retired photographer from Omaha, although sorely lacking in his command of the Spanish language, managed to date more attractive señoritas than anyone. His easy-going, confident personality and sense of humor made Anderson a magnet for the ladies and the envy of many fellow quads and paras. Present at the 1980 Clubhouse robbery.

Oscar Anderson—Early Quadalajara resident and one of many to attend Joe Miller's 1963 wedding reception for newlyweds Ernie and Hortencia Chavez. Pictured in the January 1964 *Paraplegia News* with the newlyweds and Alfred Hanson.

Jerry Andrews—Raised in a South Carolina orphanage, Andrews was easy-going and personable. He was a mainstay, and often times banker, at the Big Game during the '70s. The quad made the most of his abilities, sometimes functioning as an almost totally independent quad both out of necessity and by choice. Andrews regularly served on the Mexico PVA's Board of Directors in the late-70s. Banker the night of the 1980 Clubhouse robbery.

“Big Earl” Annis—The five hours Big Earl spent at Casa de Vida Nueva before heading back to the airport and returning to Boston should qualify him as the record holder for the shortest stay in Quadalajara.

Tatsumi “Gato” Aragaki—One of Quadalajara’s early Pioneers. Gato spent many years living by Jalisco’s famous Lake Chapala. Gato was one of the Mexico Chapter PVA’s most generous donors, especially for the Children’s Christmas posadas. Gato was rumored, according to Quadalajara folklore, to keep a coffin that he would fill with empty Tequila bottles for later burial.

Oran Arms—Mexico PVA member who resided in Colonia Chapalita during the ’70s.

Larry Bagget—“Married a tall good looking girl from Patino’s” (from Joe Miller’s High Society column, *El Sombrero News*).

Arlene Bailey—Arlene met future husband Bill Bailey when she left New York and visited Patino’s Place in 1971. The couple married in 1972, moved to a home of their own, and had one daughter.

Bill Bailey—Married to Arlene, Bill was one of many Muscular Dystrophy survivors to call Las Fuentes home.

Bill Bailey—**Founding Member of the Mexico Chapter PVA**—One of the very early Quadalajara Pioneers, Bill was originally from Lewiston, Idaho and Baker, Oregon. In 1958, he became the first gringo wheeler to marry one of Quadalajara’s pretty señoritas. He was also the Mexico Chapter’s president before National PVA’s charter accepted the Mexico PVA as its only chapter on foreign soil. Known for his signature cigar, “Don Guillermo” could kick your butt in everything from chess to whatever card game you dared challenge him to. He and his wife, Maria Elena Cruz de Bailey, were extremely generous with financial support and the giving of their time to help both the Mexico PVA and their local community.

Bill Baker—Bill was a very interesting storyteller. The double amputee para with the black cowboy hat claimed to have bought into an early theory—according to some in the medical community—that legs on a para or quad were no longer necessary, and that one could function more independently without them. Though it was a good theory, few opted for this surgical procedure.

Dick Baker—The quad from Indiana joined the "Poker Wars" for a short time around 1974. He then married a local señorita and moved back to Indiana.

Jerry Baker—Jerry was a family man who lived in Colonia Chapalita with his wife and daughter. He was the former resident of Hawaii who first mentioned Quadalajara to fellow Islander, Jerry Fesenmyer.

Bob Barrett—**Founding Member of the Mexico Chapter PVA**—Barrett lived down the street from George Ray's Place, and especially enjoyed playing Pinochle with Bill Bailey and Joe Miller. He was responsible for first suggesting *El Sombrero News* as the official title of the chapter's monthly newsletter.

Clayton Bawden—Bawden is one of the few Mexico PVA members to have never visited Quadalajara.

Werner Begall—The German citizen visited Quadalajara in the late-70s while staying at Cubilete. Werner participated in the Mexico PVA's 1980 Chess Tournament.

Bob Beilsmith—The quad from St. Louis, injured in his teens, found his way to Quadalajara in 1962. A successful gambler, Beilsmith was also active in the Mexico PVA, serving as chapter president in 1968. He married his long-time novia, Teresa, in 1967, and eventually returned stateside to settle in Phoenix, Arizona in the early-70s. The Beilsmith's were among many to revisit this unique Mexican city for extended vacations. Photographed during the 1971 Clubhouse robbery.

Jim Beletti—Beletti was one of a number of guys to show up late for the party. The friendly para who first made the scene in the late-70s was one of the few unfortunate gringo wheelers to be murdered in Quadalajara.

Greg Benisch—Benisch was a blond quad from the Midwest who was injured in his mid-teens. He found his way to Hacienda Las Fuentes in the '60s. Greg's passion was cars—fast cars. Benisch, Bill Kahler and a few friends were enjoying a late night drink in an after-hours cantina when a man walked over and shot another man dead. Benisch and Kahler shared another memorable event while checking out Quadalajara's famous pyramid. Having left their wheelchairs and attendants behind one evening, the adventurous young men soon found Greg's car stuck in the sand off the highway with no way to get it out of the pyramid's mystical sand trap. The two quads spent the night in the vehicle with only a six-pack of cerveza and an eight track tape of "Janice Joplin & Big Brother and the Holding Company" to get them through the night until a passing truck spotted them the following morning. Benisch moved to the San Diego area during the Northern Migration.

Tom Berry—Berry was one of those featured in a 1972 *Ebony Magazine* article (see Appendix B, pages 329, 333-334) of Black-American veterans living in Quadalajara. The para from New York resided in Mexico with wife, Shirley.

Claudio Bertoli—Bertoli was one of a number of New Englanders from the West Roxbury VA who stayed at George Ray's Place in mid-60s. Bertoli later stayed at Patino's in the early-70s.

Bob Beske—**Founding Member of the Mexico Chapter PVA**—The combat injured veteran married a Mexican lady and purchased a home in Quadalajara. Unfortunately, Beske's injuries prevented him from enjoying a more active life and confined him to living at home for many years.

Jack Black—Jack was a post-polio, avid poker and bridge-playing para from Chicago who quickly jumped into Mexico Chapter politics. He served as chapter president in both 1971 and 1975. As chapter president, he led an unpopular effort to sell the PVA Clubhouse in fiscal year 1975 (June 1974 – June 1975). He and wife Teresa had two sons, and eventually moved to Phoenix, Arizona in the mid-70s.

Larry Blinn—The heavy-set resident of George Ray's Place soon gained the moniker Larry "Blimp" from Joe Miller's High Society column in the monthly *El Sombrero News*. Blinn was elected to the chapter Board of Directors in June 1965.

Herb Bloom—The post-polio quad from Massachusetts called Casa de Vida Nueva home for a few years before moving into his own apartment and hiring an attractive Mexican lady as his caregiver.

"Captain" Ben Borish—Captain Ben was Quadalajara's answer to Lawrence Welk. An entertainer turned quad, Borish often supplied the Mexico PVA with local talent to entertain chapter members and guests both after Friday night BINGO and at chapter fiestas. He also wrote and sang his own songs, "Mariachis in the Moonlight" being among them. Borish was voted an Honorary Member of the Mexico PVA at the November 1966 Board of Directors meeting. Captain also ran his own poker game in the mid- to late-60s. In 1968 Borish teamed up with Mexico PVA life member Jack Lastor to found "Free Wheelers," a project to provide used wheelchairs to needy disabled Mexican citizens. The project quickly gained support from the Mexico PVA, and chairs were soon donated to two Mexican children, "both of who have never walked nor used a wheelchair before" (*Paraplegia News*, February, 1969).

Leo Bourdosis—One of the forgotten ones, at least by his relatives, Leo was a regular at the Big Game. Leo's trademark bald head rested atop a man completely paralyzed by Multiple Sclerosis. Although Leo had returned to Quadalajara after some time spent in Sepulveda, California, he was originally from Taunton, Massachusetts. He had a contagious personality and a love for playing poker and Gin Rummy, and he spent many afternoons playing Gin Rummy with Gil Turetsky at Cubilete. Leo and Gil were inseparable for a time, often sharing a taxi from Cubilete to the Big Game at the PVA Clubhouse in Ciudad Granja. That was until a wild, sexy young English-speaking señorita named Mercedes showed up at Cubilete. The jovial fifty-seven-year-old man and the eighteen-year-old sex kitten from Quadalajara struck up a physical relationship. Leo once confided that if he ever met a woman who could make him "experience sexual performance again," he would marry her. A few months later, to the surprise of many and the delight of others, Mr. and Mrs. Leo Bourdosis tied the knot in the spacious front room at Cubilete. After moving back to Sepulveda, Leo would return to Cubilete a couple of years later a widower—having lost his wild and sexy young wife to a drug overdose. Leo spent his final years (and money) with a very unattractive young woman whom he called "Sweetie." It seemed that the now visually impaired man simply wanted female companionship and the satisfaction of dying penniless, knowing no long-lost uncaring relative would inherit a cent.

Freeman Bradshaw—One of the original Pioneers, Bradshaw spent his final years living by Lake Chapala. He passed away there in 1969.

Joe Branigan—Mexico Chapter PVA member who frequented membership meetings in the mid-60s.

Bob Brassfield—A U.S. Air Force veteran, the reverse quad from Iowa—Brassfield could actually move his legs and stand with assistance while being totally paralyzed above the waste—was reportedly injured in a freak accident when a helicopter blade struck him in the back of the neck. Brassfield was a regular member of the Mexico PVA's Board of Directors throughout the '70s. The extremely likable and respected "helpless" quad could always be counted on and, despite his disability, was one of the most responsible and dependable PVA members and friend one could hope to know. Brassfield's conservative nature served him well whenever he attended the Big Game, translating into more winning than losing evenings.

Don Bush—Don Bush was a goateed quad from the Bay area. His limited income forced him to rent rooms from a number of his fellow residents during the '70s.

Joe "Candy" Candalaria—Candalaria, originally from Colorado once roomed with Pioneer Ray Foland.

Dave Carlson—Carlson penned a monthly column titled "Chaplain's Corner" in the chapter newsletter in the late-70s. The Northern Migration took Carlson to Tucson, Arizona.

Richard Carlson—Mexico PVA member elected to the chapter's Board of Directors for fiscal year 1966.

Dale Carr—Elected to the chapter's Board of Directors in May 1965, Carr later married and took his bride to Oregon for a thirteen month "visit."

Mary Lou Carroll—Mary Lou rented a room from Eileen Van Albert. She later married Quadalajara resident Joe Fox and the couple returned to live in the States in the '70s.

Eugene Carter—Carter was a quad from Mississippi who was featured in the 1972 *Ebony Magazine* article (see Apendix B, pages 328, 330-331) on Black veterans living in Quadalajara. He was also a former law student with a passion for writing. Carter served as chapter secretary in 1975, and volunteered his time to assist the Mexico PVA service program.

Joe Cella—Cella was a walking quad from Philadelphia who showed up in the mid-60s via the Richmond VA Hospital. Joe was a Cadillac kind of guy, often returning with the "snowbirds" driving a brand new Caddy convertible. When not at Motel Chapalita or shooting the breeze at Cubilete, Joe could be found at the Big Game and also proved himself to be a very good chess player. Cella was the only member present at the 1980 Clubhouse robbery not to lose his wallet. Cella bought a home and moved to Jupiter, Florida in the late-70s.

Charles Ceska—**Founding Member of the Mexico Chapter PVA**—Ceska was elected Mexico PVA's first vice president in June 1964. Ceska would later hold the position of chapter service officer. He was responsible for assisting fellow PVA members with benefits, medications and supplies, hospital visits, and more.

Ernie Chavez—A resident of Quadalajara from 1962 to 1968, Chavez participated in the Alliance for Compassion's successful effort to take some three hundred children from the Hospicio Cabañas orphanage to a picnic at one of the famous recreational swimming spots. He then went on to serve Zia Chapter PVA (New Mexico) as *Roadrunner* editor and chapter president, and later served in the National PVA as service director. Chavez received the 2004 Paralyzed Veterans of America's "Speedy Award" for services rendered to the organization and fellow veterans. Chavez was pictured in the January 1964 *Paraplegia News* with his bride Hortencia, flanked by Alfred Hanson and Oscar Anderson.

Jim Chew—A para from the Baltimore area, Jim and his wife lived a somewhat secluded lifestyle. He built quite a hacienda in Tesistan, a small town about ten miles outside of the city. Chew eventually visited the PVA Clubhouse, became a chapter member, and enjoyed the chapter's fiestas. He was a jovial man who liked to joke around with his fellow gringos.

Bill Christensen—"Officer and a gentleman." Bill Christensen served as Mexico PVA president in 1969. He was a well-respected quad from South Dakota. "Chris," as he was often called, was an avid collector of everything from coins to antique firearms. He and fellow collector Joe Anderson often ventured outside the Quadalajara area hunting down leads on firearms they could add to their respective collections. Chris was a man of many interests, as was Anderson, playing poker and practical jokes among them. The South Dakotan and Nebraskan were inseparable from the late 60s until the early-70s when Chris married and returned stateside in 1973. The two pranksters had their own favorite targets—each other. During the 1969 lunar landing, Anderson happened to stop by to visit his buddy. When Joe entered his friend's house, he found Chris intensely watching the simulation shown on TV that explained to the viewers the events taking place. When Anderson asked what was going on, he was quickly shushed by Chris. After a moment of eerie silence, Chris told Anderson, "They found bones on the moon!" "What kind of bones?" Anderson excitedly inquired. "They don't know yet," Chris seriously replied. With the stunning news of this monumental discovery, Anderson left to finish his rounds and spread the news. An amused Bob Beilsmith, basking in the sunshine in front of his home, fondly recalled being the brave soul who burst Joe's bubble. With that, Chris had successfully pulled off one of the best practical jokes of the Quadalajara era.

Joe Cicero—One of the early Bronx VA Hospital "escapees," Cicero talked fellow patient Charlie Newbold into giving Quadalajara a try in November 1964. He later married Cliff Gulick's sister-in-law. Joe Cicero had the distinction of being the last Mexico Chapter PVA president. Cicero and wife Teresa raised two daughters and still live in Guadalajara some forty years later.

Joe Clark—Friend of Joe Cicero from the Bronx VA, Clark and Norman "Mousie" Frisk first visited Quadalajara in the '60s. Clark, a former Air Force sergeant, and Frisk rented a house together. Clark married a Mexican nurse and eventually moved to California.

Cornelius Clifford—Cornelius was the father of Ray Clifford. The elder Clifford developed Multiple Sclerosis sometime after Ray was injured on the battlefield in South Vietnam. The debilitating disease ironically qualified the veteran for membership in the Paralyzed Veterans of America as a non-service connected member. Cornelius and Ray Clifford were, quite possibly, the only father/son tandem in PVA history.

Ray Clifford—Ray was a kind, gentle giant originally from Illinois. The para first arrived in Quadalajara in 1968 after rehabilitating in the Hines VA Hospital in Chicago. Ray wasted little time becoming active in chapter activities, and was possibly the only Mexico PVA member to hold every chapter office—president, vice president, secretary, treasurer, Board of Directors member, service officer, and Mexico Chapter PVA executive director. One of PVA's most tireless workers, Clifford was truly the chapter's Jack-of-all-trades. Ray bypassed the Big Game in favor of helping out and playing BINGO on game nights. He never complained about the hand life dealt him, and one would be hard-pressed to find a soul who would utter an unkind word about him. Clifford and Tom Kirch were the only two "lucky" enough to have been present at both the 1971 and 1980 Clubhouse robberies (see Appendix B, pages 333-334).

Bill Coe—Early Quadalajara Pioneer, and proprietor of Bill Coe's Place from the early- to mid-60s, Coe was famous for running a "loose ship." He carried an on-going feud with neighbor and rival gimp camp operator, Larry Kegan.

George Connoly—George was a para from New England who rehabbed at West Roxbury VA Hospital back in the day when canteen staff would stop by each ward selling the patients anything from shampoo to cigarettes. He stayed at Casa de Vida Nueva where he met Jimmy Lietz and attendant Miguel Lopez. The three drove to Cape Cod where they spent the summer of 1971.

Arnold Conrad—New Yorkers Conrad and Chuck Deverjanck first visited Quadalajara in 1961. While staying at George Ray's Place the two were, in Ray's words, "Taking their time deciding when to go home."

Bart Corbett—Corbett was another West Roxbury alumnus and active PVA member in the '60s. He represented the Mexico Chapter, along with Eddie Lucier, as a delegate to the National PVA's 1965 Annual Convention in New York. In December 1966, Corbett was responsible for organizing one of the Mexico Chapter PVA's successful Christmas Posadas to aid poor school children and give them school supplies, candy, fruit, and an all-around festive afternoon.

John Coughlin—Coughlin was a para who spent time at the West Roxbury VA. He lived in Florida and visited Quadalajara, where he became a Mexico Chapter member in the mid-70s.

Ed Creegan—Participated in the Mexico Chapter PVA's annual Christmas party in 1966.

Joe Darichuk—Joe D. was a high level quad who resided at Larry Kegan's Hacienda Las Fuentes in the early-60s. Darichuk thrived on conversation and sunshine. Kegan's Place was the ideal fit for the man from Taylor, Michigan. Joe D. married a Mexican señorita and relocated stateside only to return to Quadalajara a "free" man in the late-70s. He later returned to the States and built a home in Chandler, Arizona in the early-80s.

Ed Davis—Davis was introduced at the February 1970 Mexico PVA membership meeting as a new "Life Member" after transferring his membership from the California Chapter PVA.

George Dean—"In memorial: The Quadalajara wheelchair community was shocked by the tragic death of George Dean in an automobile accident. George had visited the Quadalajara area several times before. A veteran of twenty years service, he had been one of the last of the flying Navy Chiefs" (*El Sombrero News*, January 1967).

George Dempsey—The well-known and respected quad from Chicago was a frequent visitor to Quadalajara.

Jim Deery—Deery was a para from Ohio who usually rented accommodations at Cubilete.

John DeRudder—DeRudder lived out of town off the Chapala Highway in the small town of Ixtlahuacan de los Membrillos. Rumor was that his spouse, unable or unwilling to care for the MS quad, took John to Quadalajara. Once there, and after securing a place to stay and getting a full-time attendant for him, she returned to the States. DeRudder then met and married a kind and caring Mexican woman and the two began a family. DeRudder would often visit the Clubhouse to attend monthly membership meetings. The couple was always accompanied by their adorable young children who enjoyed dining on hamburgers, french fries, and soft drinks from the Clubhouse kitchen. The last sighting of DeRudder was at the U.S. Consulate where he was attempting to secure visas for his wife and children for a return to live stateside. Because of legal red tape involving the validity of his Mexican marriage, Consulate officials initially refused to grant John's request. The rest is a mystery…

Chuck Derevjanik—**Founding Member of the Mexico Chapter PVA**—Chuck D. was a frequent target in Joe Miller's High Society column in the *El Sombrero News*. His main feat was a five-day, five-night visit to one of Quadalajara's better-known cantinas. The marathon record of "five days and nights without leaving the saddle" was set with the help of his favorite adult beverage, some attractive Mexican ladies, as well as the proprietor, bartender, bouncers, and some gringo dollars.

Bruce Diaso—An honorary member of the Mexico PVA, Diaso volunteered to help with the chapter newsletter. He made Quadalajara folklore when he and a fellow quad decided to finish their marathon chess match at one of the city's better know cantinas—having the ladies help by moving the pawns and pieces on the chessboard.

Gary Dier—Dier was a Mexico PVA member and came in second to Jack Myrick in vice presidential balloting in May 1967. He was elected to the chapter's Board of Directors at the same meeting. Dier also lost an opportunity to serve as chapter president, losing by a single vote to Bill Christensen in 1969. From Joe Miller's High Society column in the chapter newsletter: "Dier got the tomahawk on Saturday, February 4. He and Bertha tied the knot."

Eddie Doody—Doody was a Quadalajara family man who played in friendly poker games with Jimmy Lietz, Richard Jaros, Ray Clifford, and other not-so-high-rollers. Eddie and his family moved to Tucson, Arizona in the early-70s. He was originally from Mississippi.

Harold "Windy" Doolittle—After six years of exploring Mexico for the perfect place to live, Doolittle found his way to George Ray's Place in Quadalajara in 1961. His dream of opening a place in Cuernavaca dashed; the Miami based Doolittle, according to Ray, "Was here for the duration" (see Appendix B, page 322).

George Dunaway—Dunaway was a para from Poplar Bluff, Missouri. Dunaway and Ralph Durain married sisters. He was elected chapter treasurer in 1973. Dunaway opted to return to his hometown in the mid-70s where he would go on to serve the Gateway Chapter PVA as its National Service Officer.

Tom Dunker—The North Dakota resident visited George Ray's Place in 1961.

Helen Dunn—Helen was one of the warmest and most kind-hearted residents of Quadalajara. She rented rooms in her Jardines Alcalde home to other disabled individuals with limited financial resources. Although living with Muscular Dystrophy, the New Jersey native was active in community affairs and spent her post-Jardines Alcalde years living in the Lake Chapala area. While there, she organized an effort to bring used children's wheelchairs and prosthetic equipment from the States to be donated to disabled Mexican children in the Chapala area. She was the recipient of the Mexico PVA's non-member category "George E. Ray Award" for outstanding service to the chapter and community.

Ralph Durain—Durain was George Dunaway's concuño for having married George's wife's sister. Durain left Quadalajara after a couple of questionably "necessary" surgeries at the Hospital Mexico-Americano.

Ronald "Dizzy" Dziekonski—Dziekonski (pronounced ja-coin-ski) was an affiliate Mexico Chapter member during the late-70s. Dizzy called the Quadalajara Trailer Park his home.

Harold Elkins—Elkins arrived in Quadalajara from Colorado in the fall of 1970.

George Embry—This amputee was rumored to have sold "papers" (six month tourist and automobile visas obtained with the help of an enterprising Mexican border crossing official) to residents of Quadalajara who were unable or unwilling to make a run to the Mexican/American border to officially leave Mexico and return from the U.S. side (said "papers" usually cost 500 Mexican pesos or $40 U.S. before the Mexican currency was devaluated in 1976—or so the rumor went). The Northern Migration took Embry to Tucson, Arizona.
Bob Enge—**Founding Member of the Mexico Chapter PVA**—An early visitor from the New York area, the red-headed para was known to have "mixed it up" with able-bodied Mexican men from time to time. Enge was not the only paraplegic Pioneer to "enjoy" a good barroom brawl.

Charles Erickson—Erickson married a Mexican señorita and returned to live stateside. The Ericksons later returned to Quadalajara, ironically, about the time of the Northern Migration.

Donald Evans—**Founding Member of the Mexico Chapter PVA**—Evans was a Quadalajara Pioneer.

Bill Fausnight—Fausnight was a wheelchair-bound arthritic. He served Uncle Sam as a mess hall sergeant. Fausnight hosted the popular Tuesday, Thursday, and Saturday poker games at his Colonia Independencia home, and enjoyed getting compliments on the food he taught his cook, Margarita, to prepare. He rented a room to Gil Turetsky for a number of years in the '70s.

Jerry Farnum—Farnum visited Quadalajara in the late-70s. He spent a few months renting a room from Herb Miller. Rumor had it that, while a patient in the Hines VA, Jerry acted as a bookie for horse races and sporting events.

Jerry Fesenmyer—Fesenmyer was a World War II veteran, originally from Iowa, who showed up in Quadalajara in 1965. The active para and former resident of Hawaii would forgo the tequila and mariachis in favor of pursuing señoritas. He especially enjoyed trips to Manzanillo and other Mexican beaches. Fesenmyer was one of the three Mexico PVA members nominated to fill the vacancy of the office of chapter president upon the resignation of George Ray in November 1967, but he opted to decline (see Chapter 14, pages 169-170).

Pat Fitzgerald—Fitzgerald was a quad from Springfield, Massachusetts. He was one of many Mexico Chapter quads to rehab at the West Roxbury VA. Health concerns limited Fitzgerald, and he would usually make his annual trek from Quadalajara to New England at the rate of two to three hundred miles per day—extending a five or six day trip by a week or longer.

Bob Flowers—Another who showed up "late for the party," Bob arrived from the Richmond VA area in December 1977, joining old friends Ray Reed and Darrell Roberson. The three quickly made up for lost time after renting a house on a spacious property in Los Pinos, which someone dubbed "The Ponderosa." Along with two American attendants, the boys from The Ponderosa soon stacked their new home with cases of beer that climbed the wall more than half way to the ceiling. Flowers was a poker player who knew a few of the regulars in the Big Game from time spent in the Richmond VA Hospital. He enjoyed beer as much as poker, and soon got under the skin of a few players by staying in hands he shouldn't have due to the over-consumption of his favorite beverage. The para from Baltimore, injured while serving with the Marines in Vietnam, soon met and married his own pretty señorita. Bob, wife Angela, and son Robert settled in Phoenix, Arizona in 1981.

Ray "Doc" Foland—Early Pioneer who was among the avid deep sea fishermen, Doc served on the chapter's first Board of Directors in 1964. Foland was chapter secretary in the mid-60s, and was active in the Mexico PVA from its inception until returning stateside in the late-60s with wife Maria and son Arturo. Doc was one of those all-around good guys who helped newcomers get adjusted to life in Mexico.

Sam Frazier—From Miller's High Society: Sam "The Supermarket" Frazier. Sam got him nickname because one of his favorite pastimes was going to the local supermarket, Rica Mesa, purchasing orange juice and vodka and watching the señoritas go by.

Norman "Mousie" Frisk—Bronx VA veteran who ventured to Quadalajara with Joe Clark in the '60s. Frisk and Clark were reunited with fellow Bronx VA alumni Charlie Newbold and Joe Cicero. Frisk shared a house with Clark before the latter married and returned stateside.

Marion Fuget—**Founding Member of the Mexico Chapter PVA**—Fuget was an early Pioneer as well as a Member of the Alliance for Compassion.

Tom Gilbert—From High Society: "Tom Gilbert, who hails from California, was here less than a week when he broke his leg in five places." Gilbert was elected to the Mexico PVA's Board of Directors in May 1967.

Charlie Gilliam—Gilliam was a high-level quad paralyzed from the neck down. Gilliam was active in the Mexico PVA from the late-60s to the mid-70s, and was elected Mexico PVA president in 1974. He eventually built a house and settled in Tucson, Arizona in late-70s.

Billy Gilly—Gilly was another West Roxbury VA alumnus who stayed at George Ray's Place in the mid-60s. Gilly made the most of his stay in Quadalajara, accompanying fellow hospital buddies Claudio Bertoli and Eddie Lucier on a junket from Quadalajara to Veracruz, and then Mexico City and Acapulco.

Kenny Ginsterblum—El Cacahuate ("the Peanut") got his nickname either from his tiny stature or from the fact that he liked the long peanuts sold at the local *tienda*. Kenny took over and ran Cubilete from the early-70s until the Quadalajara era came to an end. The Muscular Dystrophy survivor from Iowa was an avid reader and chess player. He also happened to be the brother of fellow resident Eileen Van Albert. (see Appendix B, pages 333-334).

Philip Gioirdano—Mexico PVA member in the late-70s and early-80s.

Tony Gomez—Gomez was one of the Quadalajara Pioneers to enjoy fishing trips to the coast with George Ray, Doc Foland, and others. Gomez was a participant in the early era of tequila, señoritas, and mariachis.

Lee Gresham—Gresham Hand Controls was one of the most well-known and used brands of controls for paras and quads who could enjoy the freedom of driving their own vehicles. In addition to operating his Michigan-based company, Gresham was a frequent visitor to Quadalajara. Ironically, as chapter president of the Michigan PVA in 1964, Gresham's official letter welcoming the Mexico PVA into the fold was the first correspondence the Mexico Chapter received from another PVA chapter.

Cliff Gulick—Gulick was one of Bill Macleary's early Las Fuentes renters. He married one of two sisters to tie the knot with Quadalajara gringos. He and Joe Cicero would become concuños.
Ken Gulrud—Gulrud stayed at La Morada (House of Rest, better known as George Ray's Place or Cubliete) while in Quadalajara, but left in 1971 to head back to Minnesota.

Tom Hale—Quadalajara Pioneer and Mexico PVA member.
Randy Hall—Mexico PVA member who resided at Cubilete in the late-70s.

Alfred Hanson—"Alfredo" was a Spanish-speaking Mexican-American (his mother was Mexican) who enjoyed driving around Quadalajara. Always willing to visit and help newcomers, a visit from Hanson would often lead to a relaxing, beer-drinking get-together and the standard "Let me introduce you to my sister-in-law" invitation. Hanson is pictured in the January 1964 *Paraplegia News* with newlyweds Ernie and Hortencia Chavez and Oscar Anderson.

Bob Harmon—The Muscular Dystrophy survivor was a business associate of the "Dennis The Menace" founder Hank Kethcum and original write for the popular comic strip. After Harmon and Ketchum parted ways, Bob moved to Quadalajara in the early-60s and married wife Suzy. The couple relocated to Phoenix, Arizona where they were reunited with former Quadalajara residents Bob and Teresa Beilsmith, Jack and Imelda Myrick, and Steve and Silvia Wilson. The Harmons returned to Mexico a few years later, as others often did, and remained until the late-70s. Harmon lived partially off his "Dennis The Menace" royalties, and was a regular at Bill Fausnight's Tuesday-Thursday-Saturday poker games.

Paul Harycki—Harycki was a former police chief from Thorp, Wisconsin.

Bob Hawkins—A resident of Patino's Place in the late-60s, Hawkins was a chess player who regularly tangled with Hines VA newcomer and future Mexico PVA chess champ Bill Kahler, while giving him

Spanish lessons on sunny afternoons in Quadalajara. He was originally from Monterey, California.

Chuck Hawkins—The non-veteran quad originally from New Jersey found his way to Quadalajara in 1978. He rented a room in Helen Dunn's Jardines Alcalde home. He also briefly rented rooms from Jack Tumidajski and Jerry Andrews. Chuck soon met and casually dated Alma, a medical student who lived across the street from Helen. Chuck also befriended many of Jardines Alcalde's quads and paras living within a few blocks of his home, and frequently enjoyed a sunny daytime or comfortable evening BS session at the home of Jimmy Lietz, Jerry Andrews, or some other gringo neighbor. An avid chess player, Hawkins was present when the PVA Clubhouse was robbed in January 1980.

Stanley Hecker—The New Yorker stayed at George Ray's Place for six weeks in 1961. According to George, "He'll be back."

Kenneth Henderson—According to Joe Miller's High Society column, Henderson would leave Quadalajara to "winter in Florida."

George Hicks—Hicks was one of a few SCI veterans who brought his family to live with him in Mexico. He was featured in the 1972 *Ebony Magazine* article (see Apendix B, page 330) on Black-American veterans living in Quadalajara.

Harris Hjelter—Hjelter was appointed the Mexico Chapter's only "Poker Chairman" by Mexico PVA President Jack Black at a fiscal 1971 Board of Directors meeting.

Raymond Hoffer—Hoffer was a Quadalajara resident of Kegan's Place in the mid-60s. Transportationally challenged, this Mexico PVA member enjoyed the popular drive-in movies of the time and he often went with Eddie Lucier or Keith Ziegler. Sometimes all three of them would go in one vehicle, according to Ziegler, and would leave one or more wheelchairs at home as few automobiles had trunk space for more than two E&Js. Hoffer later married his attendant's daughter and they purchased a home in Quadalajara.

Doyal Holt—A World War II veteran, Holt was active in the Mexico Chapter PVA, and was elected vice president in 1971. Quiet and reserved, Holt later married George Ray's widow, Taeko. The couple lived in a spacious Ciudad Granja home. Present during the 1971 Clubhouse robbery.

Rose Horowitz—Rose and sister Sylvia were originally snowbirds from New York who resided at Hacienda Las Fuentes, or Patino's Place as it was more commonly known, in the early-70s and later became permanent residents of the Las Fuentes area.

Sylvia Horowitz—Sylvia and sister Rose, who first stayed at Patino's Place, would become full-time residents of Quadalajara and mainstays in the Las Fuentes community.

Matt Huly—Huly came to Quadalajara from Michigan, according to High Society.

John Humphries—Humphries moved to Quadalajara from Alabama in the '70s. He formed a strong bond of friendship with Buddy Pinnsonault that continued when Humphries moved back home a few years later.

Bob Jackson—**Founding Member of the Mexico Chapter PVA**—While living at George Ray's Place in the mid-60s, Jackson once found himself on the receiving end of a few Bob Enge punches. Jackson served on the chapter's Board of Directors in 1964 and 1965. He later married and moved to Ciudad Granja with wife Laura. The couple enjoyed planting orchids. They moved to the Lake Chapala area in the '70s.

Russ Jacobson—Jacobson was a family man who, along with wife Juanita, had three daughters. He regularly enjoyed Friday BINGO nights with family and friends. The Jacobsons moved to Tucson, Arizona during the Northern Migration to raise their growing girls. Russ served on Mexico PVA's Board of Directors in 1969.

Richard Jaros—The Vietnam veteran quad from Webster, Massachusetts first arrived at Villa del Sol in the late-60s. Almost always cold, the quad who rehabbed at West Roxbury VA often carried a flask of brandy. Jaros was close friends with Jimmy Lietz and Peter Mirche, and enjoyed basking in the Quadalajara sunshine with the guys from Villa del Sol. After marrying and moving to Tucson, Arizona for a few years, Richard returned to Quadalajara. An occasional participant in the Big Game, he eventually left Mexico during the Northern Migration, and the family settled in San Diego, California.

Tom Johnston—A practical joker from California, Johnston was rumored to have pulled out a squirt gun in a Mexican bank. (No one else saw the humor in it.) Johnston was appointed American Legion and Disabled American Veterans liaison in 1980.

Lorenzo Jones—The happy-go-lucky spinal cord injured amputee from Wisconsin found his way to Quadalajara in the mid-70s. Jones's smile was only matched by the yellow smiley button he often wore. Lorenzo rented a room from Herb Miller in the late-70s and joined in on the almost daily sunny afternoon and cool evening BS sessions in Jardines Alcalde's north side.

Jimmy Jordan—Jordan was a quad from the Hines VA. After being placed on bed restriction for continuing to break the hospital alcohol consumption rule, Jordan told the social worker to get him a one-way ticket to Quadalajara. He arrived at Villa del Sol shortly thereafter and convinced fellow hospital roommate Jerry Maurer to join him one year later. Jordan married a local señorita and moved to the nearby town of Aguas Calientes for a few years. He was rumored to have eventually relocated to Vera Cruz.

Meyer Kabot—A quad from the Bronx VA, he flew to Bill Coe's Place a couple of years after his friends, Joe Cicero and Charlie Newbold, left in search of an alternative to institutional living. Kabot returned to Quadalajara later, but this time he brought an automobile. He became a yearly "snowbird" who mostly resided in the gimp camps of Las Fuentes. Meyer married a Mexican señorita and returned to New York in the mid-70s.

Bill Kahler—A quad from Joliet, Illinois, Bill Kahler roomed with Ray Clifford, Jim Adkisson, and Tom Kirch in the late-60s in the same Jardines Alcalde house that later became Helen Dunn's home. One by one, Tom, Jim, and Bill turned in their bachelor cards, Kahler becoming a concuño of Keith Ziegler by marrying Keith's wife's sister, Graciela. Regular Mexico PVA Board of Directors member and chess champion. Around 3 a.m. on one memorable night, Kahler was enjoying an adult beverage with roommates Kirch and Clifford, along with Bob Beilsmith and Greg Benisch, in an after-hours cantina when a Mexican man walked over and shot another man seated at a nearby table. Another memory which stood out was accompanying Greg Benisch to check out Quadalajara's famous pyramid. The adventurous young men soon found the car stuck in the sand off the highway without attendants and no way to get it out of the pyramid's mystical sand trap. The two quads spent the night in the vehicle with only a six pack of cerveza and an eight track tape of "Janice Joplin & Big Brother and the Holding Company" to keep them company until a passing truck spotted them the following morning. The Kahlers were among many to move to Phoenix, Arizona in the early-80s (see Appendix B, pages 333-334).

Larry Kegan—After being injured in a diving accident as a teenager, Kegan's father pushed him to make it on his own. He made his way to Quadalajara in the early-60s and opened Hacienda Las Fuentes, which was commonly referred to as Kegan's Place. He married and moved to Florida in 1967 only to return to the Twin Cities years later. There he became an advocate for education in the relatively unknown field of spinal cord injury (SCI) sexuality. He resumed his interest in music and formed "The Mere Mortals" and hooked up with childhood friend, Bob Dylan, on concert tours. Kegan had befriended fellow music lover Robert Zimmerman (Bob Dylan) at age thirteen, and the friendship continued until Kegan's death on 9/11 (see Appendix B, page 323).

Pat Kenny—Kenny was a Wisconsin quad who resided in Las Fuentes for part of the year. Kenny served on the chapter's Board of Directors in the late-70s. He was a member of what some referred to as "The God Squad," or the bible study group. The Northern Migration would take Kenny to Southern Texas.

Josephine "JoAnn" Kirch—The lady from Hastings, Minnesota married the skinny quad from Kellogg, Minnesota, and the two quickly became one of Quadalajara's most respected couples (see Chapter 14, pages 162-165).

Tom Kirch—Tom was everyone's best friend. After a seven-year long distance courtship, he finally married his life-long love, JoAnn. Present at both the 1971 and 1980 Clubhouse robberies.

Ron Kovic—The Vietnam veteran, who later turned anti-war activist, visited Quadalajara for a while before returning stateside and writing the book that later became the box office success *Born on the Fourth of July*.

Bob Krekeler—**Founding Member of the Mexico Chapter PVA**—Krekeler was a colorful character few people would or could forget. Krekeler roomed with fellow Pioneer Lee Schyler and later spent part of his time at Casa de Vida Nueva.

Florence Krieger—Florence flew down from New York with Sandra Otinsky in the early-70s to stay at Patino's.

Lewis Landstra—Landstra was from Michigan, according to Miller's High Society.

Jack Lastor—The tall Texan and World War II pilot resided in Quadalajara until the end of 1972. He was a serious poker player whose game was Five Card Stud. He married his tiny girlfriend, Teresa, and the couple moved stateside to live in Texas. In 1968 Lastor teamed with friend, neighbor, and Mexico PVA honorary member Ben Borish to found "Free Wheelers," a project that provided used wheelchairs to needy disabled Mexican citizens. The project quickly gained support from the Mexico PVA, and chairs were soon donated to an 11-year-old boy and a 14-year-old girl, "both of who have never walked nor used a wheelchair before" (*Paraplegia News*, February, 1969).

Robert Lawrence—Lawrence was a Mexico PVA member, and was elected to serve as chapter secretary in 1974. In October, however, he resigned the position at the general membership meeting. Might this be the same Robert Lawrence who National PVA President Harry Schweikert sent to Mexico in 1959 to verify claims that were made, both pro and con, about the highly publicized resort San Jose del Tajo?

Jim Lawson—Lawson was voted honorary membership into the Mexico Chapter PVA at the November 1966 Board of Directors meeting.

Jimmy Lietz—"Elvis" dropped out of the University of Maryland and soon found himself in Vietnam. The combat-injured quad spent time rehabbing at Walter Reed Army Hospital before arriving at Villa del

Sol in 1969. He served the Mexico Chapter PVA as vice president in 1974 and as a Board of Directors member for a number of years before being elected chapter president in 1978. He was originally from Washington, DC (see Appendix B, 333-334).

Gary Lomprez—The Mexico PVA member served on the chapter's Board of Directors in 1975.

Norman Looney—Norman was a New Jersey quad who rented a home with Steve Woosley. A disagreement caused a split between the two, resulting in the following tidbit in a late-70s *El Sombrero News* scandal sheet: "Norman Looney and Steve Woosley got a divorce. Steve got the house, Norm got the van, and another good friendship got the shaft!"

Eddie Lucier—**Founding Member of the Mexico Chapter PVA**—After rehabbing at the West Roxbury VA, Lucier arrived at George Ray's Place in December 1963 and quickly became active in the Quadalajara community. He was named as a delegate to the National PVA Annual Convention in New York in 1965. Lucier was chapter picnic chairman, and later chapter fiesta chairman from the mid-60s to late-70s. Lucier, fellow West Roxbury buddy Art Wheaton, and Bob Powell left Ray's Place and rented a three-bedroom house together for eight years. Lucier was the chapter's perennial treasurer throughout the 1970s. Originally from Warwick, RI, Eddie built a home in Tucson, AZ in 1980, but continued his Quadalajara "snowbird" lifestyle (see Chapter 14, pages 155-159).

Paul Lynton—The cigar-smoking bridge player was a member of Quadalajara's Duplicate Bridge Club and an active member of the Mexico Chapter PVA in the early-70s, serving on the chapter's Board of Directors.

Bill Macleary—One of the earliest of the Pioneers, Macleary personally accompanied Bill Bailey, Patrick Wolf, and others to Quadalajara in the late-50s. Macleary teamed with fellow Pioneer George Ray, before a falling out caused Macleary to open his own gimp camp in Las Fuentes in 1959. Macleary would later lose both his novia and Las Fuentes gimp camp in the early-60s to Bill Coe.

Roselyn Mahowald—Roselyn was from New Market, Minnesota, and first visited Quadalajara in 1964 with JoAnn and Luella Raway. She wrote for the local newspaper. After returning to Minnesota, Roselyn decided to go back to Mexico, this time with Mary Margaret Sommers. Roselyn passed away in Las Fuentes a couple of years later.

Gerry Maurer—A poker playing para from Indiana, Maurer first called Villa del Sol home around 1970. Gerry was a regular at both the Big Game and the Tuesday-Thursday-Saturday games at Bill Fausnight's home. He did more than his share of dealing cards for those quads who couldn't. Maurer also served the Mexico PVA as chapter secretary more than once. He remained in Quadalajara long after the Northern Migration, managing to find poker games through members of the American Legion and, later, through American businessmen who opened shop after The North American Free Trade Agreement (NAFTA) was passed. Amidst all that poker, he somehow found time to date many a pretty señorita.

Dave McDonald—McDonald resided at Kegan's Place in the mid-60s. In 1966 he left to rent one of five wheelchair accessible apartments in a complex in Ciudad del Sol with neighbors Bill Christensen and Charlie Newbold. He was elected to the chapter's Board of Directors in May 1967. McDonald later married and moved to Texas in the early-70s.

Jim McGlynn—Stricken with Amyotrophic Lateral Sclerosis, McGlynn was a married man with three children. He was a winter visitor from the Montreal area, and soon made Kegan's Place his home when his illness dictated going into a nursing home his only viable Canadian alternative. He passed away in the early-70s at the Hospital Mexico-Americano.

Hugh McLeod—"Cannuck Hugh McLeod welcomed two winter visitors from Winnipeg," from High Society.

Donald "Cookie" Meinberg—Cookie was an early Pioneer from the Hines VA Hospital. In the early-60s he roomed with Bob Beilsmith and Frank Vertinelli. During a Hines VA Hospital visit in the mid-60s he persuaded future Mexico Chapter PVA President Bill Christensen to leave the safe confines of the Chicago area hospital for the first time—Christensen returned to an ovation of approval from both hospital patients and staff.

Jim Melican—Melican left the New York area to check out Quadalajara for himself, found Villa del Sol to his liking, and decided to stay.

John Melin—Melin was appointed to fill a vacancy as chapter treasurer for fiscal 1970. He had the misfortune of being robbed of his own funds, as well as some Mexico Chapter funds he was tardy in depositing. He was reprimanded by some irate members at the November membership meeting for carelessness, but kept his position and wasn't required to repay the chapter.

JJ Meyer—Meyer was elected to the Mexico Chapter Board of Directors in May 1965.

Asa Michael—A Mexico PVA member who passed away in the late-70s.

Ray Michaud—"Porky" joined the gang at George Ray's Place in the mid-60s. He rehabbed at the West Roxbury VA along with fellow New Englanders Eddie Lucier, Paula Veilleux, Richard Jaros, Dick Veilleux, and others who would call Quadalajara home.

Charles "Joe" Miller—**Founding Member of the Mexico Chapter PVA**—Miller was one of Quadalajara's original Pioneers. He shared a home with George Ray in 1957 before going into business on his own later that year. He opened a place in Colonia Independencia, later moving to a nearby locale that accommodated eight renters. Miller served as the chapter's first official president in June 1964. He later penned *El Sombrero News*' regular "High Society" column. Joe, who mentioned the comings (newcomers to Quadalajara) and goings (those returning stateside for visits or health-related issues) of PVA members, residents, and visitors to the increasingly popular south-of-the-border utopia, spared no one as he reported the most scandalous of activities to reach his "department."

Herbie Miller—Herb went from renting out apartments in a Miami complex to renting an apartment in Quadalajara. A Muscular Dystrophy survivor, Miller remained friends with many in the Las Fuentes community long after purchasing a home on the other side of the city in Jardines Alcalde. He once opined that there were no actors with visible disabilities on TV shows or in commercials. Even though his comment was dismissed in the late-70s by those present, Herb was ahead of his time.

Richard Millman—Millman was a member of the Arizona Chapter PVA who visited Quadalajara in the summer of 1969. Millman attended the Mexico Chapter's August BOD meeting and, after the meeting, was able to query members present about wheelchair living in Mexico.

George Milne—Milne arrived at George Ray's Place from Connecticut. He was elected to the Mexico Chapter PVA Board of Directors in May 1970.

Pete Mirche—The quad from New York arrived at Villa del Sol in 1969 after "two years of drunkenness at the Bronx VA." He highly enjoyed Quadalajara, stating "My first year was a blast. I mostly drank, learned Spanish, and became acquainted with Mexican food." On a typical sunny Quadalajara day, Mirche spotted an extremely attractive Mexican señorita walking on the opposite side of the street. "Take me home with you," Pete called out from his Villa del Sol sanctuary. "If you can make it across the street," responded the girl in fluent English. Pete and Maria Mirche were married in 1971. "We rented a house in Colonia Chapalita with three bedrooms and a fish pond in the living room for the same $120 per month that I paid at Villa del Sol." Mirche enjoyed "playing chess, the Mexico PVA (where he served on the Board of Directors in the early-70s), calling BINGO on game nights, and looking at some very beautiful girls." Pete and Maria moved to San Diego, California in 1975. Mirche later taught computer classes at Grossmont College, was a founding member of the Cal-Diego PVA, and served as the Cal-Diego chapter president in 2003.

Louie Morini—Morini was a West Roxbury friend of Eddie Lucier who also ventured to George Ray's Place in the mid-60s. The "snowbird" from New England later stayed at Patino's in the early-70s.

Dick Morrisroe—From the October 1979 *El Sombrero News*: "The members of the Mexico PVA send a special 'Hello' to Dick Morrisroe who has been undergoing medical treatment at the Audi Murphy VA Hospital in San Antonio, Texas." Unfortunately, Morrisroe passed away shortly thereafter.

Bernie Muñoz—Muñoz was a quad from California whose grandparents were born in Mexico. He befriended some of his fellow Long Beach VA patients, including Tom Kirch, who called Quadalajara home. Muñoz gave Mexico a try and rented a home in Colonia Chapalita. He served on the Mexico PVA's Board of Directors. Muñoz and his wife, Nellie, returned to the Golden State to raise their daughter, Adriana.

Tom Musker—Musker, from the Boston area, visited George Ray's Place in 1961. His one month stay was lengthened to three, and according to Ray, "He returned home with a beautiful bride."

Jack Myrick—This quad from Louisiana found his way to Quadalajara via the Long Beach VA Hospital in the mid-60s. After communicating with Bill Coe for his south-of-the-border move, Jack received the following telegram: "DO NOT DELAY, JESUS IS ON HIS WAY!" Jack got a ride to the San Diego/Tijuana border crossing from one of the hospital nursing aides. As promised, Jesus (an attendant from Bill Coe's Place) was there to meet him. Myrick was soon on his way for a three-day car trip from the international bridge crossing in Tijuana to Bill Coe's front door, and it didn't help that Jesus spoke little English and Jack spoke little Spanish. Myrick soon enjoyed every aspect of the tequila, señoritas, y mariachi lifestyle that awaited him—except for the night when he and his attendant stopped to rescue two damsels in distress. Jack found himself dragged from his vehicle and left by the side of the road, his attendant beaten, and the car taken. The supposed damsels had their accomplices waiting in some nearby bushes—so much for being a Good Samaritan. As PVA membership officer, Myrick would later oversee a large increase in the ranks as more and more gringo newcomers found their way to this magical Mexican city. Jack married Imelda and returned stateside in the early-70s to raise a family in Phoenix, Arizona.

Abe Nadel—The quad from West Roxbury VA Hospital visited Villa del Sol around 1970.

Vinnie Nash—God doesn't make them any more unique than Vinnie. The spastic stuttering quad from Massachusetts rehabbed at the West Roxbury VA, checked out Quadalajara for eight months in 1971, returned stateside a married man (never to find his Mexican bride again—parents find a way of protecting their daughters from men they

don't approve of). Nash returned to Mexico where he claimed that a quad could "live like a King on $500 a month." He met and almost married a woman named Alida—once or twice. Vinnie "left for good" in 1974 after a newly hired maid took his wallet, money, and important papers. He returned in 1981 and "settled" in the Lake Chapala area for a couple of years. Vinnie dropped out of sight after being asked to leave both the San Diego and Long Beach VA rehab centers for refusing to obey non-smoking rules.
Ralph Nelson—Nelson was an early Quadalajara Pioneer who resided at Joe Miller's Place along with Doc Foland in the late-50s/early-60s.

Bob Nemac—The Chicago area quad roomed at Kegan's Place in the mid-60s, later married a woman named Felipa, and settled into their Jardines Alcalde home to raise their two daughters.

Charlie Newbold—Charlie was a tall quad from New York via the Bronx VA who arrived in Quadalajara in November 1964 with hospital buddy Joe Cicero (see Chapter 14, Pages 160-162).

Harry "Fig" Newton—The cigar smoking para enjoyed going to Quadalajara's drive-in movies.

John P. Nichol—**Founding Member of the Mexico Chapter PVA**—Nichol and his wife were mid-60s neighbors of Bronx VA buddies and roommates Joe Cicero and Charlie Newbold.

Les Nickleson—Nickleson was a member of Mexico PVA's Board of Directors in 1970.

Art Nieland—"Returned to his Colonia Independencia home," from High Society.

"Nick" Nixon—Nixon called Quadalajara home starting in the mid-70s. He survived a rollover accident on a trip to Manzanillo in 1978. Nick was among those who continued to live in Mexico even after the Northern Migration.

Sandra Olitsky—Sandra was from New York. She visited Patino's Place with friend Florence Krieger in the early-70s.

Ken Palmer—The quad from Sioux Falls, South Dakota decided to try Quadalajara after fellow South Dakotan quad, Bill Christensen, first visited the Mexican city in 1966. Palmer married and later divorced a Mexican señorita, but returned to visit Quadalajara on a regular basis throughout the '80s.

Jack Parisea—Parisea spent a few years during the '70s renting a room at Cubilete from Ken Ginsterblum. He returned to his Midwestern home and family with his attendant in the late-70s.
Tom Paterson—Paterson was a social worker from California and the Long Beach VA Hospital who stayed at George Ray's Place in the mid-60s. He returned to Mexico in the mid-70s, married a Quadalajara widow and moved his new family to Albuquerque, New Mexico.

Paul Patino—Patino took over the reins of Hacienda Las Fuentes when boss Larry Kegan married and moved back to the States. Throughout the '70s, Kegan's Place/Hacienda Las Fuentes was merely referred to as Patino's.

Ken Perry—**Founding Member of the Mexico Chapter PVA**—Perry was a para from the Long Beach, California area and was a licensed pilot.

Bob Peters—Peters visited Quadalajara from St. Paul, Minnesota in the early-60s. He eventually married a Mexican lady and returned to live in Minnesota.

Walter "Buddy" Pinsonnault—Buddy dropped out of Sienna College and took a chance on Mexico in the early-70s. Buddy was from Plattsburg, New York, and was living with a form of Muscular Dystrophy. He met wife Teresa while living in Las Fuentes. After their marriage, the couple moved to Jardines Alcalde, where Buddy was reacquainted with friend Helen Dunn. He also befriended Jimmy Lietz, and was soon a mainstay at the afternoon and evening BS sessions on Jardines Alcalde's north side. One of a few non-drinkers among the guys, Buddy enjoyed the camaraderie he found there. Buddy could make anyone laugh about anything. He and Teresa gave Roswell, New Mexico a try before moving to the San Diego area during the Northern Migration.

Don Porpara—Porpara was a Mexico Chapter PVA member who frequented membership meetings in the mid-60s.

Bob Powell—**Founding Member of the Mexico Chapter PVA**—Powell was the longtime roommate of Eddie Lucier and Art Wheaton. Powell left George Ray's Place in 1966 to rent and share expenses with his two friends from Cubilete. At the April 1970 membership meeting, upon the passing of George Ray, Powell suggested that an award in honor of the Pioneer and founder of the Mexico PVA be given each year to the "Outstanding Member for Services Rendered to the Mexico Chapter PVA." Powell's suggestion was adopted. The annual "George E. Ray Award" was subsequently changed to include two categories: the Outstanding Member and Outstanding Non-Member for Services Rendered to the chapter and community.

Stanley Prucnal—**Founding Member of the Mexico Chapter PVA**—Prucnal was a big quad from Pennsylvania. The "snowbird" and Pittsburgh Steelers' fan enjoyed traveling. He would stop by on BINGO nights to socialize and grab a bite to eat from the Clubhouse kitchen.

Evert Rabuck—Rabuck served as Mexico Chapter secretary from June 1971–June 1972.

Luella Raway—Sister of JoAnn Raway Kirch, Luella first visited Quadalajara in 1964. She earned a college business degree and worked for the State of Minnesota. Besides Mexico, the woman from Hastings, Minnesota also traveled to Hawaii, Europe, and Canada.

George Ray—**Founding Member of the Mexico Chapter PVA**—The man most influential in informing others of the benefits Quadalajara had to offer, George served the chapter in every way possible, including as chapter president in 1967. He was best described by Joe Cicero, who simply referred to him as "Boss" (see Appendix B, page 320).

Ray Reed—Originally from the Boston area, Reed found his way to Quadalajara from the Richmond VA after unwelcome health issues dictated hospitalization and depressing medical treatments. Reed's former hospital buddy, Jerry Andrews, was enjoying life south of the border, so Reed decided to spend the time he had left as best he could.

Ray Reed would soon be joined by fellow Richmond friends, Darrell Roberson and Bob Flowers. The three friends eventually rented a house on a spacious property that was nicknamed "The Ponderosa."

Charlie Reno—A Quadalajara Pioneer, Reno was the first chapter delegate to the National PVA convention in Santa Monica, California in July 1964.

Herbert Rhoton—A life member of the Mexico PVA during the '70s, Rhoton lived in the Lake Chapala area.
Darrell "Robbie" Roberson—The second of the "Ponderosa" boys from the Richmond VA Hospital to look for independence in Quadalajara, Robbie made the trip from his North Carolina home with younger brother and attendant, Frank. An avid fisherman, Robbie left Quadalajara when the Ponderosa boys split up. He later married and moved to an ocean-side home one ferryboat trip away from Baja, Mexico.

Byron Rogers—Byron was a "snowbird" from California.

John Rogers—Rogers was an adventurous quad from Lennox, South Dakota. John showed up "late for the party" in the late-70s, but made up for lost time by frequenting the Big Game and being elected to the Mexico PVA's Board of Directors. The bearded Rogers looked as if he had just jumped off the front of a box of Smith Brothers' cough drops. Rogers was interested in fishing trips to Manzanillo and participating in the annual Christmas posadas for the poor school children, and was quick to volunteer to help haul the Christmas goodies in his van to the various locations. He was one of a few quads anywhere to qualify to be pilot of an ultra light aircraft. Slightly tipsy on the night of the 1980 Clubhouse robbery.

Alan Roth—Another of Quadalajara's residents to marry the sister-in-law of a fellow Mexico PVA member, Roth and Richard Jaros became concuños. The brothers-in-law would eventually relocate their families to Tucson, Arizona.

Rosemary Russell—Rosemary resided at Kegan's Place. She received a visit from her mother, Toddy Russell, in the fall of 1970.

Paul Saine—The wheelchair-bound arthritic called Boise, Idaho home. Saine arrived in October 1972 and immediately realized Quadalajara would become more than just a home-away-from-home. Shortly after arriving, Saine joined the already overcrowded ranks of players interested in the Big Game. He was present during the Clubhouse robbery of January 1980. Saine became an honorary member of the Mexico PVA, and later contributed by assisting the depleted core of chapter workers with kitchen and other Clubhouse duties during and after the Northern Migration. He married a woman named "Cuca" (Maria de Refugio), and purchased a home close to Colonia Chapalita.

Domingo Santos—Born in Puerto Rico, Santos rehabbed at West Roxbury VA Hospital after being injured in the line of duty. Being fluent in Spanish only served to help Domingo blend in with the local community more easily than his North American gringo counterparts. The easy-going quad wasn't much into Clubhouse activities, but he stopped by frequently on game nights to grab a bite to eat and socialize with friends. Santos was robbed at home by El Comandante and friends shortly before the Clubhouse robbery of January 1980.

Roland Schellenberg—Scellenberg assumed the reigns of La Morada after the passing away of founder George Ray in 1969. Schellenberg would eventually pass the baton to Kenny Ginsterblum who ran George Ray's Place for over a decade. The original gimp camp located on Avenida Cubilete #147 would later be referred to as simply Cubilete. Schellenberg left Quadalajara in the early-70s for the seaside town of San Blas.

Lee Schlyer—**Founding Member of the Mexico Chapter PVA**—Schlyer was a high level quad who ventured to Quadalajara after hospitalization and rehab at the Long Beach VA. Schlyer enjoyed all aspects of his Quadalajara experience, from Quadalajara-after-dark to active participation in the Mexico PVA. Roomed with fellow founding PVA member Bob Krekeler in their Colonia Independencia home.

Pete Schwenk—Pedro Pica Piedra (Fred Flintstone), as most of the attendants referred to him, was a huge quad from California. Part American Indian and part instigator, Schwenk delighted in teasing fellow PVA members and residents. Although much of his teasing was done with his tongue firmly implanted in his cheek, Pete did manage to rub a few folks the wrong way. An on-again, off-again participant in the Big Game, Pete enjoyed the PVA Clubhouse kitchen food as much, if not more, than the poker wars. Pete's interests varied from pursuing señoritas y señoras to, along with Captain Ben, securing a wheelchair for a poor paralyzed Mexican man whose family and friends were transporting him on a wooden plank. (Many acts of kindness went unnoticed or unrecorded.) Schwenk had to leave town in a hurry after, rumor had it, he slept with a neighbor's innocent daughter. The news didn't set well with Pete's girlfriend, and the girl's father wanted to kill him.

Tom Schwenk—Tom visited Quadalajara for a brief time, but the personable and remarkably independent quad soon returned stateside to live with his father in Tucson, Arizona.

James Seybold—Although there is no record of Seybold actually exploring Quadalajara, the active PVA member's contributions—both as one of Mexico's earliest Explorers as well as National PVA Research Director—certainly warrant his inclusion (see Chapter 12, pages 133-136 and Appendix B, pages 318-319).

George Seyfried—Seyfried was a quad who rented rooms by word-of-mouth at an apartment complex in Colonia Seattle during the '70s. Some of Seyfried's renters included Jerry Fesenmyer, George Dempsey, Pat Fitzgerald, and Herb Bloom. Seyfried married and moved to Phoenix, Arizona in the late-70s.

Vigil Shippe—"The Mexico PVA extends its sympathy to the family of Virgil Shippe who passed away here on May 30, 1971" (*El Sombrero News*).

Lee Sherrell—The quad who rented a room at Cubilete in the '70s was always building something with his hands. Sherrell left the safe confines of the centrally located gimp camp and ventured out to the small town of Tesistan, some ten miles from Quadalajara.

Jerry Sills—According to George Ray's letter in the August 1961 *PN*, "Attorney Jerry Sills was here for a time but the mile-high altitude interfered with his respiratory condition."

George Small—**Founding Member of the Mexico Chapter PVA**—Small served as chairman for the Alliance for Compassion and was an original member of the Mexico Chapter PVA's Board of Directors, but preferred to shy from the limelight. Small was one of Quadalajara's first paraplegic residents who, upon his death, left money specifically to Mexico's poorest children.

John Sniffen—Sniffen was an amputee whose 1962 propane-powered Chevy stood out as much as he did. Described as "happy-go-lucky" by friend Bill Christensen and as a "clown" by Keith Ziegler, Sniffen was known to have loosened his prosthetic leg and extend it a foot or two in his pant leg to the shock of approaching señoritas at Tlaquepaque's famous beer garden. Other times, he'd twist the device and put his leg over his shoulder—again drawing double-takes from those passing by.

Mary Margaret Sommers—Mary Margaret visited Kegan's Place, a popular spot for fellow Minnesotans in the mid-60s. The woman from Hibbing, Minnesota would reside for a few years in Quadalajara after her friend and traveling companion, Roselyn Mahowald, passed away.

Bill Spencer—Spencer and wife Marian resided in Quadalajara in the mid-60s. Active in the Mexico PVA, serving as both chapter secretary and *El Sombrero News* editor, Spencer was an extremely talented wood carver. He donated a wooden plaque of the official PVA logo "Speedy," featuring a man in a wheelchair speeding along complete with Sombrero, which hung on the Clubhouse wall for over fifteen years.

Bill Stanley—Miller's High Society stated, "Wild Bill Stanley is trying to corner the local vodka market as an investment."

Frank Stocker—Stocker was a non-veteran from the East Coast who roomed with Chuck D. The two regularly made Miller's High Society newsletter column for prowling Quadalajara-after-dark. Stocker eventually married and opened a gimp camp in Vallarta San Jorge in the early-70s.

Frank Stoppiello—Unofficially the youngest Mexico PVA member throughout the '70s, Stoppiello actually arrived at Villa del Sol in 1969 with two friends named John and Wayne. Neither of his friends stayed more than a month or two. Stoppiello, on the other hand, met his future bride and hit the Spanish language books as few others ever had. He was soon fluent in Spanish and, more importantly, a married man.

Stoppiello (along with Ray Clifford and Gerry Maurer) was one of the most active PVA chapter paraplegics during the ’70s, often being called upon to crank out *El Sombrero News* on the chapter’s antiquated mimeograph machine. Both Stoppiello and Clifford shared the same reason for their paralysis and eventual move to Quadalajara—they had each received Purple Hearts for being injured on the battlefield in Vietnam (see Appendix B, pages 333-334).

Greg Stephenson—A lanky para and former highway patrolman from the Pacific Northwest, Stephenson kept a low profile while spending part of his Quadalajara experience living in a small town outside the city.

Carroll Stogel—**Founding Member of the Mexico Chapter PVA**—From High Society: “Carroll Stogel hooked a sailfish in Manzanillo two kilos under the record, but it wouldn’t have counted anyway because he needed help reeling it in.”

Wayne Stroup—Stroup was a para from Pennsylvania who rented a room from Herb Miller in the popular Jardines Alcalde North neighborhood in the late-70s. One glance at Stroup’s wheelchair sticker—Pawn Power—told everything; he was a very serious and successful chess playing “rookie.”

Ernie Swanson—The well-liked quad was an early visitor to Quadalajara. A Mexico PVA member, Ernie enjoyed traveling and making trips to Las Vegas. He later married and lived a more secluded lifestyle.

Pete Tanno—A Korean War Veteran from Ohio, Tanno arrived in Quadalajara around 1970. His battlefield injury left him an incomplete quad; he was able to walk and retain some functions that most quads and paras lost. Extremely likable, Tanno enjoyed telling bar room jokes from his vast repertoire. Pete also liked to drive and was always traveling somewhere; from Florida to California. He would eventually return to Quadalajara every winter with the “snowbirds.” Tanno made occasional appearances at the Big Game, but mostly liked to socialize and enjoyed trips to Manzanillo and other Mexican beaches.

Clyde Throop—A family man and a Mexico PVA member, Clyde was meticulous in everything from his beautiful home and magnificently landscaped yard to the repairs and details of the chapter Clubhouse he undertook as Bob Brassfield's assistant Clubhouse chairman in the late-70s. Clyde's own troop kept getting bigger and bigger, so the Throop's headed north to Tucson, Arizona at the time of the Northern Migration.

Junior Thompson—According to High Society (1970), "At Hacienda las Fuentes (Lonely Hearts Club of Quadalajara) Junior married Gretchen Klinefelter." His father "flew down to meet his new daughter-in-law, approved, and the whole family returned to the States."

Vern Thorsen—An extraordinarily good quad, Thorsen helped Keith Ziegler and fellow PVA member Jack Myrick into his car after their attendants left the drinking buddies in an unnamed Quadalajara drinking establishment.

Lou Torres—Torres was a para from Southern California. He was Bill and Maria Elena Bailey's compadre. Serious and private, Torres was one of a few members to stay at Motel Chapalita. He later owned and built upon a large piece of property outside of Quadalajara on the road to Lake Chapala.

Manny Trujillo—One of the early settlers, Trujillo was among a group of Quadalajara enthusiasts, including George Ray, Tony Gomez, and Ray Foland, who frequently made successful deep sea fishing trips to Manzanillo.

Jack Tumidajski—The quad from Pawtucket, RI belatedly took on the challenge of telling the story of Quadalajara. He typed all but a few pages of the original manuscript himself, using only one typing stick from the original set of two he received during Occupational Therapy at the West Roxbury VA in 1970.

Gil Turetsky—A New Yorker who first resided at Bill Coe's Place in the '60s, Turetsky's passion was playing cards, including poker and Gin Rummy. After initially staying at Bill Coe's Place, Gil spent time renting a room in Bill Fausnight's Colonia Independencia home, and later settled at Cubilete. Turetsky teamed up with fellow MS survivor Leo Bourdosis for near daily games of Gin Rummy. Gil and Leo often shared taxi expenses for trips to the Mexico PVA Clubhouse for the Big Game. Turetsky was present the night of the January 1980 Clubhouse robbery.

Jerry Vale—According to Miller's High Society, Vale allegedly once "misplaced his car."

Eileen Van Albert—One of Quadalajara's first female Pioneers, the writer from Iowa had been married to fellow resident, Bob Harmon. She later married *El Sombrero News* editor Ken Van Albert, and continued to assist the Mexico PVA with its monthly newsletter for many years after her husband's death. She was named a Mexico Chapter honorary member in the mid-60s.
Ken Van Albert—Kenny was appointed *El Sombrero News* editor in May 1967, and served as chapter secretary in the mid-60s. Kenny was married to Eileen.

Dick Veilleux—The quad from Maine ventured down to Quadalajara in the late-60s along with fellow West Roxbury VA alumnus Richard Jaros. Although he was from the same town as another West Roxbury friend, Paula Veilleux, Dick and Paula were not related. He married a woman named Juanita and returned stateside to San Diego in the '70s.

Paula Veilleux—Popular Paula maintained a close friendship with Eddie "The Teddy Bear" Lucier. Paula Veilleux had the distinction of having two paras, Jim Deery and Ray Clifford, fight nearly to the death (of Clifford) over her. Paula served the Mexico PVA as chapter vice president under President Clifford in 1972.

Frank Vertinelli—Verinelli was an early visitor to Quadalajara, and roomed with fellow Pioneers Bob Beilsmith and "Cookie" Meinberg in the early-60s.

Barney Vigil—The quad from Wyoming visited a few times before leaving the Hines VA and making Quadalajara his permanent home in 1978. After renting a room from "Chico" Wilson, he met the señorita of his dreams. Barney and Alicia struck up a friendship that would blossom into marriage. With financial backing from friends, the couple soon built a home in the Lake Chapala area where they raised their daughter.

Frank Villani—"At Bill Coe's, the troops in Las Fuentes were all shocked the other day when Frank Villani pulled up in a Canadian-made belching 1946 Chevy."—High Society. Villani was one of

Quadalajara's more colorful personalities, and cars were one of his passions. It wasn't unusual to bump into Villani in a classic all-white Caddy parked in front of a popular downtown night spot. The quad from New Jersey seemed to bounce around from gimp camp to gimp camp. Some of his "friends" allegedly once rented a donkey from a street vendor and locked the animal in Villani's bedroom. On another occasion, according to High Society, these same "friends" went so far as to bring a group of Mariachis into his room to cure a hangover. Villani met an unfortunate death at the hands of one of his Mexican attendants.

Everett Vorrie—The Multiple Sclerosis survivor from Iowa first made Las Fuentes his home in the early-70s, and often frequented the PVA Clubhouse. He married a woman named Isabel, and the couple had one child. They returned stateside to live in Green Valley, Arizona.

Dick Wacholz—Wacholz arrived at Mrs. Cartlidge's Sun Haven in 1977 after spending time at Craig Rehabilitation Hospital in Colorado. He briefly picked up the moniker "Wolfman" for his trademark hair and beard. Dick found trips to Manzanillo to his liking. With the Northern Migration signaling the end of the Quadalajara area, he headed north to the small coastal fishing town of San Blas (close to Tepic, Nayarit). Richard Wacholz married Marta Sanchez, and the couple eventually divided time between their beach home in San Blas and their apartment in the Phoenix, Arizona desert.

Fred Weihe—The Michigan resident, according to George Ray in the August 1961 *PN*, "Arrived last week and plans to stay six months to a year."

Sandy Welborn—An affiliate Mexico PVA member from New Jersey, Welborn was among those of scarce economic resources who rented a room from Helen Dunn. Welborn returned to New Jersey, but not before having a bullet graze his arm and lodge in his attendant's back during a cowardly robbery at Helen Dunn's home in 1980.

Art Wheaton—West Roxbury buddy of Eddie Lucier who called George Ray's Place home until he, Lucier, and Bob Powell rented their own house in 1966. He later married and moved to his own home. Wheaton was elected to Mexico PVA's Board of Directors in May 1965.

Charlie Whestine—Whestine was a '50s Pioneer, and probably the first Quadalajara American wheeler to return stateside after marrying a Mexican señorita. Prior to moving to the Los Angeles area, the Whestines stayed with fellow newlyweds, Bill and Maria Elena Bailey, in 1959.

Davy White—This Mexico PVA member was one of many to rehab at West Roxbury VA Hospital. White met an untimely death in the early-70s after experiencing a grueling car trip from New England to Quadalajara.
Ralph Willard—Early visitor to Quadalajara and Mexico Chapter PVA member.

Harry "Chico" Wilson—Chico arrived in the mid-70s from New Jersey after an industrial accident rendered him a paraplegic. Chico had a contagious laugh, a wide mustache that grew wider with his smile, a typical '70s Afro, and muscles on top of muscles. Eventually, neighbor Jimmy Lietz successfully coaxed him into getting out more and meeting new people. Chico frequented the PVA Clubhouse for a time, and eventually tried his hand at poker. Although he was not accustomed to the stakes in the Big Game, Chico held his own—until he lost a hand of seven card stud, holding four Kings to neighbor Jerry Andrews' 5, 6, 7, 8, and 9 of Hearts. With that, Harry had enough of poker. He reverted back to being a homebody and pursuing his main hobby—Bar-B-Queuing. Those lucky enough to feast on Chico's specialty raved about his cooking talent and were eager for their next invite to break bread and eat ribs with the personable muscleman from the Garden State. He eventually moved to the Chapala area, married, and later relocated to McAllen, Texas with his wife and daughter.

Norman Wilson—Norman was among those of meager financial means to rent a room from Helen Dunn in Jardines Alcalde during the late-70s.

Steve Wilson—Wilson was a big para who made Quadalajara home in the mid-60s. He roomed with Keith Ziegler on a Ciudad Granja farm for the purpose of going into the pig raising business. "The pigs all died," according to Ziegler, and Wilson and his roommate parted company. Wilson later married and returned stateside to Phoenix, Arizona.

Judy Winfield—Judy was a popular blonde quad from Canada. She rented a home in the Chapalita neighborhood close to George Ray's Place, and was briefly married to a Mexican man. She eventually returned to Vancouver in the late-70s.

Jack Winkler—Winkler participated in Mexico Chapter PVA meetings in the mid-60s.

Kurt Wintermyer—Wintermyer, a Mexico PVA member, rented rooms in his Fraccionamiento Monrass home in the late-70s and early-80s.
Patrick Wolf—Wolf and fellow Pioneer Bill Bailey arrived in March 1958 at George Ray's Place. They were personally escorted to Quadalajara by Bill Macleary, George Ray's partner at the time. The group of four quads and paras went their separate ways after Bailey married in October 1958 and Macleary departed to open his own gimp camp in Las Fuentes.

Mark Woods—Woods was a cowboy from Oregon. According to Mark, legendary jockey Bill Shoemaker once told him, "Woods, you'd make a heck of a jockey if you were ten pounds lighter!" Woods was a short, slightly built para who was one of a handful of Quadalajara residents to carry a concealed weapon. The "secret" was confirmed after a night playing in the Big Game when a slightly tipsy Mark Woods rolled off the PVA Clubhouse ramp—Woods, his wheelchair, and seat cushion going one way, and a few uncollected poker chips and a small caliber handgun going the other. Mark, with wife Aurelia and son Albert, moved to Southern Texas during the Northern Migration.

Steve Woosley—A resident of Villa del Sol in the late-60s, the PVA member married a señorita named Guillemina in the early-70s. Woosley visited and socialized with fellow members and friends on BINGO nights. The Northern Migration took him to the Los Angeles area.

John Zackowski—Zackowski was nominated to the Mexico PVA Board of Directors in May 1968, but declined the nomination.

Keith Ziegler—After marrying and settling in Ciudad Granja a few blocks from the chapter Clubhouse, the quad from Colorado became active in the Mexico Chapter PVA. Ziegler, who served the chapter as service officer and *El Sombrero News* editor for a number of years, was first elected chapter president in May 1969. Ziegler would go on to hold the office of Mexico PVA president various times throughout the '70s and into the early-80s. After the chapter was dissolved in 1983, Ziegler was left in charge of literally closing the door behind him and turning out the lights of the chapter Clubhouse. Keith, wife Josefina, and daughters Blanca and Ana moved to Phoenix, AZ in the early-80s (see Chapter 14, pages 165-169 and Appendix B, pages 333-334).

Founding Member of the Mexico Chapter PVA—Refers to the original nineteen quadriplegic and paraplegic veterans who, in 1964, initially petitioned the Paralyzed Veterans of America (PVA) for a PVA chapter in Quadalajara.

Appendix A

Correspondence and Documents

PVA

PARALYZED
VETERANS
OF AMERICA

HAROLD STONE, VICE-PRESIDENT / 77 PHEASANT HILL STREET / WESTWOOD, MASSACHUSETTS 02090

April 7, 1964

George Ray
Cubilete #147
Col. Chapolita
Guadalajara, Mexico

Dear George:

Bob Webb wrote to me a few days ago with welcome news. He said that you were interested in establishing a P.V.A. Chapter in Guadalajara. With 10-20 permanent residents, who can be the source of your officers and committees, you have a sizable group. Others, who come for visits or vacations, can add to your membership and assist you while they are there. Most of your members probably will be members of other P.V.A. Chapters, so you will have many with experience and know-how to assist you.

It is very easy to start a chapter and meet the requirements for affiliation as a P.V.A. Chapter. The requirements are as follows:

Ten or more members.
The election of officers.
A set of bylaws.
A written report of meetings and evidence of activity.
The payment of dues to National P.V.A. of $3.00 per service connected, $1.00 per non-service connected member.

The above information and your request for affiliation will be submitted to our Board of Directors for its approval.

If you become affiliated before our convention in July, your chapter will be eligible to send a delegate there at National P.V.A. expense.

Under separate cover, I am sending additional information.

Keep me posted on your progress. Let me know how I can assist you. Feel free to write about any questions you may have.

Lots of luck; hope to see you at the Convention.

Sincerely,
Hal
HAROLD STONE

HS/lap

April 24, 1964

Harold Stone, Vice President
77 Hill Street
Westwood, Massachusetts 02090
USA

Dear Hal:

Tuesday, April 21st at 8:30 PM eighteen paraplegics and quadraplegics met at 147 Cubilete, Colonia Chapalita, Guadalajara, Jalisco, Mexico to discuss the forming of a PVA Chapter here. All eighteen were very enthusiastic about the prospect and all have pledged membership as soon as we can get a charter. I am going to enclose their names for your information, and as soon as we can get our charter I will forward the money to National.

We agreed to use the set of by-laws listed in "How to Run a PVA Chapter". We agreed to meet at Cubileto 147 every third Tuesday of each month. We will be called the Mexico Chapter. At all meetings of the membership of the Corporation, 10 voting members shall constitute a quorum. The Board of Directors shall consist of no less than 3 nor more than 15 members. It shall be the Board's duty to appropriate money from the General Fund not to exceed forty dollars without approval of the membership. A special meeting may be called at the request of three members of the Board of Directors. Four members of the Board of Directors shall constitute a quorum. Annual dues shall be $8.00 dlls. for all members.

The following officers were elected until the end of the fiscal year ending June 30: President, William M. Bailey; Vice President, Charles J. Miller; Secretary-Treasurer, George E. Ray; Board of Directors appointed Charles J. Ceska, Lee Schler, Stanley Prucnal, and Donald Evans. Board of Directors meeting follows regular meeting.

The pledged members are as follows: Wm. Martin Bailey, Charles J. Miller, Robert F. Krekeler, George E. Ray, Edward G. Lucier, Donald L. Evans, Carroll F. Stodgel, Lee C. Schlyer, John P. Nichol, Stanley J. Prucnal. Charles J. Ceska, Robert T. Barrett, Robert Beske, Charles Derevjanik, Robert Enge, Kenneth Perry, George E. Small, Marion Fuget, Robert Powell.

If there is anything wrong with the above procedure we would certainly welcome any suggestions and advice you might offer. Also if you could send us a book of Robert's Rules of Order we would reimburse you by return mail. If you have any membership application blanks we would appreciate about a hundred because we have many more potential members that haven't been contacted as yet.

We will keep you posted as to our activities and are really going to try to turn out a good Chapter.

Sincerely yours,

George E. Ray

MEMORANDUM

from .. HAROLD STONE, *Vice President*

DATE 5-10-64

to George

SUBJECT affiliation

Dear George,

Please pardon the note, I have been extra busy. Allow me to congratulate you on the fine job you have done. Soon the Directors will be asked to vote for your affiliation as a P.I.A. Chapter. As a PIA Chapter, you will be entitled to send a delegate to the Convention in Los Angeles at National expense - details later.

Will send Roberts Rules.

Sincerely,
Hal

MEMORANDUM

from .. HAROLD STONE, *Vice President*

DATE 5-25-64

to Bill

SUBJECT Convention

Dear Bill,

Your request for affiliation is in the hands of the Board of Directors. Since their decision will bring us very close to Convention time, I am sending the enclosed in order to give you ample time to prepare. Naturally, I assume that you will be accepted.

More later.

Sincerely
Hal

P.S. Congratulations on your election!

PVA

PARALYZED
VETERANS
OF AMERICA

HAROLD STONE, VICE-PRESIDENT / 77 PHEASANT HILL STREET / WESTWOOD, MASSACHUSETTS 02090

June 2, 1964

Mr. William M. Bailey
President, Mexico P. V. A.
c/o La Morada
Cubilete #147 Colonia Chapalita

Dear Bill:

It looks good; all the votes so far have been to accept your Chapter. Unfortunately, there is no majority yet.

I have mailed membership recruitment material and membership cards. The proper procedure with the cards is as follows:

> Have the dues expire June 30, 1965. Give the first card to the member. Usually the V. P. is the Membership Officer and signs it. Keep one card for your Chapter file. Send the National card to me, along with the $3.00 for S. C. and $1.00 for N. S. C. members. Send the other card to Bob Webb, the P. N. Editor.

Your members will receive the P. N. free once you become affiliated and have sent cards to Bob Webb.

More later.

Sincerely,

Hal

Harold Stone
Acting President

Forming a PVA Chapter in Mexico

June 10, 1964

MINUTES OF PVA MEETING OF GUADALAJARA? MEXICO

1. Meeting was called to order at 6:30 P.M. by pres. Bill Bsiley.

2. There being no minutes from a previous meeting all correspondence pertaining to the forming of a PVA chapter was read. It was unanamouisly agreed to form a chapter and it was agreed that Wed. June 17th at 6:00 P.M. would be the day for electing officers.

3. Nominations were opened for officers. Joe Miller was nominated by George Small for president. Chas. J. Ceska was nominated by Geo. Small for vice-president. George Ray was nominated by George Small for Sec-Treas. Nominated for Board of Directors were Bob Jackson by George E. Small, Stanley Prucnal by Chas. Reno, Doc Foland by Stanley Prucnal, Bill Bailey by Bob Beske, Lee Schlyer by Geo. Ray, And Bob Beilsmith by Bob Jackson. Nominations were closed.

4. A motion was made by Geo. Ray and seconded by Chas. Reno to accept into the PVA of America the Great Northwest Chapter covering the states of Minnesota, Iowa and South Dakota. The motion was carried.

5. It was agreed that Sec-Treas. George Ray should attend the National Convention in Santa Monica July 21 to 29, 1964.

6. There were three resolutions discussed and are to be drafted for consideration at the June 17th meeting. 1. To try to bring into Mexico duty free wheelchairs, beds, airconditioners, and all things that apply to the handicapped. 2. A resolution to get contracts for Mexican aides for the handicapped both here and in the states for a period of two years. These aides would have to fulfill their contracts or return to Mexico. They would not be eligible to migrate to the U. S.
3. A resolution to have aides travel with handicapped at Gov't expense when traveling to foreign countries under available transportion rules. This would apply to the service connected

7. There were 15 attending the meeting and 14 join the chapter and paid their dues for 1964-1965.

8. The meeting was adjourned at 8:15 P. M.

by George E. Ray
Sec-Treas- Actg.

First Official Meeting of the Mexico Chapter PVA

Minutes of:
June 17 '64 Meeting of Paralized Veterans of America

The meeting was called to order by President Joe Miller on Wednesday, June 17 at 6:15 P.M.

The Minutes of the May 20 meeting were submitted and read by Secretary-Treasurer George E. Ray. Charles Reno moved to accept the minutes and the motion was seconded by Robert Beske.

Motion was made by George Small to accept all nominees for Board of Directors as follows: Bob Jackson, Stanley Prucnal, Ray Foland, Bill Bailey, Lee Schyler, Bob Beilsmith, and the motion was seconded by Bill Bailey.

It was unanimously decided that a copy of the by-laws be presented to all members immediately upon their availability.

Member George Small proposed that all paralyzed persons not eligible for PVA Membership be admitted as honorary members. George E. Ray seconded the motion.

The meeting was honored by the presence of Miss Gloria Augustinson.

Secretary-Treasurer George E. Ray was authorized to pay $4.00 to Hal Stone for the copy of Robert's Rules of Order (revised) which will be the property of PVA Mexico Chapter.

The meeting was adjourned at 6:45 P.M.

Respectfully submitted,
July 15, 1964

George E. Ray
Secretary-Treasurer

First Edition of Mexico PVA's "El Sombrero News" May 1966

EL SOMBRERO NEWS

PARALYZED VETERANS OF AMERICA

MEXICO CHAPTER

Here we go--our first news bulletin for the Mexico Chapter. It was voted at our last regular meeting to purchase a mimeograph machine and put out a bulletin. A new A. B. Dick mimeograph was purchased and is now in our possession at a cost of $3,098.75 pesos or $247.90. With the machine we received a goodly supply of paper stencils and ink, but no one to operate it. So let's see what happens--see if we can come up with something of interest and benefit to our chapter and others.

MEMBERSHIP

This year, according to membership chairman Jack Myrick, our future is very bright. As of now we have 40 members mailed to National, 28 service connected and 12 non-service connected. This surpasses any previous year and is only the beginning. We expect many more on the arrival of the snowbirds. We have received several renewals from the states from members who expect to be down later. Let's keep it that way--once a member of the Mexico Chapter always a member. Bart Corbett sent a check for his dues last month even though it was stated in the PN that he was a member of the New England Chapter. Ken Gulrud from Wisconsin sent his dues this week and will be down in January. We really expect to get the Mexico Chapter off the ground this year and the surest way to do it is through a strong membership. So let's everyone serve on the membership committee and sign 'em up. Get the hold-outs and grab them as they pull into town or get off the plane. We have really been going to town signing new members. Here is a list of the new ones--Ken Van Albert, Bob Kinch, Meyer Kabot, Don Schmidt, Vern Thorson, Joe Anderson, Bill Stanley, Bill Fausnight, Paula Veilleux, Jerry Fosenmeyer, Jerry Baker, Joe Darichuk, Mario Fuget, Manuel Trujillo, Ray "Porky" Michaud, Steve Wilson, Carrol Stodgel, and John Wilson.

SERVICE REPORT
by Ceska

Sixty-nine letters were written last month. Thirty were written to Harry Scott, Veteran's Affairs Officer, American Consul Bldg., Mexico City for permission for service connected veterans to receive medicine, hospitalization,and dental care. This permission is good for six months only and is then renewed by the service officer. Seventy-five miles were traveled to visit and assist the sick and hospitalized. Several hours were spent with the officals at the American-Mexican Hospital to install a hosptial bed and mattress and bowel care equipment so that there is less likelyhood of breaking down while hospitalized. So if you have any problems drop by Cubilete #147 and see "Buck". As they say in Mexico, "Para servirle".

B -LINE-BARRETT

It has beenbrought to the attention of this chapter that things are not going well with us at the Mexican-American Hospital. Members have been complaining about having to make many trips in order to get their medicine orders filled. Others have complained that without long advance notice itis difficult to get an appointment at 4:00 to 4:30 P.M. which are the times originally set aside for the paraplegics. We are contacting Mr. Harry Scott, Veteran's Affairs Officer to see if something can't be done to see that this situation does not exist in the future. So, if you are having problems of this nature just hold your horses for a few days and I think we can straighten this out to everyone's satisfaction.

CONVENTION NOTES AND LEGISLATION
by Ray

Past president Joe Miller and myself made the great trek to Detroit in July to attend the National Convention of the Paralyzed Veterans of America. We made this 5000 mile trip to try to learn somethong about the PVA, to determine what could be done on the chapter level and, frankly, to see what type of organization we belonged to and were representing. We went, we saw, and believe me for an organization of only 4300 members I have never seen suchdedication at terrific personal inconvienience, such work load carried by the national officers, and such a group of downright good fellows. They were a wonderful bunch of people that knew exactly what they were doing and how to do it.

I cannot praise highly enough the past and present national and chapter officers whom I met in Detroit for the great work they are doing. All the above also applies to Lee Gresham, president of Michigan PVA, his charming wife, and the committees who set up and masterminded the intricate details which go into making a convention operate smoothly. So if you notice a little more enthusiasm, a little more hustle bustle in our local chapter you can attribute it to the fact that the national convention opened our eyes to the good that is being done by the PVA for all handicapped people.

The 1967 national convention is being held in Houston, Texas, and I would like to see a large turn-out from our chapter since it is so close to us. I can guarantee that anyone who goes will a rewarding experience for which he will never be sorry.

I will skip lightly over legislation as most of the pertinent laws affecting PVA are thoroughly covered in the P.N. However, on Sept. 19, 1966 the House of Represenatives passed H. R. 17488 which concerns increases in pay for the non-service connected, their children and widows. Since this bill would greatly help most NSC we should support it by getting our letters in to the Senate Committees on Finance. This could mean over $100.00 per month for some NSC veterans. For a copy of the complete bill and names of the committeemen see Chas. Ceska at #147 Cubilete. He will also help you with your letters if you need assistance.

NEW NATIONAL OFFICERS

The new officers elected for 1966-67 are: Pres. Les Burghoff of New England PVA, Vice-Pres. Leonard Chrysler of Bay Area (San Francisco), Sec-Treas. Howard Bennett of Virginia who was later named Executive Secretary to replace retiring Harry Schweikert. National Executive Committeemen are Robert Rohrer of the Vaughn chapter, Wayne Capson of Calif., and Sandy Weinzimer of Eastern. Bob Webb was re-appointed editor of Paraplegic News, Bill Green still heads our service program, and Ernest Sawyer was approved by the Board of Directors to replace Bennett as Sec-Treas on Nov. 1st when the latter goes to the Washington office. With a team like the above we can't help but have a good season.

ACTIVITIES AND ENTERTAINMENT
by Lucier

CLUBHOUSE PICNIC Fun buffs from Acapulco to Vera Cruz are already buzzing over the Mexico Chapter PVA's clubhouse picnic slated for Sunday, Oct. 23, at Granja Pavitos, Las Fuentes at Circunvalacion Sur #81.

Festivities commence at 12:00 noon with no bets on when the soiree will be over.

The gastronomical line-up would make patrons of a Roman orgy envious.

AIR MAIL

February 19, 1968

Mr. William L. Spencer
Public Relations, Mexico Chapter
Paralized Veterans of America Inc.
Privada de Las Rosas 416
Col. Chapalita
Guadalajara, Jalisco, Mexico

Dear Bill:

Thanks for your recent letter informing us of your appointment as publicity and PR director for the Mexico PVA.

Your chapter has been one of the most active in supplying us usable items and photos, and I'm sure the output will increase now that you've been officially appointed to the job. We like short items of all kinds on chapter activities, and welcome clear photos (preferably black-and-white) to accompany them.

Regarding feature material, I have been intending to contact someone in your chapter about putting together a big feature about "life in the gringo wheelchair colony" in Guadalajara, but I haven't known who specifically to contact. I hope you have solved my problem.

What I would like to do is this: a big feature on the U.S. wheeler population, not a commercial for Guadalajara but a good cross-section piece on the life and doings of the colony. Ideally, the piece would include material (and pics!) on PVA chapter activities, life at all three boarding house operations (Kegan, Ray, Coe), downtown Guadalajara scenes and activities, examples of bachelor house living, examples of family living where U.S. wheelers have married local girls, some coverage of paraplegics living in outlying areas such as Lake Chapala, Ajijic, etc., and such ....

As I'm sure you can see, this could be a great feature for the PN. If it turns out to be too much for a single issue, we can break it into two or more parts. We would, of course, edit and (if necessary) rewrite the material here, so the writer needs only to supply us an interesting and factually accurate story. We will be happy to handle all questions of grammar, punctuation, and the like.

I look forward to hearing your thoughts on the feature project -- and to many general news items from G-Town.

Cordially,

Robert L. Webb
Editor/Publisher

PARALIZED VETERANS OF AMERICA INC.

MEXICO CHAPTER

The Mexico Chapter of the Paralyzed Veterans of America would like to have you and your friends become acquainted with our clubhouse facilities located in Ciudad Granja. For this reason we are inviting you to attend the Beer Party and Raffle that we are holding there on Sunday, April 14, 1968. On that day, from 4 p.m. to 6 p.m., there will be free beer, entertainment, and the drawing for the prizes of the holders of the raffle tickets.

Among the entertainers who will appear are the Rondalla Combo from the Hilton Hotel, Jane Sans Munoz, and Antonio Velasco.

The prizes to be awarded in the drawing are a combination AM/FM radio and taped recorder, a Travel Bar, Canned Hams, a bottle of Scotch, and an electric Cardshuffler.

We are enclosing one book of tickets for this raffle. The price of the tickets are 10 pesos each, or 100 pesos for the book. The unsold tickets, ticket stubs, and the money may be returned to the Mexico Chapter PVA at Las Palmas 226, Ciudad Granja, or to Bob Beilsmith at Circunvalacion Mungia 2075, Jardines del Country, or to Ray Foland at Arbol 329, Colonia Chapalita.

Yours truly,

Robert Beilsmith, Pres.

PARALYZED VETERANS OF AMERICA, INC.

MEXICO CHAPTER

Las Palmas #226
Ciudad Granja
Guadalajara, Jalisco
Mexico

Dear Friends:

The Mexico Chapter of the Paralyzed Veterans of America would like to invite you and your friends to attend the picnic that we are going to have at our clubhouse on the afternoon of November 3, 1968. If you happened to attend our last picnic or have talked to anyone that did I am sure you heard that a good time was had by everyone.

On the afternoon of the picnic beer and soft drinks will be served to holders of raffle tickets from 1 to 5 pm., and other drinks and a special dinner will be available for those who want them at a low price. Our entertainment chairman is lining up an afternoon of top entertainment to be presented from 1 tO 4 pm., which will be headlined by Chamaco Guerrero and his orchestra, and the Tapa Trio.

We are enclosing one book of tickets for the picnic and raffle. The price of the tickets are 10 pesos each or 100 pesos for the book. The unsold tickets or the ticket stubs and money may be returned to : Mexico Chapter PVA at Las Palmas #226, Ciudad Granja, To Bill Christensen at Avenida Las Maestros 596, Col Normal, or to Ray Foland at Arbol #329, Col. Chapalita.

You are welcome to use our clubhouse facilities at any time. We are open everyday except Sunday and Monday. On Wednesday and Friday evenings we have Bingo games starting at 7 pm., and on Fridays we usually have some type of live music following the Bingo games.

In case that you have not heard of our organization, we are a group of veterans who all have spinal cord injuris and most of whom are confined to wheelchairs. The main purpose of our organization is to help our members to live a fuller and more productive life, and on the local level to help other handicapped persons in any way that we can.

I hope to see you at the picnic.

Yours truly,

Bill Christensen, President

PARALYZED VETERANS OF AMERICA
CHARTERED BY THE CONGRESS OF THE UNITED STATES

November 5, 1979

Jack Tumidajski, President
Mexico PVA
APDO 5-382
Guadalajara, Jalisco
Mexico

Dear Jack,

Just wanted to take a moment to congratulate you on becoming the new Mexico PVA president. As I'm sure you are by now aware, it is a great challange to be a chapter president and a lot of hard work.

After reading your recent October edition of the El Sombrero News, I'm quite sure that you will meet the challange. I congratulate you on the improvements in this newspaper which make it much more interesting and informative. The pictures are a welcome addition.

I was very pleased to read that the Mexico Chapter was somewhat responsible for the addition of handicapped parking spaces outside the U. S. Consulate office. Please continue to keep up the hard work and I'm sure that the Mexico Chapter will benefit greatly in the months to come through your administrations efforts. Please give my regards to Director Raymond Clifford and the other officers and members of the Mexico Chapter.

Very sincerely yours,

Michael F. Delaney

Michael F. Delaney
Senior Vice President
5646 McMillan
Dearborn Hgts., MI 48127

QUADALAJARA: The Utopia That Once Was

As a former resident of Guadalajara (1962-1968), I found the following editorial to be very interesting. It was taken from the Mexico Chapter PVA El Sombrero News and we congratulate the editor on a well-written and perceptive article.

It may be of interest to *Roadrunner* readers who have been to Guadalajara or considering going there.

Ernest T. Chavez, Editor
Zia Chapter *Roadrunner*

QUADALAJARA — The Utopia That Once Was
Jack Tumidajski

At some point in the history of this ever-growing city, someone cutely gave it a nickname that—at the time—seemed quite appropriate. By replacing the letter "G" with the letter "Q," Guadalajara became Quadalajara. Remember all those old advertisements which appeared in the *Paraplegia News* and elsewhere? QUADALAJARA: 365 days of sunshine, low cost-of-living, skilled personal care attendants for those needing assistance, etc., etc. It sure did make Quadalajara seem like an attractive alternative to US institutional living, or living with ones' family for those newly injured quadriplegics and paraplegics—victims of auto mishaps, swimming and diving accidents, and those whose lives are permanent reminders of the war in Southeast Asia.

Quadalajara wasn't exclusively for veterans nor young quads, for that matter, but in the late-60s through early-70s, it would not be an exaggeration to say that some sixty to eighty quadriplegics alone rolled around in the sunshine of this attractive city. It is estimated that the entire North American (and European) wheelchair community grew to between 120 and 160.

Time has changed Quadalajara. A decade ago—when Quadalajara was at its apex—those who roamed this Utopia were, for the most part, Korean War veterans in their early thirties and young Vietnam veterans fresh from the VA hospital system. There were daily card games. Poker games were as easy to start as breaking open a fresh deck of Kem cards. One could go downtown in the evening and find plenty of "action." Everything was cheap—compared to stateside prices, and everyone who needed a personal care attendant, maid/housekeeper, house/apartment had one. In short—everything necessary for carefree and easy living.

What was a decade ago no longer exists. At least, not to those who lived it. TIME—that great changer—took care of that. No longer will you rent a house for 800 pesos/month (or find one at all), hire a maid for 500, a driver/attendant for 1000 or less. Inflation, devaluation of the peso, the tremendous influx of people to the cities, and the emergence of a "middle class" in Mexico have all contributed to this change. Multiplying the above mentioned figures by a factor of five, you arrive at a fairly representative average of what the "basic" cost of living for your average quad consist. "Basic"—not to mention food, utilities, entertainment, and the always elusive "miscellaneous."

One might ask: "What happened to the participants of the Quadalajara era?" Well, they're still here—but not in such numbers. Many have found San Diego, Phoenix, Tucson, Miami, Albuquerque, Southern Texas, and their old home towns more attractive. This great Northern Migration has left a number of "family men" who have adopted Quadalajara as their new home, and a number of "fence-sitters" who put off the inevitable move back to the States or search for a new Utopia. Then there are the "left-behinds" who have felt the effects of these drastic changes the most—non-service connected veterans and non-vets whose fixed incomes cause them to continually have to tighten their financial belts. But with continued runaway inflation of some 30% annually, it's only a matter of time before something has to give.

This raises an interesting question: what will these fixed income "left-behinds" do and whose responsibility are they? They came to Quadalajara financially stable by Mexican standards. They have been away from family and home for many years. Many have become, through the years, Quadalajaranized, spoiled maybe, but with nowhere to retreat to. Families who could barely care for these individuals a decade ago—well, add ten years and you'll find that nursing homes would seem to be the alternative for many.

The future for "left-behinds" is not bright. Not all of us, fortunately, have experienced nursing home care first hand. But, if it's anything like the image that this alternative projects—one of staffing shortages, poor food, insensitive employees, isolation, etc., combined with the special needs of a quadriplegic—and the picture looks uglier still!

Who or what is to blame: societies' attitude toward the handicapped, the economic situation in the States, the economic situation here, those—who for financial gain—advertised and hyped Quadalajara and brought down the majority of the "left-behinds," or the individual himself? It's a tough question to ponder. One might answer that the individual is responsible. Sometimes one is backed into a corner and takes a chance—one that he has to live with if it fails or when it comes to an end.

History will write the bottom line of this editorial. In any event, it is safe to say that we can drop the letter "Q" from Quadalajara and reinsert the letter "G." Quadalajara—the Utopia that once was—is gone and gone forever. But rather than feel bitter about what no longer is, maybe we should be thankful for what once was. The memories, experiences, and lessons learned will remain with us for the rest of our lives.

The original editorial appeared in the October 1979 edition of *El Sombrero News*

Zia Chapter
paralyzed veterans of america, inc.

833 GIBSON BLVD. S.E., ALBUQUERQUE, NEW MEXICO 87102
Telephone (505) 247-4381/82

January 18, 1980

Jack Tumidajski, Editor
Mexico Chapter PVA
APDO 5-382
Guadalajara, Jal., Mexico

Dear Jack:

I wish to compliment you on your editorial wisdom in selecting "The Night Before Christmas" (NOCHE Buena) story that appeared in the December, 1979 Zia Roadrunner. Its always flattering when another chapter reprints your articles.

Let me say further, I was very impressed with your front cover on your January, 1980 issue.

Hope to meet you sometime.

Fraterally yours,

Ralph

Ralph Markward
President

RM:dlm

cc: Ernie Chavey
Editor, Zia Roadrunner

CHRISTMAS IN JANUARY!!! **Editor**

Well, not exactly, but the following poem which appeared in the ZIA Chapter's Roadrunner (December 1979) arrived a few days too late to appear in our last newsletter. We thought you might appreciate it since so many of our members are "fluent" in Spanish. Besides, what's wrong with letting the Christmas spirit carry over into the new year?

THE NIGHT BEFORE CHRISTMAS

(Noche Buena)

'Twas the night before Christmas and all through the casa,
Not a creature was stirring. Caramba! Que Pasa?
Los ninos were all tucked away in their camas,
Some in long underwear, some in pajamas.
While Mama worked late in her little cocina,
El viejo was down at the corner cantina
Living it up with amigos, Carracho!
Muy contento and poco borracho!
While hanging the stockings with much cuidado,
In hopes that old Santa would feel Obligado
To bring all the children, both buenos and malos,
A nice batch of dulces and other regalos,
Outside in the yard there arose such a grito
That I jumped to my feet like a frightened cabrito.
I ran to the window and looked out afuera,
And who in the world do you think that it era?
St. Nick in a sleigh and a big red sombrero
Came dashing along like a crazy bombero!
And pulling his sleigh, instead of venados,
Were eight little burros, approaching volados.
I watched as they came, and this quaint little hombre
Was shouting and whistling and calling by nombre
"Ay, Pancho! Ay, Pepe! Ay, Cuca! Ay Beto!
Ay, Chato, Ay, Chope! Maruca Y Nieto!"
Then standing erect with his hand on his pecho,
He flew to the top of our own techo.
With his round little belly like a bowl of jalea,
He struggled to squeeze down our old chimenea
Then, huffing and puffing, at last in our sala,
With soot smeared all over his red suit de gala,
He filled all the stockings with lovely regalos,
For none of the ninos had been very malos.
Then chuckling aloud, seeming very contento,
He turned like a flash and was gone like the viento.
And I heard him exclaim - and this is verdad -
Merry Christmas to all! Feliz Navidad!

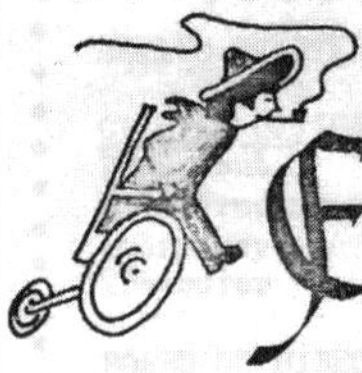

El Sombrero News

Paralyzed Veterans of America, Inc.
Mexico Chapter

MONTHLY NEWSLETTER — JANUARY 1980

The purpose of this organization shall be charitable and non-profit; to provide a closer, friendlier and more fraternal relationship among its members; develop their ethical consciousness; improve their personal welfare and, in general, to do everything in its power of a civic, educational, charitable and/or benevolent nature to better living conditions for all people suffering from spinal cord injuries or diseases and those affected directly or indirectly thereby.

* *

El Sombrero News is the official publication of the Mexico Chapter PVA

Editor: Jack Tumidajski

A NOTE ABOUT OUR COVER PAGE — Editor

The familiar paragraph that appears on our cover page is reprinted from the chapter by-laws (ART II, Section 1). It appears as a constant reminder of what the purpose of our organization is. I would like to thank Wayne Stroup for his assistance in lettering the cover page.

El Sombrero News January 1980

PARALYZED VETERANS OF AMERICA

MEXICO CHAPTER
APDO 5-382
Guadalajara, Jalisco, MEXICO

Mr. R. Jack Powell, Executive Director
Paralyzed Veterans of America
4350 East West Highway, Suite 900
Washington, D.C. 20014

February 1, 1980

Dear Mr. Powell,

On Monday, January 28, 1980 four men (one carrying a semi-automatic weapon) entered and robbed the Mexico Chapter PVA clubhouse and 10 of the members who were present at the time.

The attachted statement of events was read and signed by eight (8) of the ten members present when the incident took place and submitted to the appropriate authorities via the U.S. Consulate here in Guadalajara. The chapter's Board of Directors unanimously agreed to report the incident and to use the U.S. Consulate as a vehicle in pursuing this matter.

This is the third such incident that has occured in the Guadalajara area during the past few months. Although the other incidents took place in private homes, it is our feeling that these incidents should be properly reported and followed up on, especially since all three appear very much to be inter-related, and, in more than one case, PVA members were physically assaulted.

I realize that this is somewhat out of the ordinary for a PVA chapter president, but do to the circumstances, I will continue to be in contact with Consulate officials on this matter in hopes that no further incidents of this nature occur in Guadalajara's wheelchair community.

If you have any questions or suggestions please contact me through the chapter's mailing address or by phone (home) 37-06-32.

Sincerely,

Jack Tumidajski

JACK TUMIDAJSKI
President
Mexico Chapter PVA

cc: Joseph Romagnano, National President
Frank DeGeorge, National Advocacy Director
Thomas Deniston, Southwest Region Advocacy Director

Attachment

February 28, 1980

Mr. Jack Tumidajski
President, Mexico Chapter PVA
APDO 5-382
Guadalajara, Jalisco, Mexico

Dear Mr. Tumidajski:

I received your correspondence of February 1, 1980 outlining the the robbery that took place in your chapter clubhouse on January 28, 1980.

We will keep this information on file and thank you for keeping us informed of these events.

Sincerely,

R. Jack Powell
Executive Director

ARIZONA CHAPTER

Paralyzed Veterans of America, Inc.

MEMBER OF
NATIONAL PARAPLEGIA FOUNDATION
WORLD VETERANS FEDERATION
International Society for the Rehabilitation of the Disabled

May 28, 1980

Mexico P.V.A.
Jack Tumidajski, Editor
APDO 5-382
Guadalajara, Jalisco
Mexico

Dear Mr. Tumidajski:

I am writing to tell you how much I enjoyed your May Edition of the El Sombrero Newsletter. I particularly enjoyed the "Chaplain's Corner", by David Carlson. I hope to see more special articles like that in other newsletters. Also, the "Quotes and Misquotes - Statements and Misstatements" was delightfully humorous.

I noted that you will be returning to the U.S. shortly and therefore will not continue to be the Editor of El Sombrero News. I hope your successor will continue the newsletter along the same lines. Good Luck.

Sincerely,

Laura D. Green, Secretary/Editor
The Desert Oracle, Arizona Chapter

Keith A. Ziegler
6945 W. Merrell
St.
Phoenix, Arizona
85033
May 13, 1987

Mr. Joe Sternberg
Comtroller
Paralyzed Veterans of America
801 18th Street, NW
Washington, DC 20006

Dear Mr. Sternberg,

Enclosed is a check for $5,000.00 which the past membership of the Mexico PVA voted to have sent to the National Office to be donated to the PVA Capitol Campaign Fund. We would like for our chapter to be rememberd with our name engraved on a brick or whatever you do to remember those who donate such an amount for the PVA National Building.

Your office will be receiving the remainder of our funds shortly which have been earmarked for Spinal Cord Injury Research. If you should have any further questions, please let me know. I would like a receipt from your office for my records in the case someone should ask to see our records.concerning these last transactions.

I thank you for your cooperation in these matters.

Sincerely,

Keith A. Ziegler

PVA

PARALYZED VETERANS
OF AMERICA

Forty Years of Service
1947–1987

May 22, 1987

Mr. Keith A. Ziegler
6945 W. Merrell Street
Phoenix, AZ 85033

Dear Keith:

On behalf of National PVA, I would like to express our gratitude to you and the other former members of the Mexico Chapter for your recent $5,000 contribution to the PVA Building Fund. Your decision to donate these funds to the PVA Building is an important expression of confidence and support for the work being accomplished by your national organization and it is deeply appreciated by the officers and staff.

As a lasting symbol of your support and tribute to the past membership of the Mexico Chapter, a recognition plate will be appropriately engraved and placed on a brick in the front lobby of the PVA Building. In this way, the Mexico Chapter will be remembered by everyone who visits the PVA Building.

Once again, thank you for your support and please convey our appreciation to the other former members of the Mexico Chapter.

Sincerely,

R. Jack Powell
Executive Director

Keith A. Ziegler
6945 W. Merrell St.
Phoenix, Arizona
85033
August 18, 1987

Mr. Joe Sternberg
Comptroller
Paralyzed Veterans of America
801 18th Street, NW
Washington, DC 20006

Dear Mr. Sternberg,

Enclosed is a check, No. 039572, From the Centennial Savings Bank for $21,393.58, which we, the members of the Mexico Chapter of the Paralyzed Veterans of America, have chosen to donate to the Spinal Cord Research Foundation of the Paralyzed Veterans of America. This is being done at the request of all of the members of the ex-Mexico PVA. This is the last of our funds after all of our assets have been liquidated and all of our financial responsibilities have been met.

Could you please send me a receipt for these funds for our records. In the event you should have any questions, please let me know.

I sure thank you for your cooperation.

Sincerely.

Keith A. Ziegler

PVA

PARALYZED VETERANS OF AMERICA

Forty Years of Service
1947–1987

August 28, 1987

Mr. Keith A. Ziegler
6945 W. Merrell Street
Phoenix, AZ 85033

Dear Mr. Ziegler:

It was a pleasure talking with you earlier in the week, and again, thank you for the check of $21,393.58 from the members of the former Mexico PVA chapter.

From our discussion and your correspondence, I understand that it is the intent of the Mexico chapter members to dedicate this contribution to spinal cord injury and disease research. As you and I discussed, the PVA Board of Directors passed an important resolution regarding PVA's future activities in SCI research (copy enclosed). The resolution provides the permission for PVA to enter in a co-venture arrangement with Yale University over the next five (5) years. The project, consisting of a physical building and SCI scientific research, will be called the Yale/PVA Center for Neuroscience and Regeneration Research. This extraordinary partnership will in large part be due to the $1.5 million commitment PVA has made to the Center over the next five years.

I have enclosed a brief fact sheet about the project and a profile on the individual who will be heading the Center, Dr. Stephen Waxman. We are currently in the contractural negotiation stage with Yale and expect to have the arrangement formalized over the next month.

You may also be interested to know that 21 of PVA's 31 chapters have pledged a total of $450,000 over the next five (5) years towards fulfillment of PVA's $1.5 million pledge. Therefore, it seemed only natural that the members of the Mexico chapter would like to join with this effort.

At this point, I hope I've provided you with enough information. Please call, if you wish, and I can answer any of your questions. I'll be in touch.

Sincerely,

Linda K. Coughtry
Director of Development

LKC:daj

Enclosure

Keith A. Ziegler
6945 W. Merrell St.
Phoenix, Arizona
85033
September 2, 1987

Paralyzed Veterans of America
Linda K. Coughtry
Director of Development
801 Eighteenth Street, N.W.
Washington, D.C. 20006

Dear Miss. Coughtry,

I thank you for your quick response and the information which you sent concerning the donation of the former Mexico PVA Chapter.

I have spoken with a number of our former members about donating these funds to the Yale/PVA Center for Neuroscience and Regernation Research. These members all agreed with me that these funds could best be used in this new project which the PVA is entering into, so you have our permission to use these funds for the above mentioned project.

It has always been the wish of the founders and members of Mexico PVA that any monies which are left in our treasury if and when the chapter should fold would be used for spinal cord research. So I think that this would be an appropriate memorial for all who were part of the Mexico Chapter.

I do thank you for your assistance and counsel in these matters.

Sincerely,

Keith A. Ziegler

Appendix B
Articles

MEXICO, A PARADISE FOR PARAPLEGICS

By JAMES E. SEYBOLD

Did you have a hard and trying winter? And you Californians; did the smog and fog drive you to distraction? Your worries are now over, for here, in Mexico City, is the *ideal retreat.* At 7,349 feet the warm, spring-like climate varies little all year long. The site of the city was once the bottom of a lake, therefore it is flat and suited to wheel chair travel.

Until you have actually seen it, it is hard to realize just how beautifully modern, and how far ahead in architectural design Mexico, D.F. is. Typical of this is University City, the national university of Mexico, which can better than equal any U.S. collegiate campus. While on the school's acreage, it's like going ahead in time a hundred years.

A few words to those who should decide to drive down: The three main highways are good all the way, except for the spots where construction is being done. The terrain is in long, level stretches or mountainous. In the mountains be extra careful, as there are no guard fences in many of the dangerous places and others haven't adequate safety precautions, as have similar spots in the States. Mexican gasoline is poor! Their Ethyl is equal to our regular. You buy gasoline by the liter and drive by the kilometer. One hundred kilometers is equal to 62 miles; 3.79 liters equal one gallon. A knowledge of Spanish is helpful in reading road-signs.

The streets in Mexico City are, generally, well planned, but the traffic system is quite poor. Mexican drivers are the worst I've ever seen. Everyday is like the Indianapolis "500" to them. For a few pesos you can save a lot of time and worry by taking one of the city's many taxicabs. (The driver gets fifty centavos over the meter reading, as this last goes to the company).

Motels are good but few and only in the larger towns. This being so, it is advisable to make reservations in advance so that you will have a place to sack-out after a long haul. The American Automobile Association and its affiliates in Mexico is a convenient and helpful organization. In addition to making accommodations for you, they plan scenic routes and obtain the best insurance for your car. Most U.S. policies are not valid outside the States. It is wise to re-insure at the border.

Since the devaluation of the peso, one dollar is worth twelve and a half pesos when entering the country. When leaving you get one dollar for every eight pesos. Thus, economy for the American tourist. However, in order to make your money last it is important to think of the pesos and centavos as you would dollars and cents.

The water in Mexico is bad but you can expect drinkable water in the better hotels and motels. Drink bottled water (Agua Ideal) or other beverages such as Coca-Cola, Pepsi-Cola, Agua Mineral and beer.

The Mexican people are, in general, a happy, carefree race. Their exotic music grows on you and virtually becomes a part of you. Speaking of exotic things; I must say a word in behalf of the lovely senoritas—WOW!

As in all places where the American tourist spends his money you will find those who have ways of separating him from it. Mexico is no exception. An example: If you should buy a national lottery ticket from one of the kids in the street, don't be surprised if it turns out to be two weeks old.

It seems that, in order to be *someone* here, one must have a uniform. Don't let it throw you by thinking that the uniforms contain officials. However, obey the uniforms with guns—they are the police.

I have found that the greatest obstacle is not the language but a siege of diarrhea which hits every visitor to Mexico. Once your system becomes adjusted to the food, you can enjoy those tasty dishes with gusto.

Activities are numerous; from bullfights, Jai-Lai and soccer to visting such nearby places as Maxmillian's Castel in Chapultepec Park, the Shrine of Gudalupe and the Aztec pyramids. As Mexico City is centrally located it can be used as a base of operations from which these side trips can be made. Some of these points of interest are Vera-Cruz, Acapulco, Puebla, Cuernavaca, Guadalajara and Taxco.

As I mentioned in the beginning, see Mexico in the wintertime. The rainy season prevails during much of the summer.

REPORT FROM MEXICO CITY

(The El Dorado of the Western Hemisphere)

by James E. Seybold

Did you just pick up your Paraplegia News after pushing your cold-rimmed wheelchair through a snow bank? Why not get away from it all? Visit Sunny Mexico!

The value of the peso is still 12½ to 1. For $100 or less, depending on the gas mileage of your car, it is possible to reach the border from almost any part of the U.S.A. Although the prices here in Mexico City, Monterrey and Acapulco have gone up slightly since the author was here two years ago, the other sections of this nation remain the same. It is advisable for anyone who plans to come for the first time and has no definite place to stay to check with his nearest travel agency for accommodations. Another thought which came to mind concerning travel agencies is that every person in a wheelchair who drives his own car should be a member of the American Automobile Association.

Highway Conditions Improving

Road conditions in Mexico are good on the main highways, and other roads to secondary points of interest are improving. Another joy to my heart was the installation of traffic lights in Mexico City along Paseo de la Reforma and Insurgentes—the two main drags.

Although a knowledge of some Spanish is helpful (any tourist guide book will suffice), one will find a lot of English-speaking people along the main routes. The people themselves are very friendly. They are not lazy as most Americans picture them to be; in fact, they are well-meaning people who know how to relax. However, if your car isn't ready at the garage on the day you were told it would be—well, that's too bad. You must compensate for these things. This situation is changing though with the commercialism which is becoming established in Mexico.

Beautiful Buildings

I never cease to marvel at the magnificent architecture of Mexico, both modern (hotels of Mexico City and Acapulco) and ancient (beautiful cathedrals, like the one I visited yesterday in Taxco). The town of Taxco is located in the mountains between Cuernavaca and Acapulco, some 5,740 feet in elevation. It is known to be the oldest mining town in North America. The great Spanish explorer, Hernan Cortes, put it in operation when he discovered silver deposits. The Church of San Sebastian y Santa Prisca took seven years to complete, 1751-1758. When one notes its position a-top the highest point in town and also sees its exquisite interior, one can readily understand why it took seven years to build.

All in all, I'm delighted to be away from the cold and the winter. The only Spanish I know, to sum up how I feel about Mexico is "Puda Viva," which literally translated, means "This Is The Life."

Paraplegia News February 1957

A PARAPLEGIC PARADISE NOW OPEN IN MEXICO

by George E. Ray

I have been living in Mexico for the past year and a half. During that time I have had but one dream: a place where paraplegics and quadriplegics could stay and receive personal services. That dream has been realized.

A vacation and retirement spot especially designed for the para and quad is now open and operating at Guadalajara, Mexico. It is a modern motel equipped with every modern convenience: confortable bedrooms, convenient bathrooms, large dining-room particularly adapted to wheelchairs, beautiful lounge and a swimming pool.

It was built by Mr. Paul J. De Lecour, a retired building contractor from Minnesota, at the suggestion of this writer.

The San Jose del Tajo has 24-hour service for the ones who need help with personal services, getting in and out of bed and in and out of cars.

Guadalajara was chosen because of its year-round temperate climate. It is never too hot or too cold for the para or quad with circulation or perspiration problems.

San Jose del Tajo is located ten minutes from the city. It is modern, clean and boasts a population of over a half million. The motel is only 30 minutes from the world renowned Lake Chapala, the largest lake in Mexico, and the picturesque artist colonies of Ajijiic and Jocotepec.

Paras and Quads Only

San Jose del Tajo is closed to the general public; catering only to paraplegics, quadriplegics and their families. No expense has been spared to make a home-like, happy atmosphere for the person who wishes to spend a vacation in colorful Mexico.

For the paraplegic who is self-sufficient cost is $120 per month (room, three American cooked meals of the highest quality, and laundry). The monthly cost to the quadriplegic is $180. He receives all that the para does, plus the 24-hour service (bladder and bowel care and medication).

For detailed information, write to: Mr. Paul J. De Lecour, San Jose del Tajo Guadalajara, Mexico.

Paraplegia News April 1959

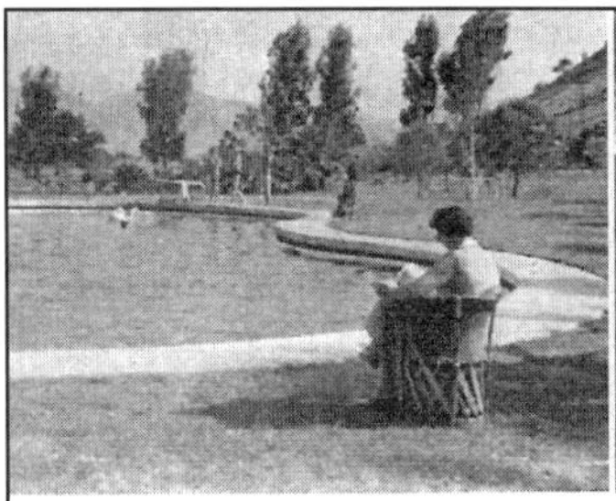
San Jose Pool.

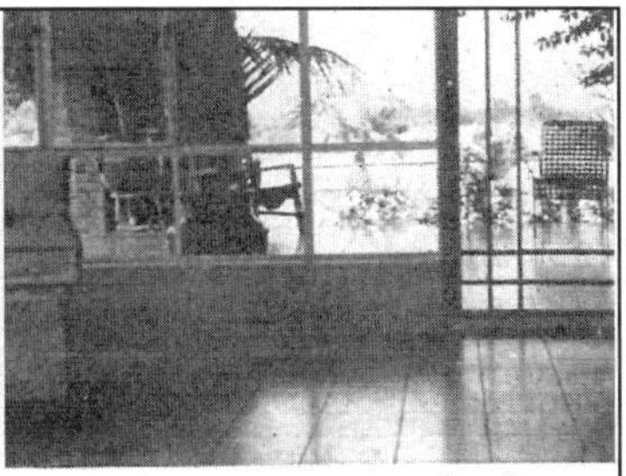
Looking out onto patio at San Jose.

SAN JOSE DEL TAJO ATTACKED AND UPHELD

A letter to the PARAPLEGIA NEWS from a Florida quadriplegic states that the article "A Paraplegic Paradise Now Open In Mexico" was misleading. And that quads would not find the place satisfactory to live in. He also stated that the food was inferior, there was no telephone and no transportation in case of sudden illness.

Harry A. Schweikert Jr., president of the Paralyzed Veterans of America, asked a PVA member to check on San Jose Del Tajo. Below is the report of Robert M. Lawrence, Glen Ridge, New Jersey:

Lawrence, a quadriplegic, feels that the climate is perfect: high temperature but humidity seldom over 10%, use of blanket at night, great ease of breathing and elimination of perspiration problem. "This writer," he says, "for example is a quadriplegic who has never breathed more freely and comfortably before, anyplace."

Food prepared pretty much as it is on the eastern seaboard of U.S. Breakfast: (9-11) juice or fruit, toast, eggs-fried or poached, dry cereals, milk and coffee. Dinner: Principal meal is served at about 1:30 P.M., roast or stew (occasionally a Mexican dish), green vegetables, potatoes, rice, rolls, Italian bread, butter, pie, ice cream, fruit, coffee and milk. Supper: (6:45), Light meal *(see books on nutrition; one "Let's Eat Right To Keep Fit" by Adelle Davis*)* usually of franks, rolls, cold cuts, potato salad, and things of that sort, dessert and beverage same as at dinner.

Accommodations

Single and double rooms: each has bathroom with shower, wash basins are proper height, always hot and cold water, comfortable beds, small chest of drawers, writing table, two-headed lamp, large window, AC current, safe drinking water delivered daily in sealed plastic containers.

"I can emphatically state," Bob adds, "that because of the altitude, the pure air and the beautiful mountain vistas, one isn't even *tempted* to be constantly seeking something to do. One becomes caught up with the rhythm of an older and more tranquil civilization than our own."

The proprietors arrange transportation for those who wish to go sightseeing or on visits to Guadalajara. The social side of life is quite friendly.

There is complete and proper care in bladder and bowel treatment for those requiring it. Women guests are welcome but this service is not available for them as yet.

Two documents are necessary: proof of recent small pox vaccination, and a travel permit obtained from the Mexican Consulate in New York City, or one of the branch offices.

"I might add," Robert Lawrence concludes, "that for the paraplegic with an automobile, a more delightful place than this, for a holiday or for an extended visit, can scarcely be found."

**Harcourt, Brace and Company.*

Paraplegia News July 1959

FLORIDA QUAD PLANNING MEXICAN VACATION SPOT

A non-service connected quadriplegic, Harold E. Doolittle, is attempting to arrange a set-up in Mexico where U.S. paras and quads can vacation or live on a permanent basis. He plans to rent or lease a place in Cuernavaca (50 miles south of Mexico City.)

Before he goes ahead with the financing of his project he would like to have an idea of how many physically handicapped would be interested. He says that he would like all persons interested to drop him a card.

Mr. Doolittle has been roaming around Mexico for the past several years, looking for the most likely spot to live. He settled on Cuernavaca because of its climate and its location. Doolittle speaks Spanish fluently.

He says he would cater to any type of disability, and welcome wives or husbands of the disabled, and any children. He is sure that he can operate by charging $120 monthly for quads who need care, and less for those who do not. His venture will be non-profit.

Schools

There are many, many things to see and do in Mexico. There are three movie houses in the city. For those with children there are numerous schools for kids of all ages. This is because of the large American colony in Cuernavaca.

The requirements for entering Mexico are simple: A six-months tourist pass can be obtained with a birth cirtificate or other proof of citizenship. Also needed is a vaccination which has been given within two years prior to entry.

If one wishes to remain longer than six months, he can be issued a new six-months pass by making a trip back to a border town. There are several other methods.

When contacting Harold Doolittle concerning your Mexican trip please include the following information about yourself: approximate length of stay (one week, a month, six, etc.) type of disability, financial status (service connected veteran, non-service connected, non-pensioners, and if the latter whether they have a source of income).

Send correspondence to Mr. Doolittle at Ward 15-A, VA Hospital, Coral Gables, Florida.

Paraplegia News April 1960

Quadriplegic teaches English to Mexican choir

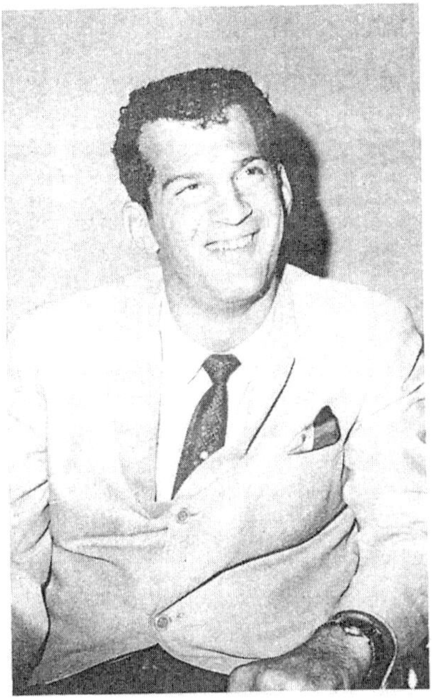

Larry Kegan

Quadriplegic Lawrence P. Kegan certainly has one of the world's most unusual and interesting avocations for a wheeler. He is the official English teacher for the Girls' Choir of the Instituto Cabanos, a home for underprivileged children and

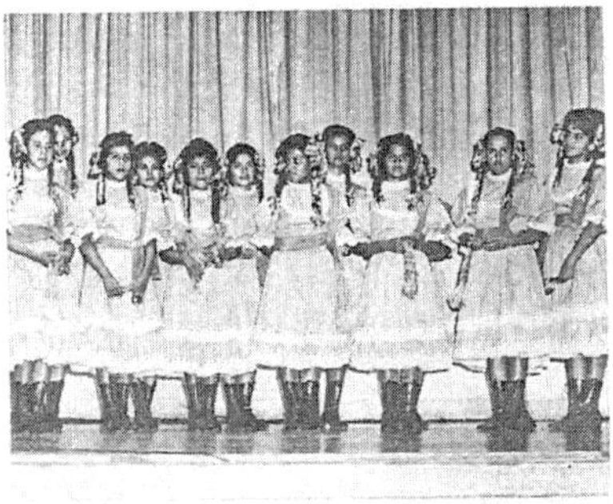

The Instituto Cabanos Girls' Choir

orphans in Guadalajara, Mexico.

Larry recently accompanied the 16-member Girls' Choir when it came to California to perform. The occasion for the trip was the biennial Downey-Guadalajara Sister City Convention, but while here the girls also performed at Disneyland, Knott's Berry Farm, Rancho Los Amigos Hospital, UCLA, Long Beach VA Hospital, and aboard an aircraft carrier.

Songs in English

Especially for the California tour, pedagogue Kegan turned showman and taught the Girls' Choir English translations of three of their traditional songs. These reportedly went over big with the Stateside audiences.

Before he discovered Guadalajara, Larry Kegan was a gringo Mid-Westerner. For the past several years he has been operating Hacienda Las Fuentes, a resort and permanent residence complex for disabled men and women located outside Guadalajara.

Paraplegia News October 1965

U.S. wheelers host posada in Mexico

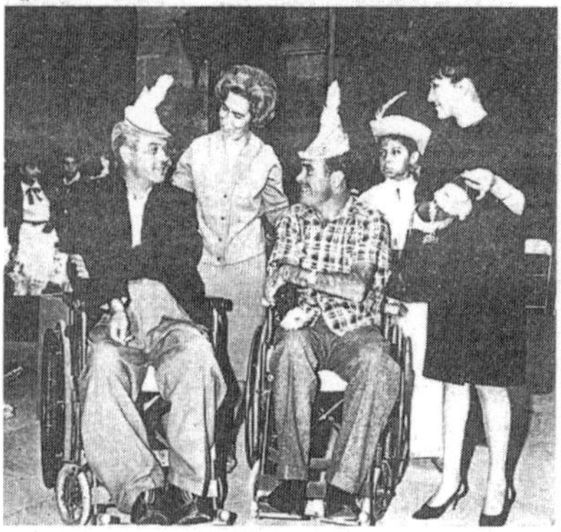

The hosts seem to be having more fun than anybody at the wheelers' Second Annual Christmas Posada in Guadalajara. (L to R) Joe Miller, president of the Guadalajara PVA Chapter; Senora Asuncion Garcia Sancho, director of the orphanage; Mario Fuget; one of the Hospicio de Cabanas orphans; and Mrs. Fuget.

GUADALAJARA, Mexico — The 400 orphans at the state home Hospicio de Cabanas had a brighter Christmas this year as a result of the Second Annual Christmas Posada put on for the children by members of Guadalajara's U.S. "wheelchair colony." 58 paraplegics and quadriplegics raised 7,200 pesos for the posada, and 34 of the wheelers attended personally to help host the affair.

All 400 of the children at the home were given Christmas presents, as were 300 other youngsters who come to the orphanage each morning under the federal school breakfast program.

Bigger next year

Joe Miller, president of the Guadalajara PVA Chapter and one of the party's organizers, says the wheelers' Christmas Posada is now a permanent tradition, and plans are already underway for a bigger one next year.

Another PVA paraplegic, George Ray, is commander of the Guadalajara Post #3 of the American Legion, which raised more than 6,500 pesos for the "Pesos for Braces" program. Proceeds from this program are used to purchase orthopedic braces for crippled children from poor families.

Paraplegia News February 1965

Needy Guadalajara children get merry Christmas

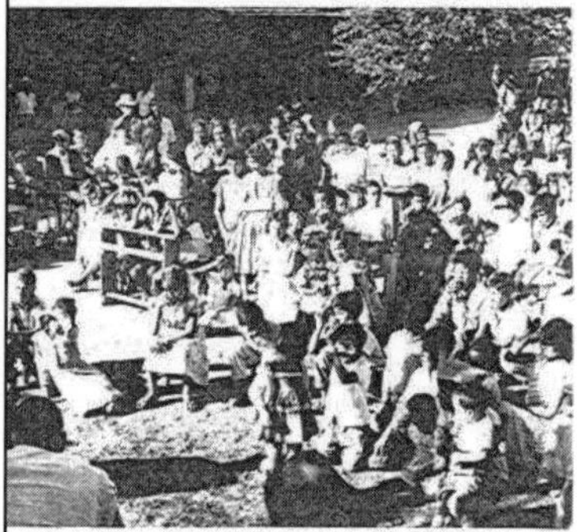

Some of the more than 400 children at the Ninos Heroes School who attended the Christmas party hosted by 60 Guadalajara paraplegics.

It was a big and unforgettable Christmas for 1,500 needy children in Guadalajara, Jalisco, Mexico, thanks to the generosity and hard work of the 60 paraplegics who raised 7,500 pesos for the biggest Christmas fund yet.

Guests of Americans

A poverty-stricken Catholic school, an equally poor public school, and all the orphans at the state Orphanage were guests of the Americans at three separate parties. Both schools received swings and teeter-totters, plus soccer, volley-ball, baseball, and other games equipment. Every child received a bag of candy, an orange, and home-baked cookies baked by American women in Guadalajara, who backed the paraplegics' traditional Christmas observance.

Ray Foland, acting president of the Guadalajara PVA, was unofficial chairman of the "Santa Claus Crusade," with Rev. Paul G. Hunter, pastor of the United Church of Guadalajara, as his executive officer and assistant.

Membership grows

Rev. Hunter said, "When I came here three years ago, there were only about 40 paraplegics in this area, and they were just looking for a way to integrate into the American community. Today there are more than twice that number, and they have become an influential and important segment of the American community. In fact, no American effort in Guadalajara is going to get off the ground without the paraplegics' support."

Paraplegia News February 1966

PVA Clubhouse A "First"

The men of the Mexico Chapter of the Paralyzed Veterans of America (PVA) are not content to just sit around.

Rather the 100 or so members, all of whom have suffered injuries or diseases of the spinal cord, have done what almost every other group in Guadalajara said they themselves would do first—they bought a clubhouse.

After three years of planning, the PVA purchased a fully accessible building with six rooms and two baths in the Ciudad Granja. The clubhouse is situated on over one-half acre of land with rooms utilized for offices, storage space and game area. There will also be an exceptionally large room suitable for meetings and bingo. The group intends to have a ramped swimming pool that can be used by all.

The purchase of the clubhouse sets a precedent in Guadalajara and serves as a further bond of unity for the men on "wheels."

The only chapter of the PVA on foreign soil, the group began to form in 1957 when a few "rebels" came to Guadalajara to "find new auras," since they "had nobody and nowhere to go," according to George Ray, president of the chapter.

The men came down to investigate the warmer climate, find cheap help and perhaps marry. According to Ray over 90 percent are disabled veterans with 75 per cent being injured while in service. After they are hurt, too many problems are created and what home life existed before, usually then fails, he said.

When the first men arrived in Guadalajara it was "almost like opening the frontier," according to Ray. Many Guadalajarians agree with this statement although they have said the men lived like it was the wild west. The group began to acquire a bad reputation as many people claimed the men came down for marijuina and cheap liquor

Members of the group admit that this is how things were but also state it was because the men here had responsibilities only to themselves. However, as more men came from the States, commercial houses were established (where the men could live and receive help) and in 1963, the chapter of the PVA was formed.

According to Ray, "In those days a few people thought it would be a good idea to have a PVA chapter in Mexico but didn't know exactly why. Since those days they have found out why and have been progressively going forward to fulfill the high ideals and aims of the National Organization."

The group, which numbers upwards of 200 in the winter months, has advanced to a solvent organization with a net worth of over $30,000 pesos. The group has a service program a special fund for anyone in financial distress and has held annual Christmas parties for over 1,000 children.

Money for the clubhouse was raised by issuing bonds in denominations of 500 pesos and upwards. The chapter has pledged itself to pay 10 per cent interest annually on these bonds.

The Colony Reporter July 29, 1967

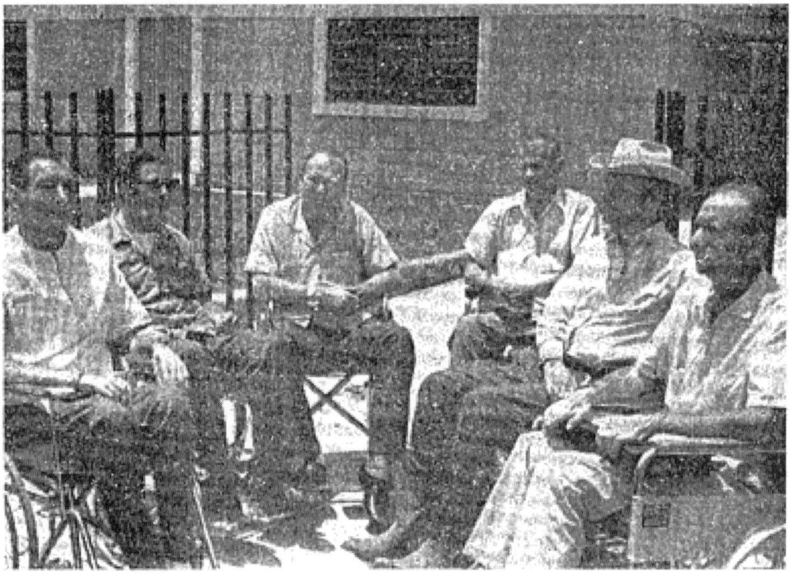

PVA members shown before their new clubhouse are (right to left) Ken Van Albert, Keith Zeigler, Carroll Stodgel, George Ray, Steve Wilson and Jack Myrick.

Colony Reporter July 29, 1967

Mexico PVA sharpens Clubhouse

Mexico Chapter PVA's Clubhouse in Ciudad Granja recently underwent alterations and improvements, according to *El Sombrero News*, the chapter's newsletter.

An arched doorway, between the fireplace and outside wall, now joins the main room with one of the game rooms, facilitating greater ease in handling crowds.

A public address system, featuring FM music from nearby Guadalajara, was installed with speakers in each room. Gas heaters also were installed.

Custom-made tables replace the former commercial tables, and new chairs have been purchased.

A bathroom and shower also have been installed in the caretaker's house.

Outside the Clubhouse trees and shrubs have been planted in the backyard. Walkways have been cleared across the center island to permit access to the other side of the street.

The 75-member chapter holds its meetings, as well as weekly bingo games and drawings, at the Clubhouse.

Situated at Las Palmas 226, the Clubhouse has a restaurant and bar open to members and their visitors.

Paraplegia News March 1968

Mexico PVA fetes multos muchachos

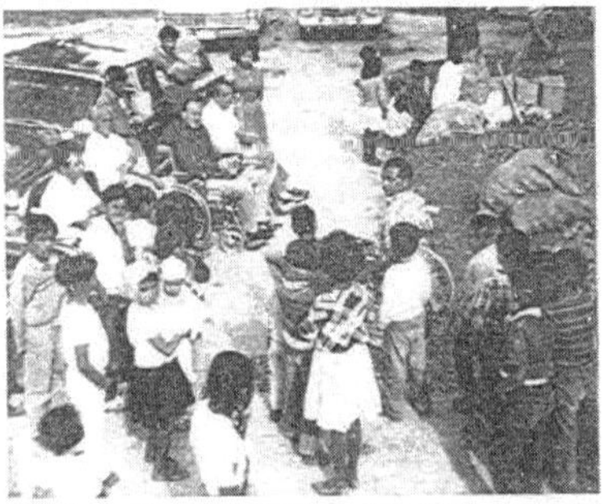

Members of the Mexico PVA join their guests at fourth annual Christmas party hosted by the wheelers for underprivileged school children in the Ciudad Granja area. Present somewhere in the photograph are PVA members Steve Wilson, Joe Miller, George Ray, prexy Bob Beilsmith, and Jerry Fesenmeyer.

The Mexico PVA chapter held its fourth annual Christmas parties for groups of underprivileged children at two schools in the Ciudad Granja area of Guadalajara. The chapter's new clubhouse is located in Ciudad Granja.

The parties featured the traditional breaking of pinatas, with candy and fruit for 1,100 boys and girls. PVA members also presented the two schools with an assortment of sports equipment.

According to chapter secretary Raymond R. Foland of Guadalajara, the chapter has now begun gathering used clothing in preparation for distribution to needy individuals in the Guadalajara area.

Individuals or groups interested in helping collect clothing may contact: *Mexico PVA, 226 Las Palmas, Ciudad Granja, Guadalajara, Jalisco, Mexico,* or *George Ray, Cubilete 147, Colonia Chapalita, Guadalajara, Jalisco, Mexico.*

Paraplegia News February 1968

1,100 Guadalajara children attend parties

Members of the Mexico PVA held their annual children's Christmas parties in the city of Ciudad Granja, the Guadalajara suburb in which their chapter clubhouse is located.

More than 800 children were feted at the local public school on Dec. 10. The following day a second party was held for almost 300 boys and girls at the Catholic school.

In addition to breaking of the traditional Mexican pinatas, each child received a Christmas bag of fruit and candy. Playthings included balls and jump ropes. Through the chapter, 60 school "uniforms" of heavy duty blue pants and a white short-sleeved shirt were donated to boys of the Catholic school. Dress material for the girls was supplied to parents.

Ed Lucier of Guadalajara was in charge of the annual Christmas parties.

Mexico PVA undertakes community project

"Free Wheelers" — that's the title of a Mexico PVA chapter project originated by honorary member Ben Borish and life member Jack Lastor, both of Guadalajara.

Purpose of the project is to provide wheelchairs for use of needy disabled Mexican nationals of the Guadalajara area. According to Raymond R. Foland, chapter secretary, the project is rapidly gaining support among the many U.S. citizens residing in the area.

Chairs have been donated to two charity hospitals which previously had no wheelchairs for use of their patients. The recipient institutions, according to the Guadalajara *Colony Reporter,* are the Zapopan and Guadalajara Civil Hospitals.

Chairs scarce

Individual chairs also have been donated to an 11-year-old boy and a 14-year-old girl, both of whom have never walked nor used a wheelchair before.

A major problem encountered by project personnel is the scarcity of used wheelchairs in Mexico, Foland said.

Interested persons may write to: *Ben Borish, Siete Colinas 1512, Colonia Independencia, Guadalajara, Jalisco, Mexico.*

Paraplegia News February 1969

The following 4 pages are from *Ebony*, January 1972

MEXICO:
A HAVEN FOR DISABLED VETS

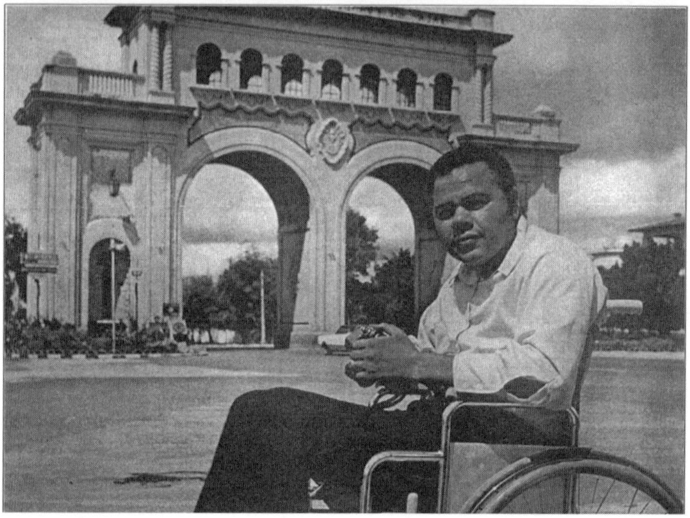

Guadalajara is favorite spot for growing number of American blacks

By Louie Robinson

IT IS only 590 miles to the U. S. border at Laredo, but for many who have chosen to make Guadalajara, Mexico, their home it is a world away—a world of difference in time and how it is used, in money and what it will buy, and in the faces of the people who look upon them in the solitary confinement in which their bodies have imprisoned them.

Lying deep inside the country, it is a tourist attraction, a railroad, trucking and cigaret manufacturing center, a repository of opal mines and granaries, a city of silversmiths, leather craftsmen and pottery makers. Its more than one million population, including some 30,000 to 35,000 U. S. citizens, makes it Mexico's second largest city.

Among the Americans are many who have battled death and achieved an uneasy truce. They will never again be the men they were, but they have at least escaped with their lives, however changed those lives may be.

These are men (and some women) who have spent time in military service of their country, and now, ironically, find life more tolerable away from their country. Some are bitter. Some are not. Some are emo-

Top photo: "Eugene Martin Cater, one of American disabled war veterans living in Mexico, sight sees near Guadalajara's Hospitality Arch which welcomes visitors to the historic city."

MEXICO *Continued*

tionally dispassionate. The demands their adopted home makes upon them are only minor inconveniences, such as learning—or acquiring at least a passable knowledge of—the language, or having to return to the border every six months for a new tourist card, or not being able to purchase property except through a Mexican national, or being deprived of U.S. television.

Some of the veterans who have chosen Guadalajara are more fortunate than others. They simply have taken to its gentle clime and low cost of living. Their minds and bodies are intact, perhaps disturbed only occasionally by some distant irritating memory.

For others, the injuries are deep and permanent. Their lives are endless days of pain, medication, sexual frustration, confinement and the indignity of having to be lifted and wheeled about. And they live each day with a dread statistic: the life-expectancy of a man who suffers spinal damage is 15 years from the day of his injury. For these men, there are no more truly good times, but in Guadalajara they seem to find the bad times just a little more bearable.

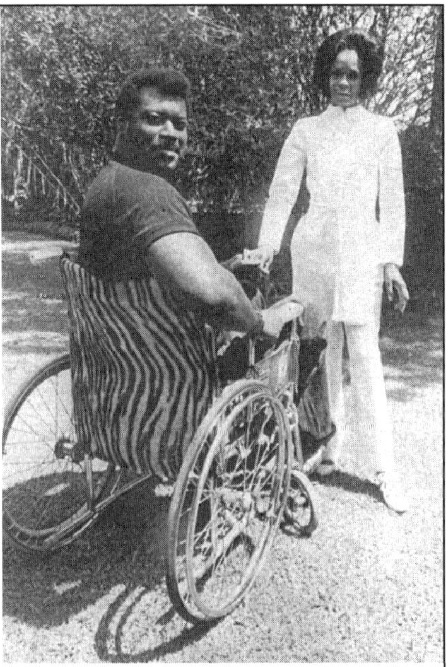

THIRTY-FOUR-YEAR-OLD Thomas Berry was a young Air Force enlistee serving at Roswell, N. M., in the late '50s when the truck in which he was riding on a flight line had a blowout and crashed. He suffered a head injury. "My actions weren't too rational after that," he says today, so he was discharged from service in 1957. Several years later, he suffered a fall that left him paralyzed below the waist.

Sixteen years ago, Berry visited Juarez, Mexico, and since then had "always planned on coming back." Later, some friends in a New York hospital where he was confined after his fall made plans to go to Mexico. Berry did not join them. But today, after two years in Guadalajara, he and his wife, Shirley, also a New Yorker whom he married five years ago, have taken over an 18-apartment complex which they have named *La Casa de la Amistad* (Friendship House) where living quarters and board are offered to people in wheelchairs for $160 a month.

Although Berry volunteered for military service at the age of 17, he says that, if he were a young man today, he "wouldn't go to war; I'd take the stand Muhammad Ali took."

Many things have happened to bring him to that opinion. "When I was first in service," Berry explains, "I was prepared to do anything they told me regarding protecting the United States. Being an American meant a great deal to me then. But I couldn't relate to the United States now—militarily, politically, racially. I'm an American, and if America really wanted me and showed it did, I'd be all for it. But I'm not going to give up my manhood, my dignity, for some place that shows it didn't want me the way I am. Down here, they have a community of people who are in wheelchairs. I get along better with them even though they are mostly white. I don't stand out down here. Back home, I used to even dress up to try not to look like a beggar. Once I had a bottle of beer in my hand and a man tried to drop a quarter in it. That bugged me."

Not only was Berry dissatisfied with what was happening to himself in the U. S., but he also disliked what he saw happening to others. "Blacks are hurting blacks in Harlem," he declares. "It's not just whites against blacks. Everybody seems to be trying to climb all over everybody else. You don't have that down here. It's no Utopia, but it's the best place I've found."

Photo top left: "Thomas Berry and wife, Shirley, enjoy Mexican sun in their yard. Unlike some paraplegics, he has not hired a personal aide to help him care for himself and to get around. 'I'm his personal aide,' his wife says."

TEXAS-BORN George Hicks, 53, who was reared in Denver and later lived in Oakland, Calif., spent only nine months on military duty during World War II. Except to say that in 1959 he underwent an operation "that didn't turn out too well," he prefers not to discuss the disability that causes him to spend the rest of his life in a wheelchair.

Hicks has lived for the last two years in Guadalajara with his two teen-age sons on a non-service-connected disability pension and Social Security.

"Money problems primarily caused me to come," confides Hicks, who was divorced from his wife after his paralysis. "My income goes a little farther down here."

For $120 a month, he and his sons, Raymond, 15, and Frank, 13, live in a modern four-bedroom apartment which Hicks admits is "really too large for us, but at the same time I have ample space for maneuvering the wheelchair."

In addition to food being cheaper (except for dairy products and meat), servants are plentiful and cheap. Hicks has a maid but he does a good deal of the cooking. Because he has good use of his arms, can drive his own car and is "pretty independent," he does not employ a personal aide, although he could hire one on a 24-hour-a-day basis for a fraction of the $400 to $500 it would cost him monthly for such help just eight hours a day in the U. S. "The things I require in the States, I couldn't afford in the States," he says.

Weather is another factor for Hicks, as it is for all the paraplegics. "In a wheelchair, you couldn't very well fight snowballs," he says, laughing as he remembers U. S. winters.

But there are other aspects of being wheelchair-bound in the U. S. which Hicks remembers. "When you're in a wheelchair and things happen to you," he says, "you can't fight it. If somebody does something you don't like, you can't walk away from him. If you want to go somewhere and there are steps, you can't climb them (There are many ramps for wheelchair-users in Guadalajara). I've been to football games in San Francisco, and after the game is over and everybody is trying to leave, people see you in a wheelchair and still they seem to try to walk right over you."

EUGENE Martin Carter, at 36 a veteran of 12 years in a wheelchair, has his own feelings about Mexico vs. the United States for those disabled like himself. "This is home," he declares as he sits in his $120-a-month, one-bedroom apartment that has a den, patio and neatly landscaped back lawn. "Here, if you have the ability, you can make it. The wheelchair doesn't matter. In the States, they throw all kinds of things at you."

Carter is a bright, studious young man who was graduated from Mississippi's Tougaloo College then studied law for three years at the University of Mississippi. An Army veteran, he was returning to his home in Leland, Miss., after a short stint with the Active Reserve in Montgomery, Ala., when the jeep in which he was riding overturned. He wound up a paraplegic.

Carter went back to school the next year, but later he forsook both his law studies and the United States for a number of reasons—some of them concerning the present U.S. administration—and came to live in Guadalajara a year ago. "I know the laws," he says. "They've been on the books, but who the hell is going to enforce them? Surely not Nixon."

In Guadalajara, Carter, who has a personal aide, cook and gardener, keeps himself busy studying (he speaks five languages), writing a history of the development of the political economy of Mexico, and outlining another book which he calls *Capitalism: Black Man's Burden*. "When you're in a wheelchair," he says, "you have to be highly motivated. Otherwise you just sit and look out the window."

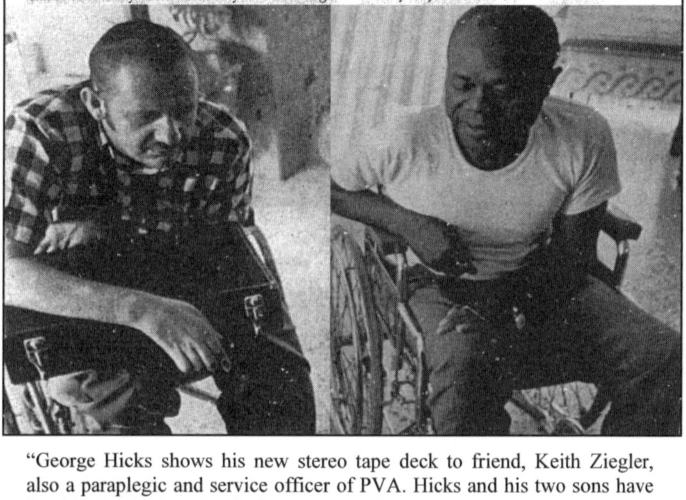

"George Hicks shows his new stereo tape deck to friend, Keith Ziegler, also a paraplegic and service officer of PVA. Hicks and his two sons have lived in Guadalajara for the last two years."

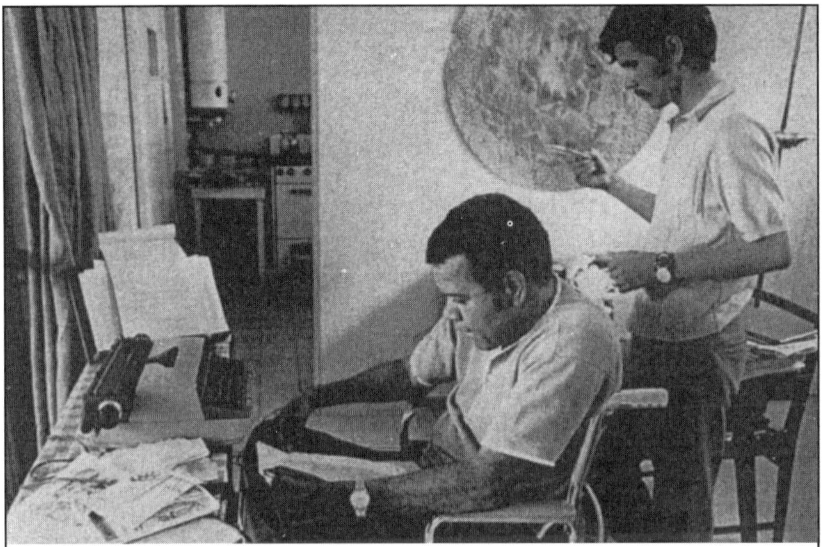

MEXICO Continued

Carter feels especially benefited by Guadalajara's climate. "Humidity drains me in the United States," he explains. He also finds medical care easier to come by in Mexico. "You can hardly get into a VA hospital at home," he says. "They're loaded with Vietnam guys."

Although he feels he could live on his pension income in the U. S., Carter admits that he had to "tone down a little." In Guadalajara he says that he manages very well but cautions: "You have to redefine what your needs are."

Gene Carter redefined his needs in other ways, too, and one, he found, was to get away from family ties. "There are 10 of us," he explains. "I knew I had to break the connection. The family wanted to help me so much that they were stifling me."

Although the general pace of life, if not that of motorists, appears to be considerably slower in Mexico, Carter seems to work and study with a fervor that is distinctly American and almost as if he is trying to fulfill some need deep within himself. But he says this has always been his style, and he chooses to minimize any effect his paralysis would have on that style. "I wasn't born in a wheelchair," he says. "I lived 24 years without it. But I know I'll be in it the rest of my life. I have no hopes of walking."

Top Photo: "Eugene Martin Carter was paralyzed when jeep overturned as he returned from Reserves training. He works on book with help of personal aide, Ernesto S. Ahor."

News stories depict life of U.S. vets in Mexico

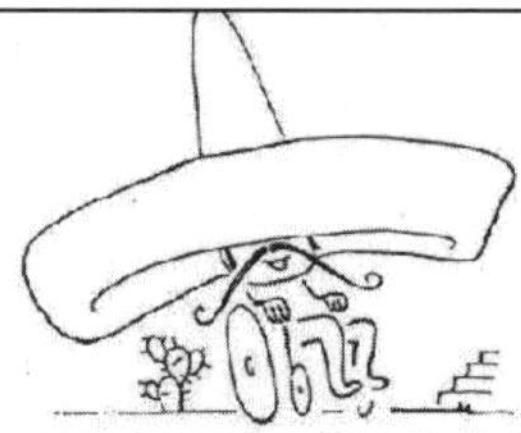

The paraplegic and retired colony of United States veterans in Guadalajara, Mexico, has received attention in U.S. newspapers during recent months.

The veterans help form one of the largest concentrations of North Americans in Mexico, living in the Guadalajara "in harmony and serve as a welcomed boom to the nation's economy," according to Associated Press writer John Platero. About 10,000 U.S. citizens, mostly retirees, live in Guadalajara, the capital city of Jalisco State. About 4,000 more reside in smaller nearby towns such as Chapala, Ajijic, and Chula Vista.

About 200 partially or totally disabled U.S. veterans live in the capital city, according to New York *Times Service* writer Richard Severo. Among them is a former WAVE, Paula Veilleux, who is quadriplegic as a result of a spinal injury sustained in an auto accident near San Francisco in 1961. A resident of Guadalajara since 1966, Miss Veilleux is vice president of the Mexico chapter of the Paralyzed Veterans of America.

Clubhouse

Since the establishment of the paralyzed veterans group after World War II, the PVA chapter has built a clubhouse in Ciudad Granja at which meetings, bingo games and other entertainments are held. The chapter also treats Mexican school children gifts and refreshments, during various holiday seasons, and has provided wheelchairs for needy disabled children of the area.

Known as the "Pearl of the West," Guadalajara ranks as the country's second largest city with a population of 1.3 million and boasts a subtropical climate that never does not vary more than 10 degrees throughout the year. It is said to resemble a big "little town," clean and quaint and with the cost of living lower than Mexico City and other tourist spots.

Dramatic evidence that the living costs are much lower than those in the United States is the fact that one can live for as little as $4 a day, according to writer Platero. At the same time, the capital city offers fine medical care, hospitals with modern facilities, and abundant cultural activities.

Spanish and English

One veteran said that the Mexican people are wonderful — "they try so hard to help and you don't have to know Spanish." The city features an English language radio station and English newspapers, its menus are in both Spanish and English, and many of the people speak both languages.

The average age of the U.S. "immigrants" is about 50 or older, it is estimated. Consul General W. B. Connett, Jr., said that many of those who retire in Mexico invest most or all of their capital within the country. Tom Germann, president of the local Disabled American Veterans group, added that disabled and paralyzed veterans probably account for about $100,000 a month of the city's economy. Less seriously injured veterans who cannot afford their own houses often live together.

Despite the sunshine and low prices, veterans are reminded periodically that they are living in a foreign country. Actually, all are on tourist status and are required to leave the country every six months. As one can imagine, such a law presents a major problem for sick veterans, who frequently must try to obtain special and possibly expensive dispensations from the Mexican authorities.

High tariff

Mexico's tariffs on imported goods also can be high. One veteran is said to have paid $150 duty on an imported wheelchair. Disabled American Veteran leader Germann told of being charged a duty of $10.24 on a cheese worth $7.75 including postage — a Christmas gift.

Veterans injured after discharge from service cannot receive remuneration for medical supplies purchased outside the United States. And if they want to work normally they would find it difficult to obtain Mexican work papers.

Paraplegia News February 1972

The following 2 pages are from *LA Times "West" Magazine* August 20, 1972

The Wheelchair Community of Guadalajara

It is a business transaction, the American, needing arms and legs, has learned that in his own country the rental comes too high. In Mexico, he can bargain for young men with sturdy limbs but scant prospects for the future.

The result is the wheelchair community of Guadalajara, where victims of automobile accidents, polio and multiple sclerosis have come to be hoisted and borne by boys of the town. For these services they pay $50 or $60 a month. North of the border, the cost would be 10 times greater assuming that the same gentle care was available in an equally temperate climate.

War casualties have also been coming here for years. Thanks to Vietnam, their number is greater now.

Over the winter months 300 or more paralyzed Americans may be renting private houses or filling such wheelchair hotels as La Morada or Hacienda Las Fuentes or Lilian's. Dr. Anthony Williams, who operates the popular Villa del Sol, claims he can predict from the first letter inquiring about arrangements which of the Americans will like it here. If they ask too obsessively about dirt or drinking water, they are poor prospects for staying on.

Frank Stoppiello, a former Marine, did not come directly to Guadalajara after he was paralyzed in Vietnam. First he tried going home to West Orange, New Jersey, hanging around old haunts scaring up afternoon poker games. But his friends were all working. No one had time for a beer at 3 p.m. Down here, Frank says, "I can always roll around the corner and find somebody to make noise with."

And Frank found a wife, a spirited Mexican girl who, for all her verve, defers to her husband. "I don't think I could marry an American girl," he says. "They're too demanding."

Among the chairborne, courage is a quality taken for granted. When Keith Ziegler goes through the contortions of slipping on the hand brace that lets him drive his own car, no one who watches is murmuring encouragement. If they think anything as they see him struggle, it is that Keith is lucky to have a hand that, properly wired, is still serviceable.

About any American living here, there are two critical distinctions to be made, but neither concerns how he was injured. Older residents often aren't sure whether the young fellow they have known for years was cut down in Vietnam or on a California freeway. What does count is whether he is a "quad"—quadraplegic paralyzed from the neck down, or a "par" (pronounced "pair")—paraplegic and immobile only from the waist.

As a par, Stoppiello can function without an aide. Keith Ziegler depends on Roberto Rodriguez to lift him from wheelchair to car seat, to light his cigarette and raise a glass to his lips when Keith hasn't strapped on his hand brace.

It also matters supremely whether the catastrophe that left the man crippled was service connected. On the outskirts of the city, Ray Clifford, Bill Kahler and Jim Adkisson share a sunny bungalow. Ray was struck by a sniper at Chu Lai. No injury is more service-connected than that. Men in that category may draw between $1,100 and $1,200 a month. One of Ray's friends, another casualty of Vietnam, reports that by living here he can save $2,000 a year.

Bill Kahler survived months on an aircraft carrier in the Gulf of Tonkin to be injured three months after his discharge in a car accident. He must make do on his Navy pension and Social Security. Febrile, funny, bitter, Jim Adkisson was shot 11 years ago, age 19, while in college in Missouri. Totally non-service-connected, Jim must live entirely on an insurance settlement, at times scraping by on $200 a month.

When a man first rolls into town, the freedom of being loose in a foreign land—or the fright and finality of having reached this port—may keep him continuously drunk. Birthdays, holidays, anniversaries, there's always an excuse for a party here, and a man can avoid sobriety for months, if that's his best answer, without much censure or good advice.

Ken Ginsterblum, who operates La Morada from a power-driven chair, sometimes questions whether the younger men might not be better off back home, trying to stay competitive with their age group. But even he grants that anyone in a wheelchair will find a warmer response among the Mexican people. "Americans don't like to get involved. They want to stay away from anybody who's different," he says.

Tom Berry, a black par, misses the excitement of New York City, where he grew up, but not the harassment over race. "The United States is a good place to visit," he says, grinning.

Jimmy Lietz, except for his chair, could have stepped off a Pepsi-Cola poster. After an ambush in Vietnam in 1967 and the subsequent years here, he decided to investigate Cape Cod last summer and see what contact he could make with other Americans in their mid-twenties.

"I found I didn't mix at all with my own generation," Jimmy says. "They knew I was hurt in Vietnam, but when they found out that I wasn't angry and wouldn't condemn the war, they shied away from me."

Since it was Wednesday night, Bingo night, Jimmy had come out to the clubhouse of the Paralyzed Veterans of America, Guadalajara chapter. The game itself he doesn't much like. "But it beats staring at the walls."

Jimmy lives alone in a house with his Mexican aide, and he knows his own temperament well enough to get out regularly. "I've always believed that being hurt doesn't change a person," he says. "I was moody before, so there are still going to be days when I wake up feeling depressed."

Truism though it is, the happiest men here are the busiest. Keith Ziegler studies the Bible by mail, works for the P.V.A. and the Seventh Day Adventists, expands a large tape collection and plays with the two impish daughters of Josefina, the attractive woman he met and married here five years ago.

Questions of sex and marriage cause some anxiety and distress in the wheelchair community, exactly as among the world's walking. Nightclubs abound at Guadalajara — the Seven Leagues, the Honeymoon, Dandy, the Afro-Casino—and there are even more brothels. The wheelchair community occasionally frequents both. "I'm lucky," one polio victim says, "because I've still got feeling below the waist. But whenever some of the unmarried boys go out to a place, all of them will probably end up bringing girls back to their houses. No matter how bad they've been hurt, just seeing that nice smooth body next to them on the sheet seems to make them feel better." —*A.J.L.*

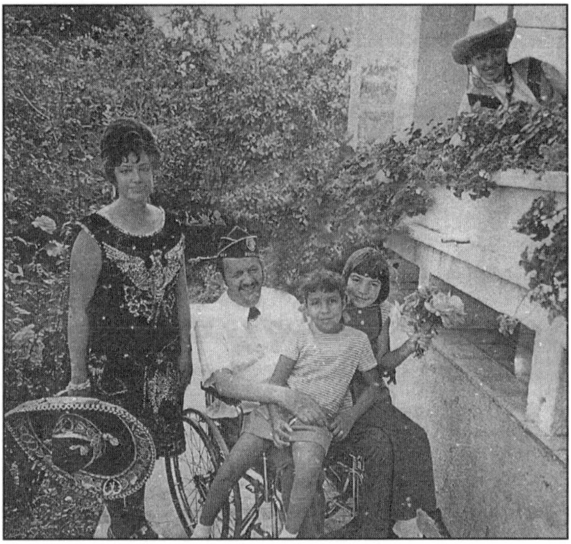

"Keith Ziegler is one of the luckier American veterans in the 'wheelchair community' of Guadalajara. Five years ago he married Josefina, a Mexican woman, (left); his new family now includes his helper, Roberto Rodrigez; he stepdaughters, Blana (holding flowers) and Anita; and his sister-in-law, Graciela Arana."

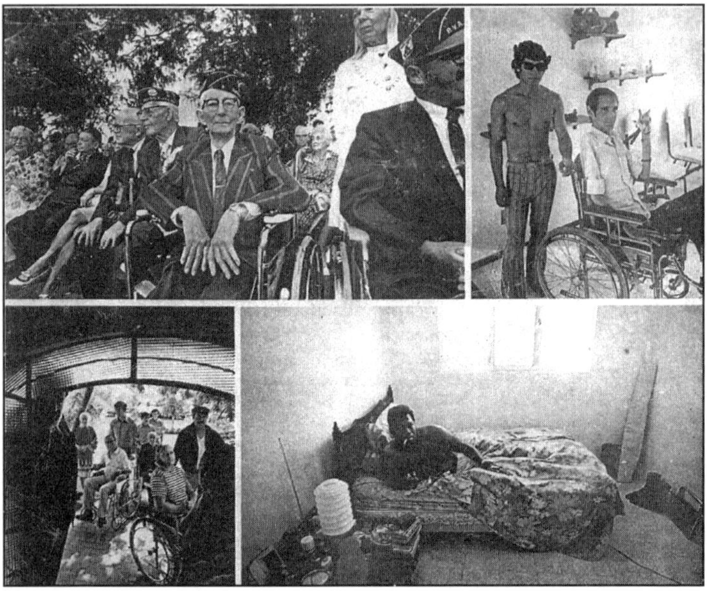

"Not all of Guadalajara's disabled Americans are Vietnam causalities. Some are veterans of long-ago wars (top left). Jim Adkisson (top right with his helper) and residents of Villa del Sol, the biggest of the 'wheelchair motels' (left), are among the non-veterans. Most, like Tom Berry (right), have no plans to return home."

Mexico PVA cited

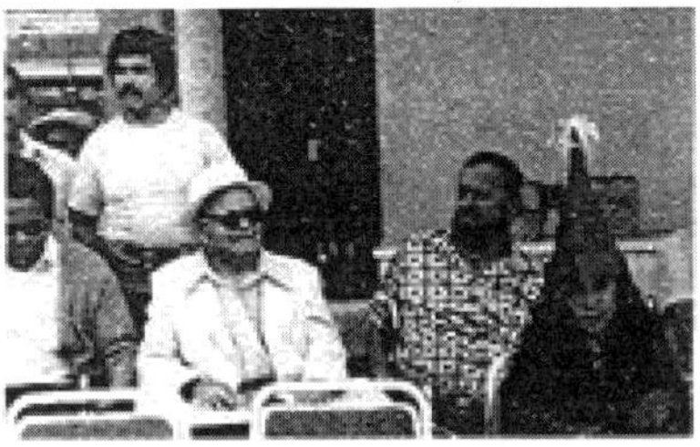

Charles Gilliam (in hat and sunglasses) and chapter president Keith Ziegler are flanked by co-chairmen Gene Carter (left of Gilliam) and Edward Lucier (far right) as Mexico PVA members view proceedings at Christmas party sponsored annually by chapter.

The Mexico chapter of PVA recently was cited in Guadalajara's English language newspaper *The Colony Reporter*, as well as the American Society's magazine *Armistad*, for its efforts in hosting Christmas parties for 1800 Mexican children in three primary schools in Jalisco.

The three schools, all located in relatively impoverished areas on the outskirts of Guadalajara, were presented with playground equipment this year. Each child also received gifts of fruit and candy in what has become a holiday tradition for the chapter and its members.

In the ten years during which the chapter has hosted Christmas celebrations at schools in the Guadalajara area, 20,000 children have enjoyed Christmas parties and treats. The project is funded almost entirely by donations from chapter members.

Paraplegia News March 1976

The following letter was received from Mrs. Sally Holmes, Public Relations Representative for the organization "Pesos for Braces" here in Guadalajara:

"Dear Commander Lietz and the Members of the PVA:

The organization of "PESOS FOR BRACES" wish to express our very sincere gratitude to you for your faithful contribution of $1,000 pesos.

Mr. Hunter told us that there are two boys who need help, one braces and shoes and the other one who needs shoes. When the boys come to the Hospital Civil for them we shall take pictures of them and you shall receive copies of them.

To date, this has been a busy year for this organization. We have two presentations a month and this is wonderful! Thank you very sincerely for your aid in this very important work."

El Sombrero News August 1978

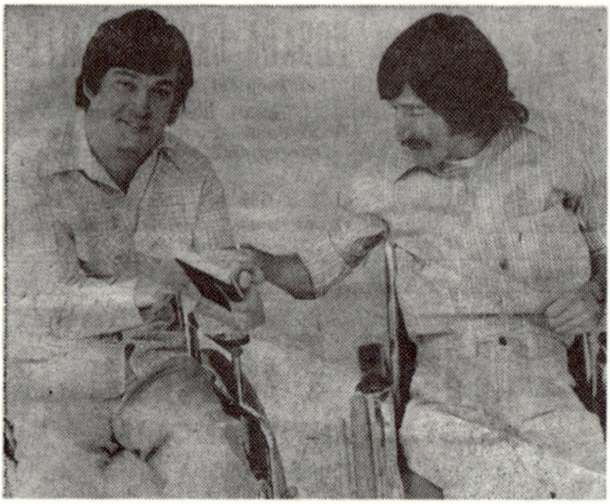

The Paralyzed Veterans of America, Mexico chapter, recently held its election of officers for the year 1979-1980. Newly-elected and installed president Jack Tumidajski (right), succeeds outgoing president Jim Lietz. (H. Croninger photo)

Paralyzed Vets Of America Install Officers And Announce Donations

The Paralyzed Veterans of America, Mexico chapter, held its installation of officers June 14 in the clubhouse, at Las Palmas 226, Ciudad Granja. Newly installed as officers were Jack Tumidajski, president; William Bailey, vice-president; Frank Stoppiello, secretary; and Edward Lucier, treasurer.

Annual donations presented at that time, totaling 11,000 pesos, went to Pesos for Braces; the Mexican Red Cross; the Associacion de Lisiados de Jalisco, A. C. (ALJAC); and the Guadalajara Blind Girl's School.

The annual George E. Ray member award was presented to both Jack Tumidajski and Edward Lucier for their service to the chapter during the previous year.

The Paralyzed Veterans of America, consisting of 69 veterans and 17 affiliate members, meet the second Thursday of each month, while the board of directors meets the last Thursday of each month, 5 p.m. at the PVA clubhouse.

The clubhouse will close for the months of July and August and will reopen in September. Regular fall hours of operation will be every Friday, from 4 to 11 p.m., with possible Monday and Wednesday hours to be added in October or November.

The Colony Reporter July 30, 1979

Photo Gallery

’50s Explorers and Pioneers

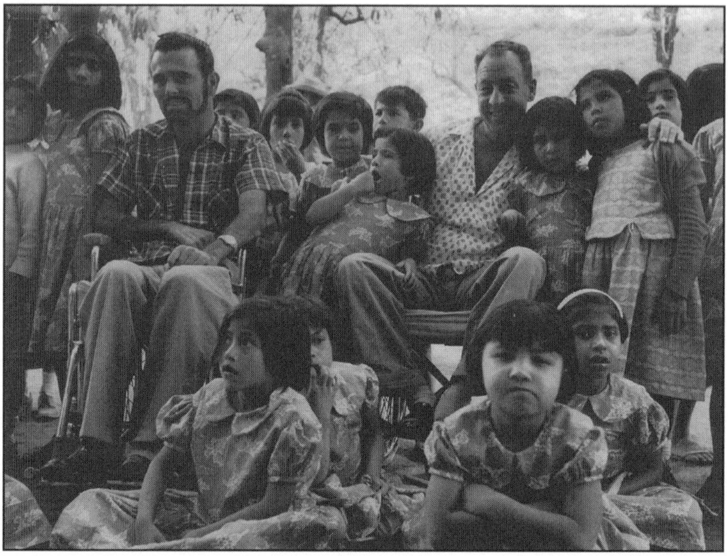

Mid-50s Pioneers Marion Fuget and George Small at the Hospicio Cabañas Orphanage in 1964

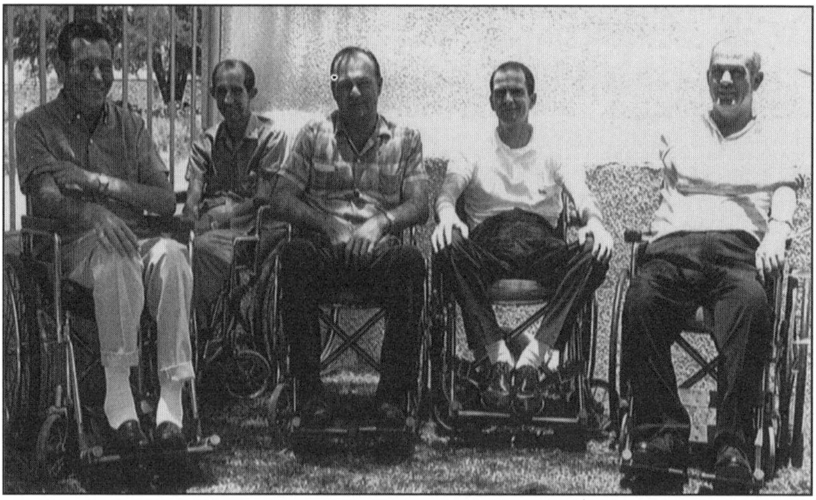

Jack Myrick (vice-president) with 50s Pioneers Ray “Doc” Foland (secretary), George Ray (president), Bob Barrett (treasurer), and Charles “Joe” Miller (immediate past president) make up the Mexico PVA’s slate of newly elected officers in June 1966

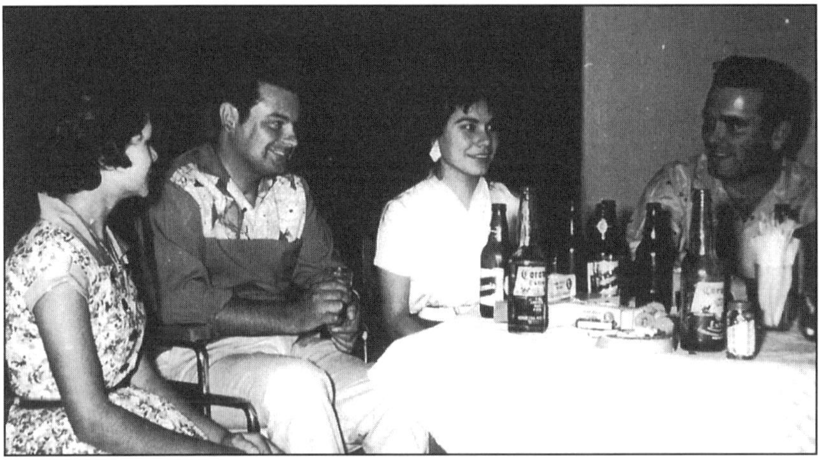

Mid-50s Quadalajara arrivals Tony Gomez and Marion Fuget socialize with some pretty señoritas

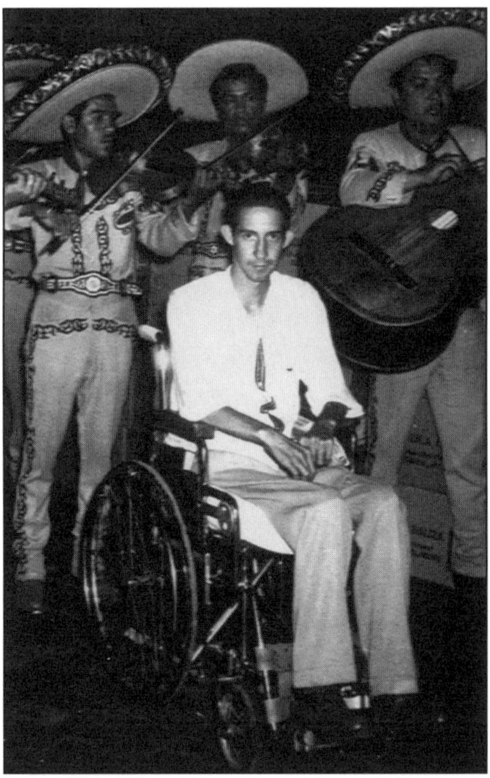

Ray "Doc" Foland with mariachis

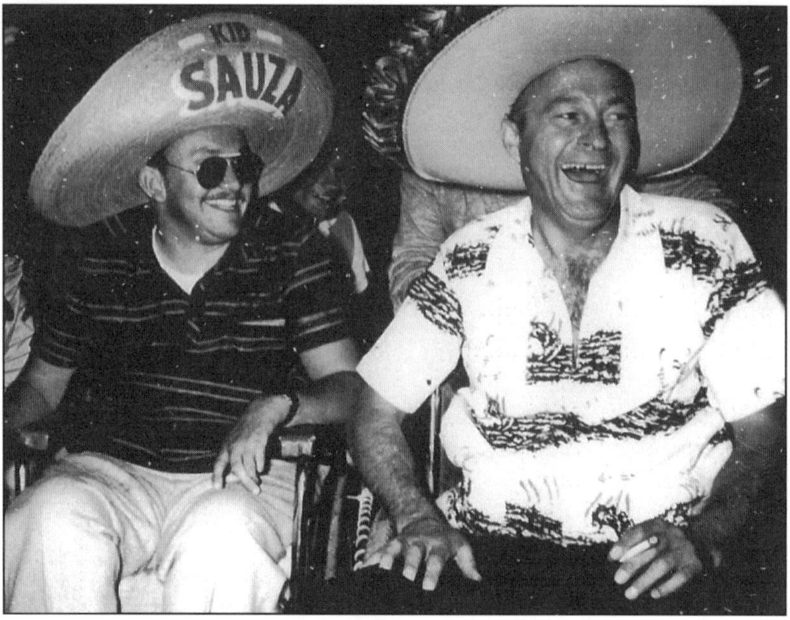

George Ray (on right) and future fellow gimp camp operator Bill Coe each arrived in the mid- to late-50s

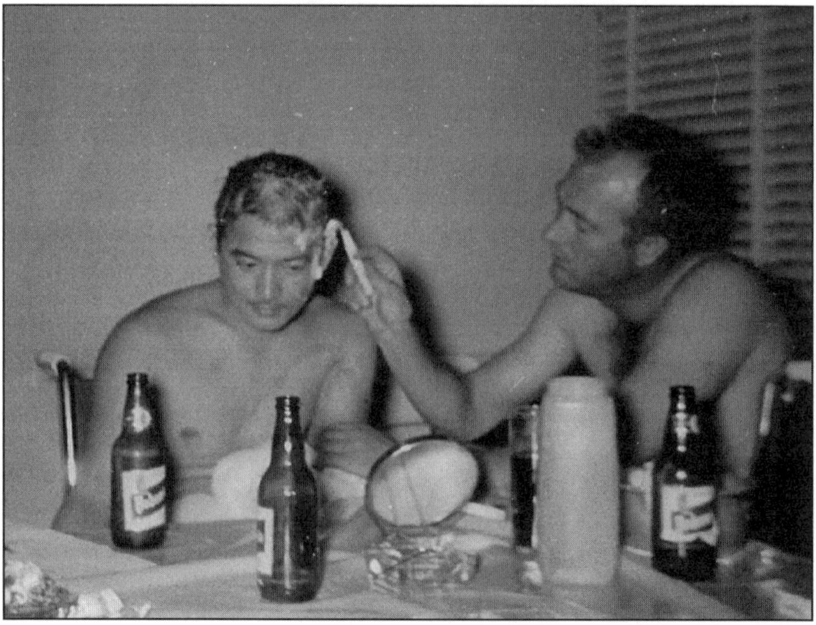

Tatsumi "Gato" Aragaki gets a trim from friend and fellow 1957 Pioneer George Ray

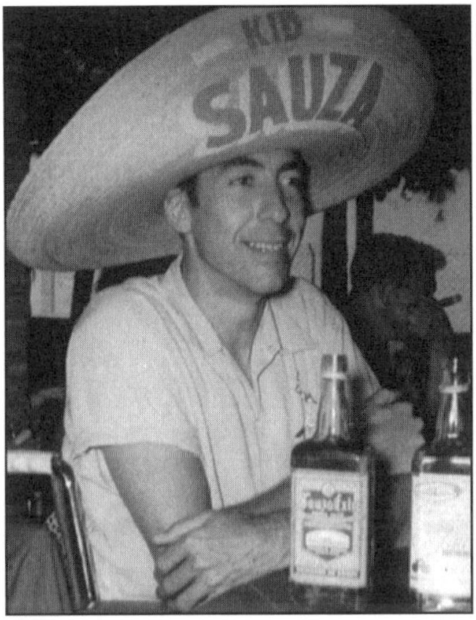

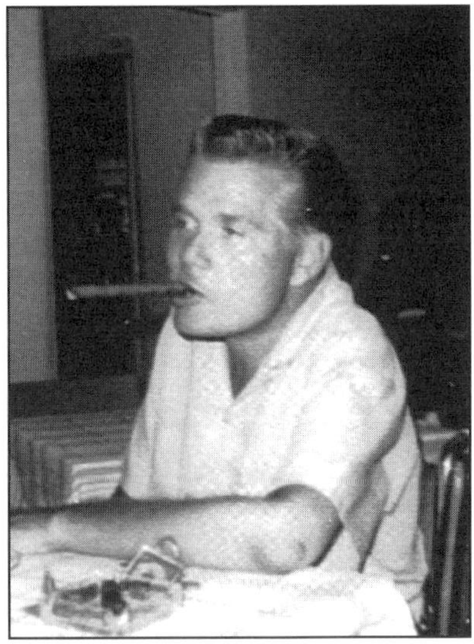

Patrick Wolf (left) and Bill Bailey found their way to George Ray's Place in March 1958

Wolf later returned stateside, while Bailey married a local señorita in October of that year and made Quadalajara his new home

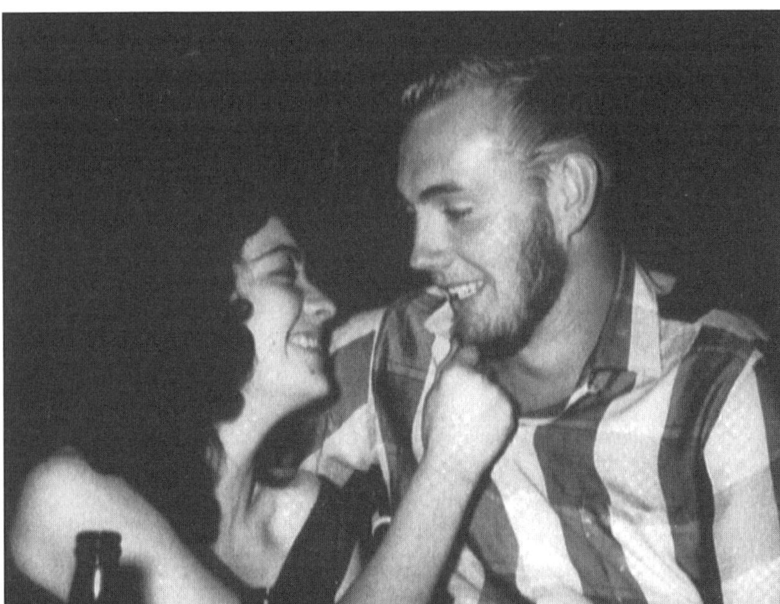

Pioneer Charlie Whestine and fiancée Anie married in 1959 and moved to Los Angeles a year later

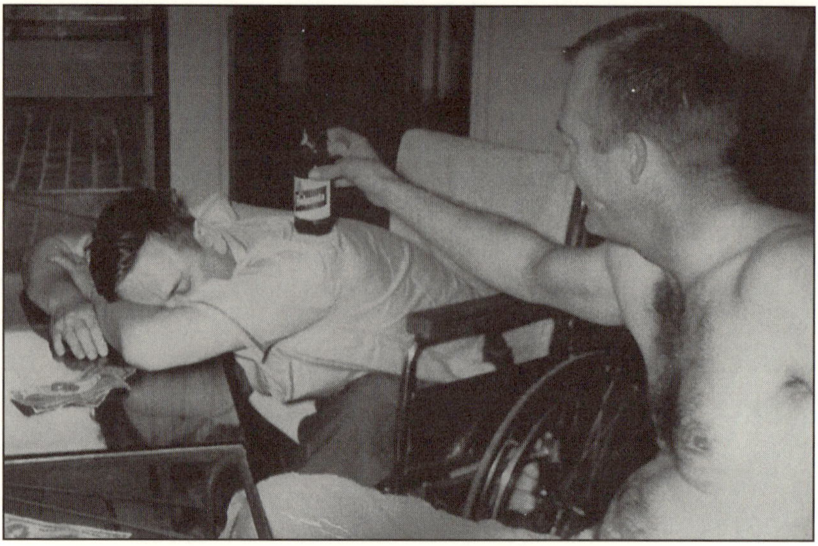

Quadalajara initiation
George Ray bids goodnight to an unidentified guest

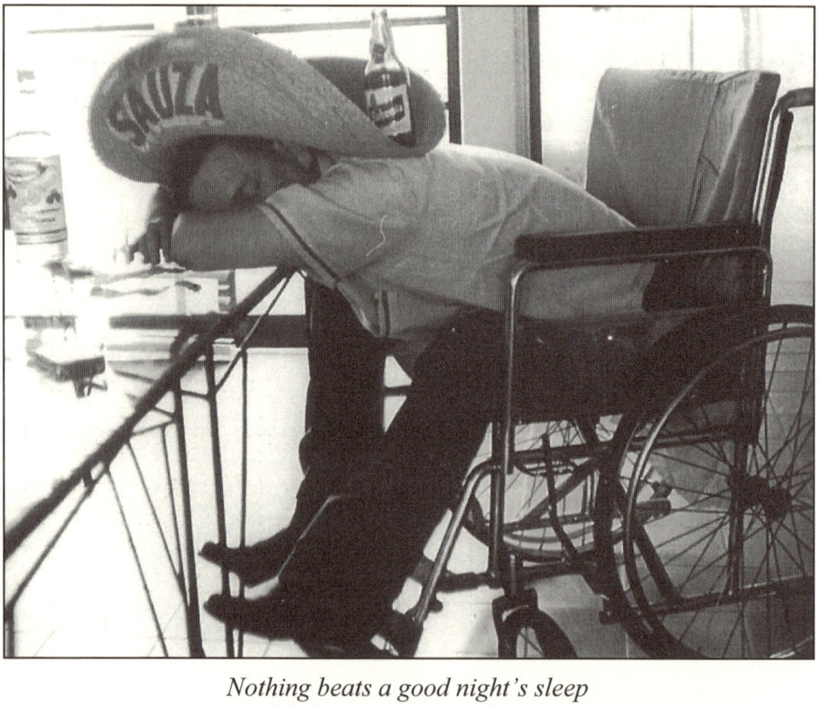

Nothing beats a good night's sleep
It is unclear if the still-sleeping guest woke up in time for breakfast

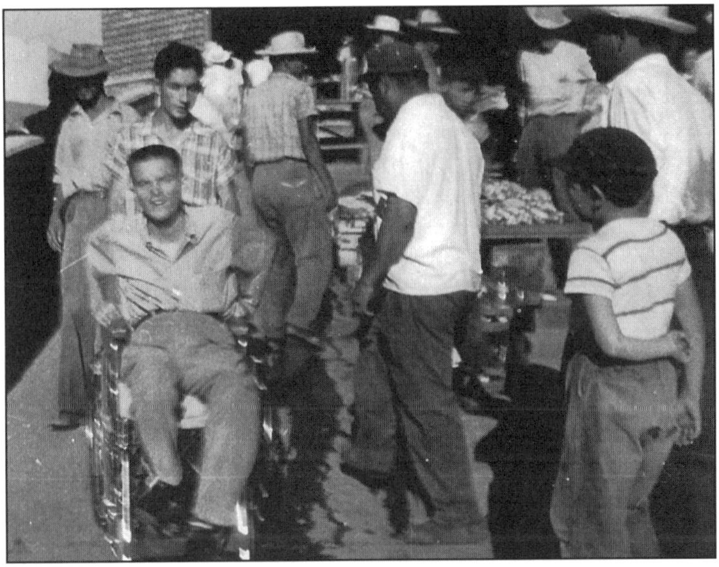

Pioneer Charlie Reno at Quadalajara's famous Mercado Libertad

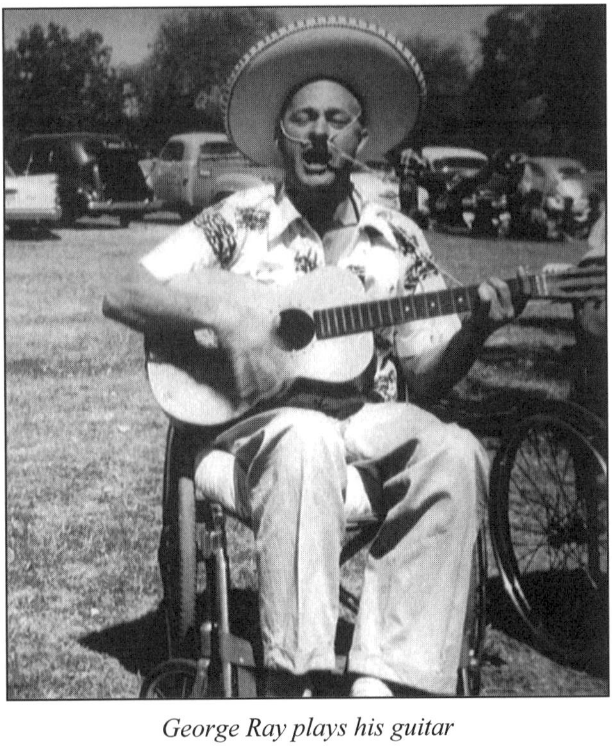

George Ray plays his guitar

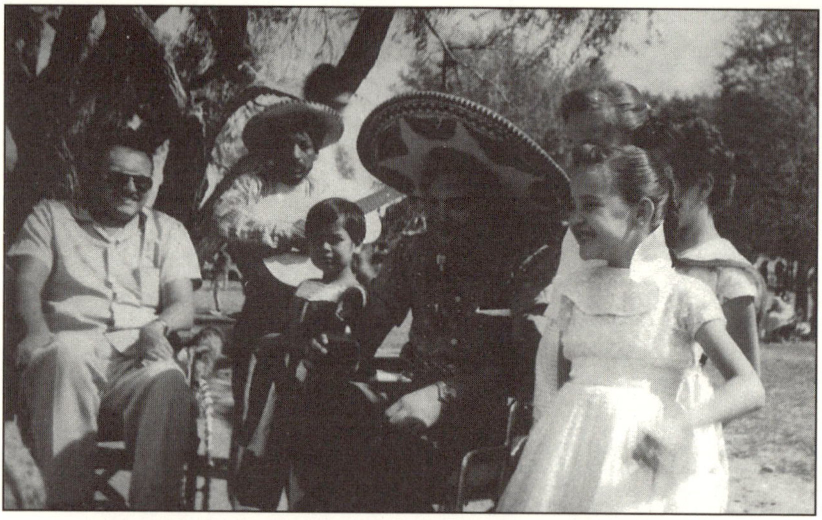

Bill Coe, Tony Gomez, and some pretty little friends

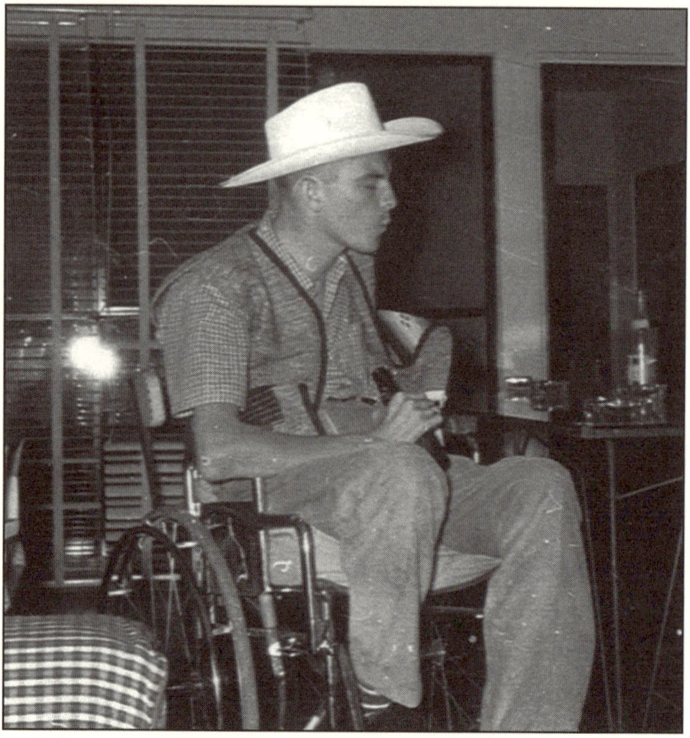

Charlie Reno "enjoys" a bit of solitude at home

'60s Pioneers: PVA and Purpose

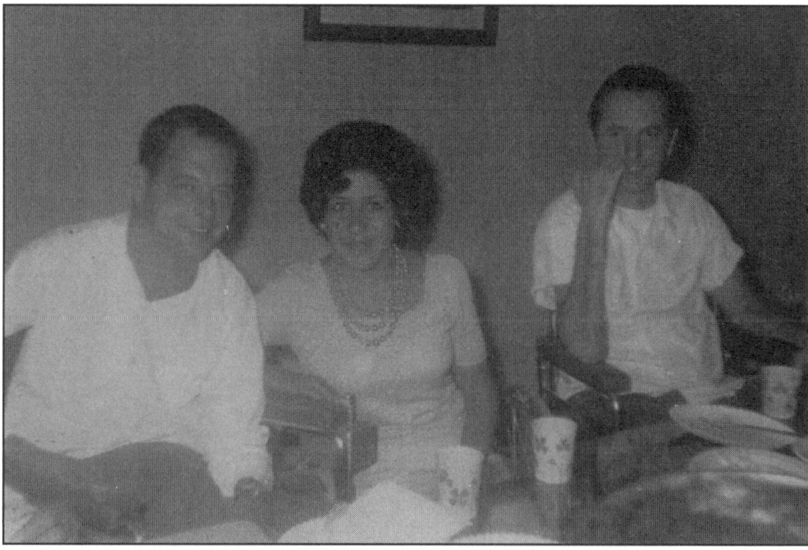

Bob Beilsmith with future bride Teresa and roommate Frank Vertinelli

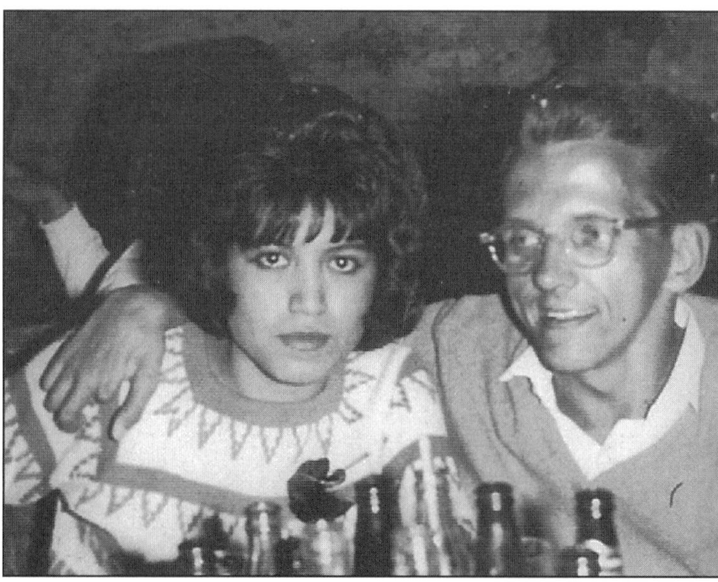

"Cookie" Meinberg with girlfriend

Meinberg, Beilsmith, and Vertinelli shared a three-bedroom house in 1962

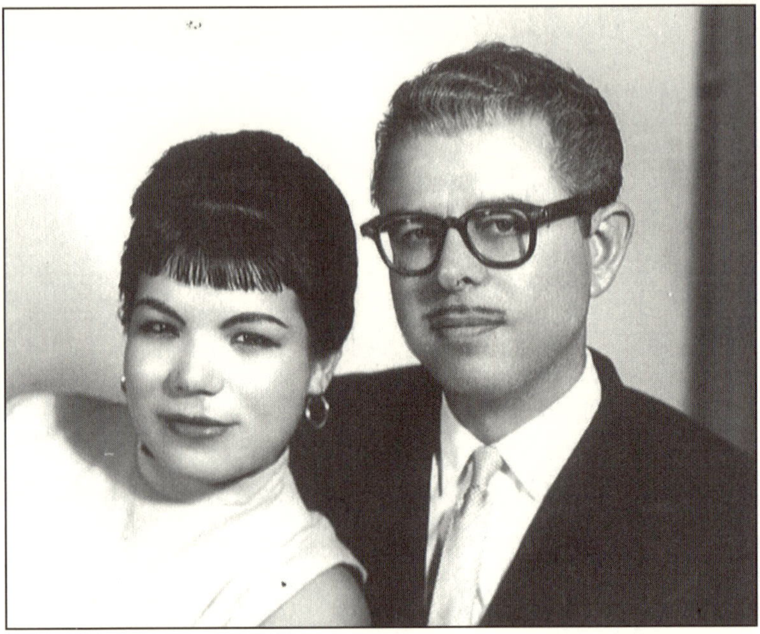

Bob and Suzy Harmon 1963
The Harmons and Beilsmiths would later live in the same Phoenix, Arizona neighborhood in the late-60s and early-70s

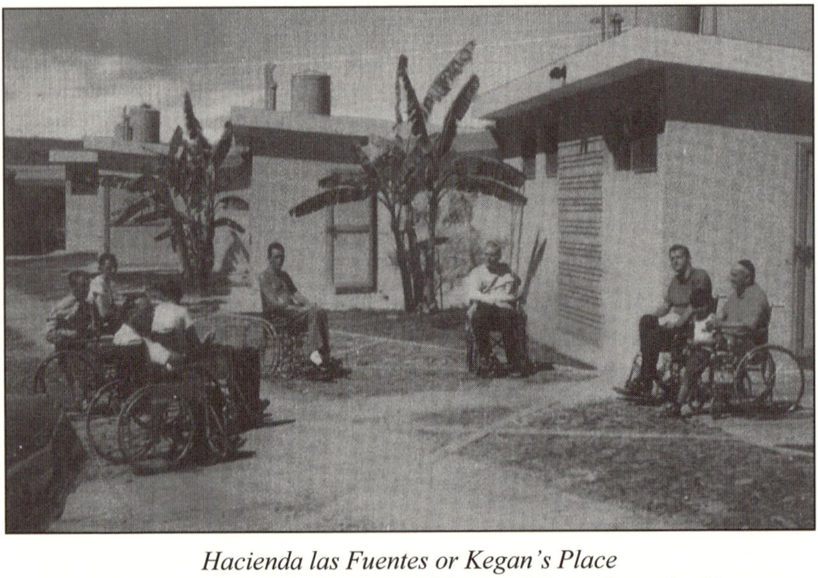

Hacienda las Fuentes or Kegan's Place
Opened by Larry Kegan (second from right) in the early-60s

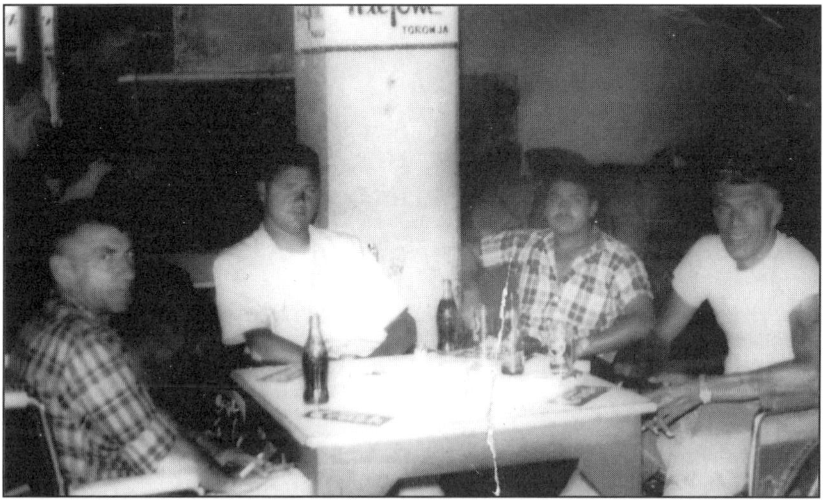

Tom (from Atlanta), Bob Enge, Gabriel Chavez, and Bob Beske, 1964

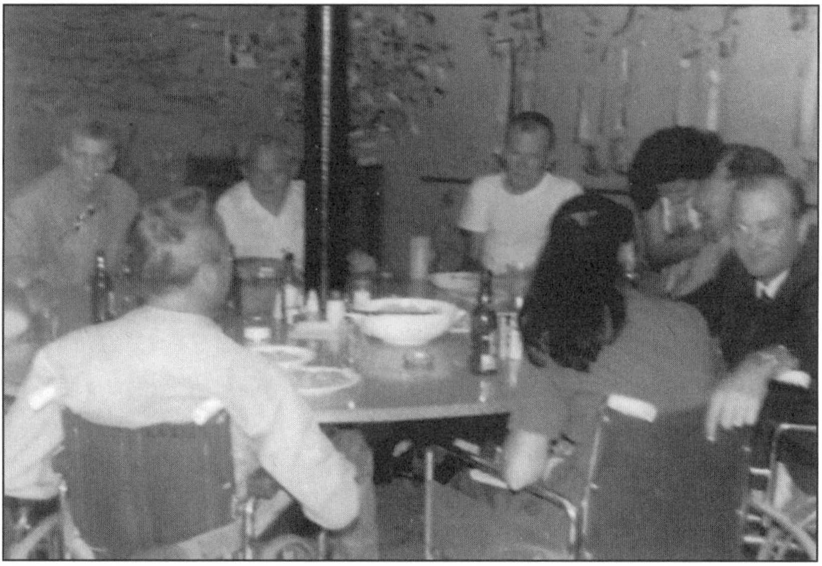

Bob Harmon (back turned), unidentified man, Charlie Ceska, Bob Powell, Eddie Lucier (whispering sweet nothings to unidentified guest), and George Ray (chatting with female guest) socialize at George Ray's Place, Cubilete #147

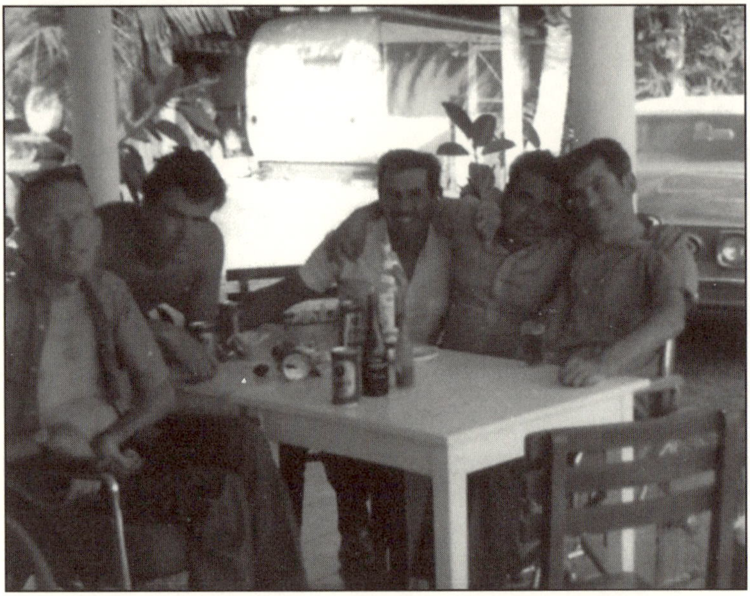

Bob Powell, Fernando, Florentino, Gabriel Chavez, and Eddie Lucier enjoy a trip to Manzanillo

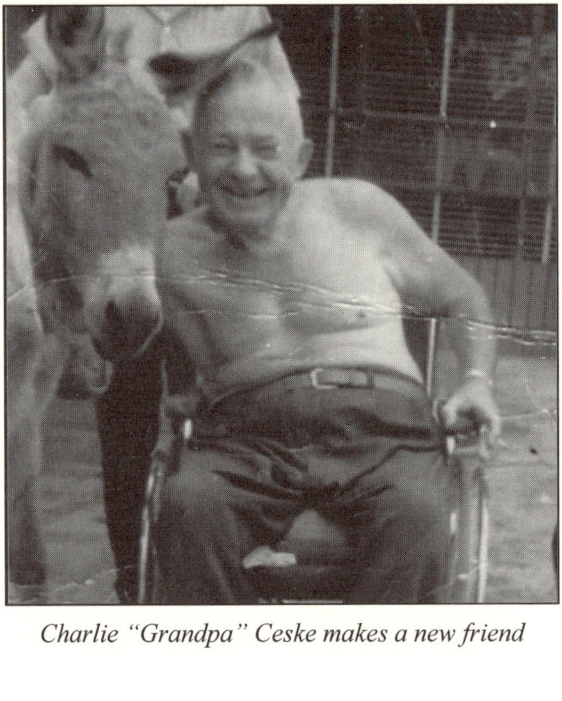

Charlie "Grandpa" Ceske makes a new friend

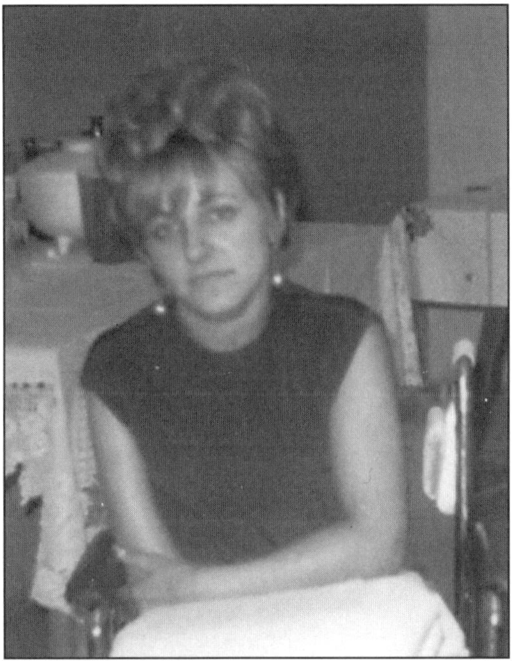

West Roxbury VA Hospital alumna Paula Veillieux

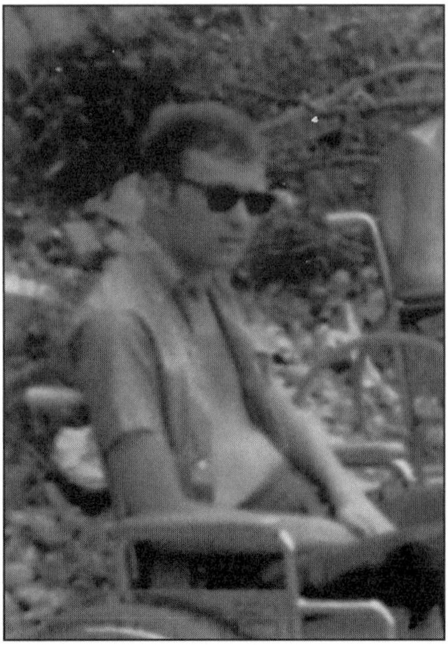

West Roxbury VA Hospital alumnus Arthur Wheaton

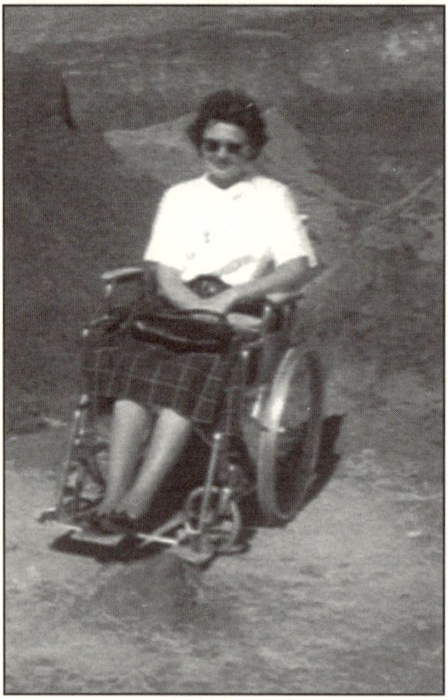

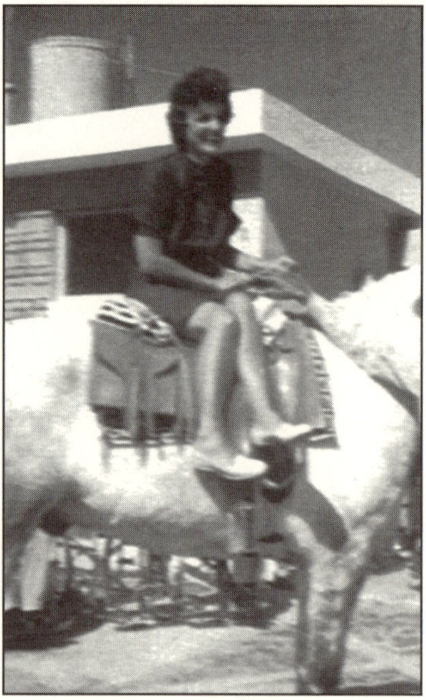

JoAnn Raway (Kirch) *Luella Raway gets a ride*
November 1964

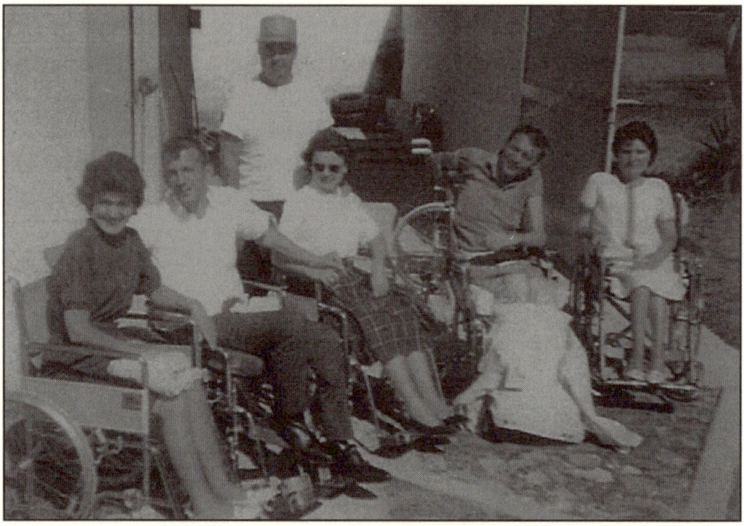

(left to right) Luella Raway, Larry Kegan, JoAnn Raway (Kirch), Tom Kirch, and Roselyn Mahowald enjoy a sunny day in paradise at Kegan's Hacienda Las Fuentes, November 1964

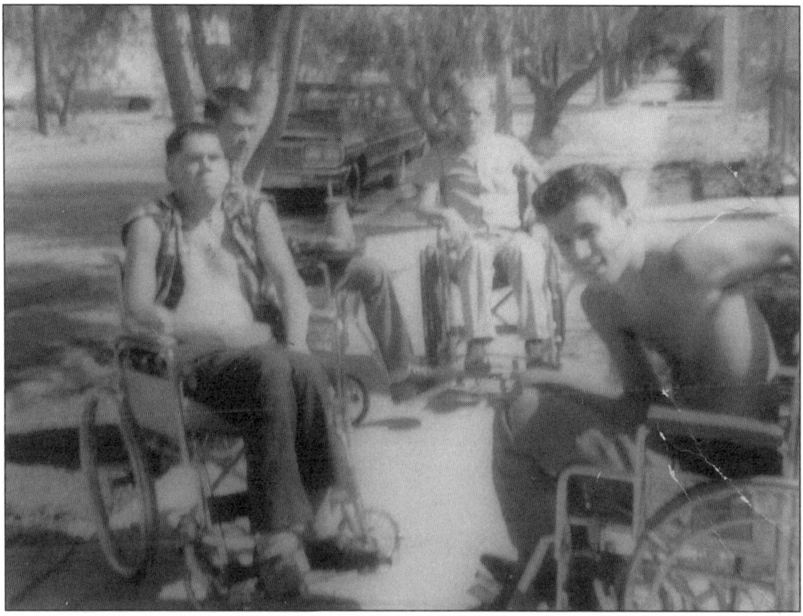

"The Men"—New Quadalajara arrivals Bart Corbett, Charlie Erickson (behind Corbett), Wisconsin's Kenny "Blanco" (nicknamed Kenny "Blanco" by the attendants because of his fair complexion), and Joe Cicero bask in the sunshine in front of La Morada (George Ray's Place), 1965

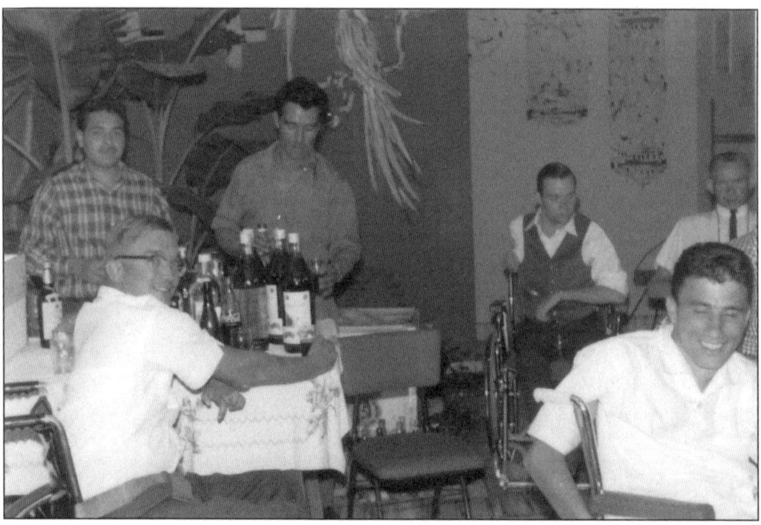

(left to right) Larry Blinn, Art Wheaton (with vest), George Seyfried (with tie), Cicero in foreground, Gabriel Chavez, and another unidentified attendant, 1965

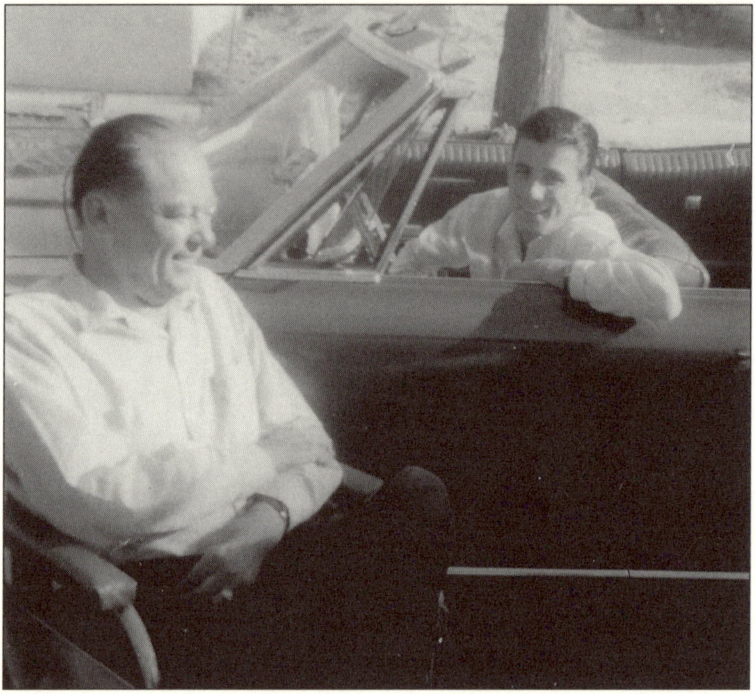

Frank Stocker receives visit from Joe Cicero in 1965 photo

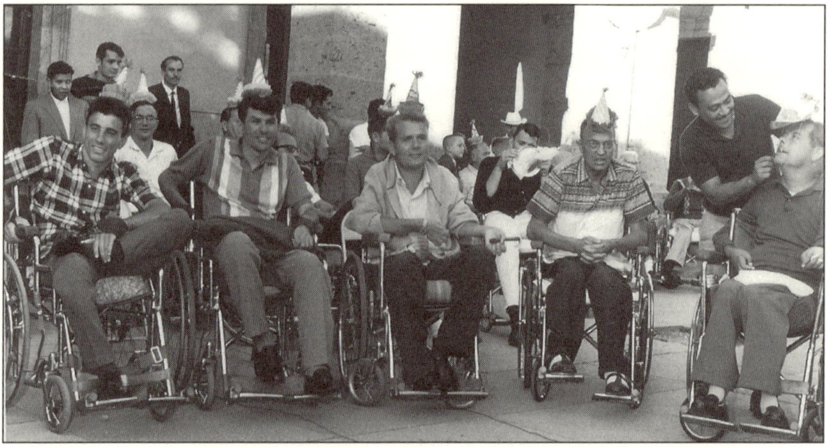

Joe Cicero, Eddie Lucier, Bill Bailey, unidentified Pioneer, and Bob Beilsmith (with others in the background), enjoy festivities at the Hospicio Cabañas Orphanage, mid-60s

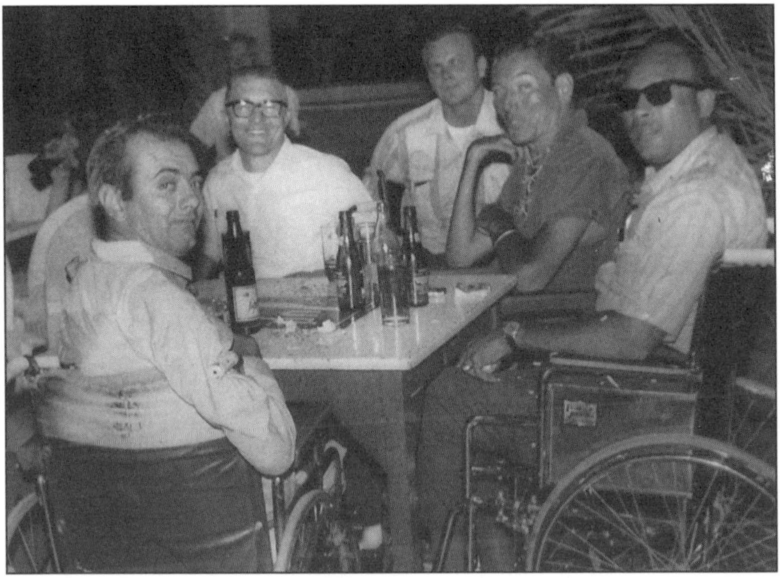

(left to right) Norman Frisk, Bill Christensen, Vern Thorson, Jack Myrick, and unidentified friend socialize in 1966

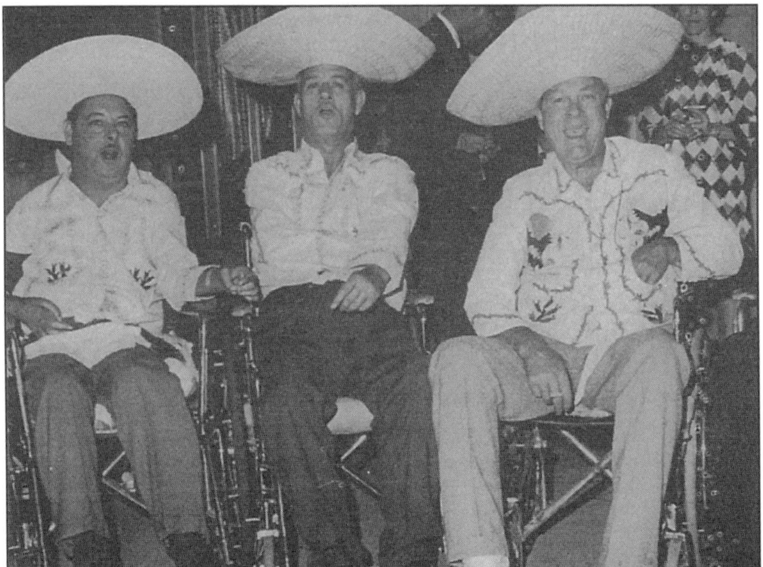

(left to right) Delegates Bob Beilsmith, Joe Miller, and George Ray from the Mexico PVA provide a south-of-the-border touch at National PVA Convention in Houston 1967

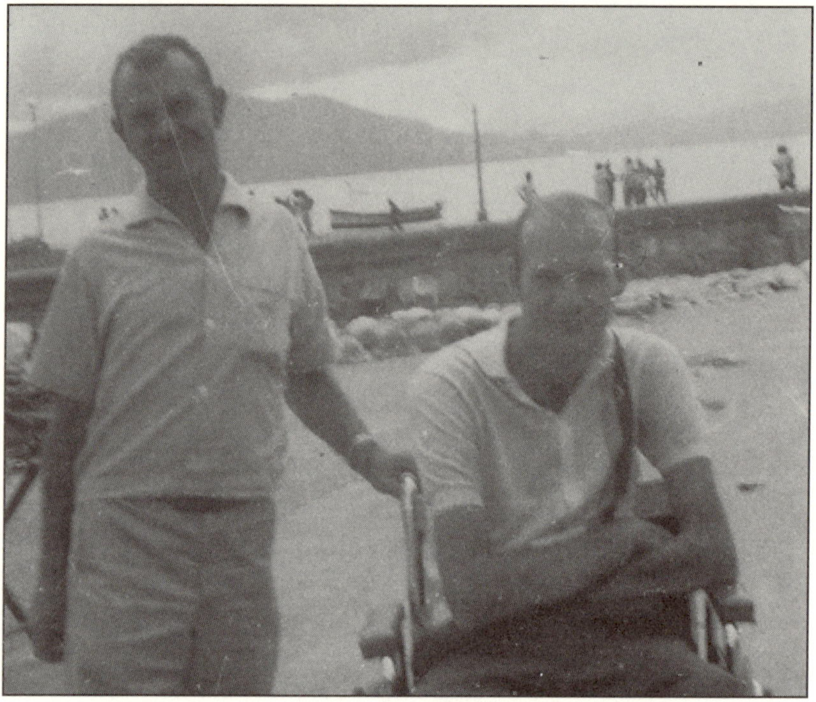

John Sniffen and Charlie Newbold with Lake Chapala in the background, late-60s

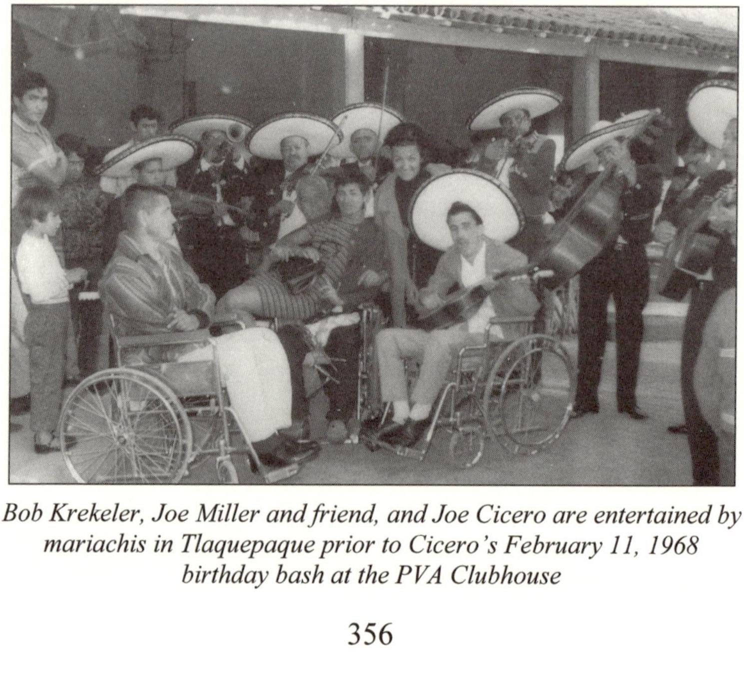

Bob Krekeler, Joe Miller and friend, and Joe Cicero are entertained by mariachis in Tlaquepaque prior to Cicero's February 11, 1968 birthday bash at the PVA Clubhouse

’70s Newcomers Mingle With Old-timers

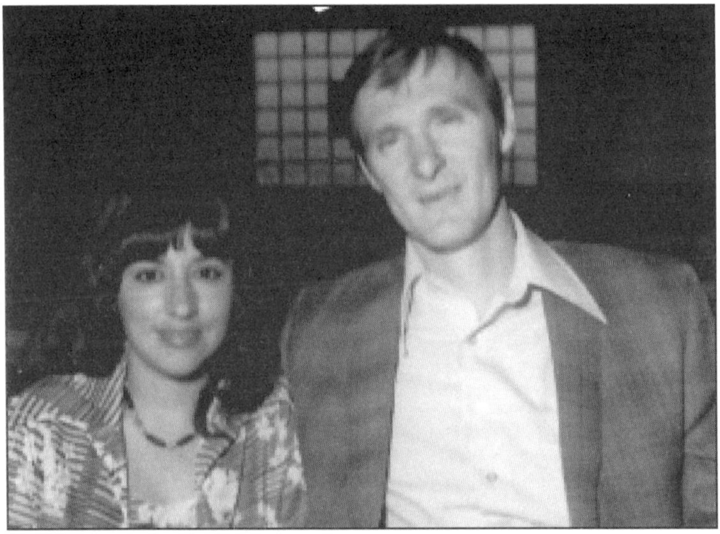

Graciela and Bill Kahler tied the know in the early-70s

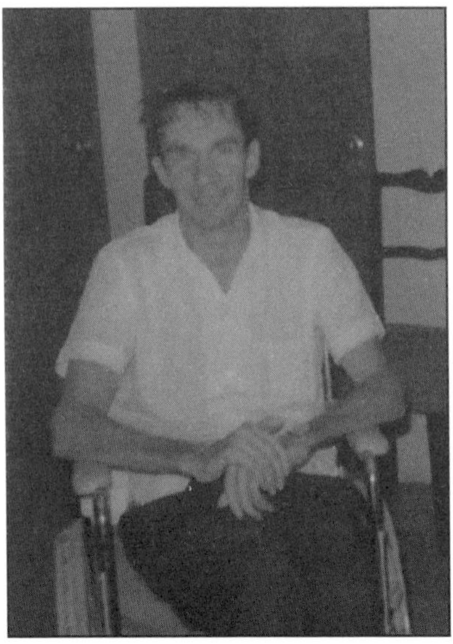

Popular Chicago area snowbird George Dempsey

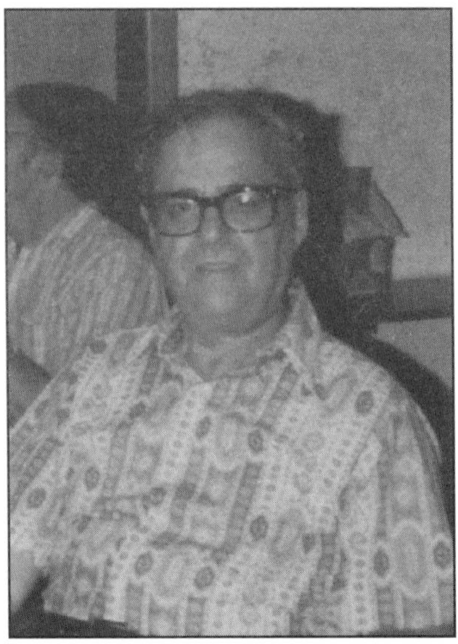

Chicago’s Jack Black was twice elected Mexico PVA president (fiscal ’71 and ’75)

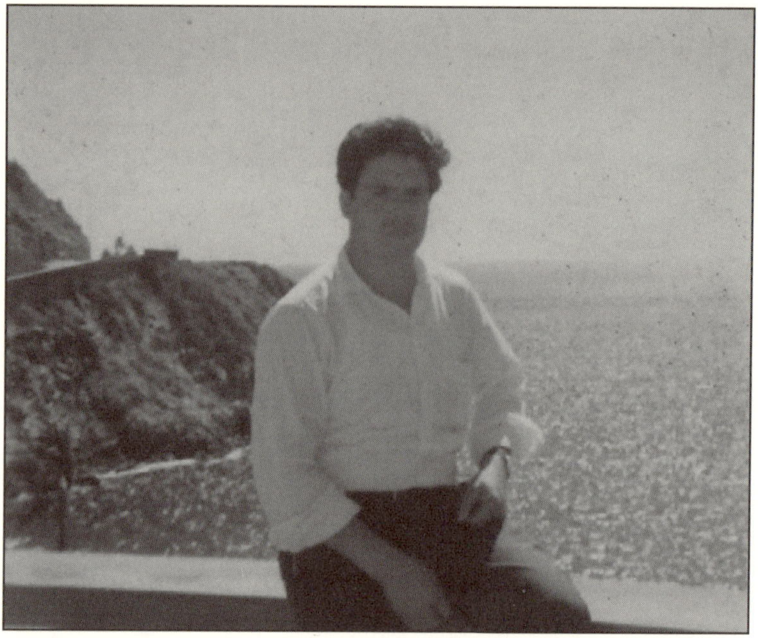

Miguel Lopez accompanied Jimmy Lietz to Acapulco in 1970
Miguel is one of very few attendants to assist quadriplegic gringos for more than thirty years, Lopez also worked for Jack Tumidajski

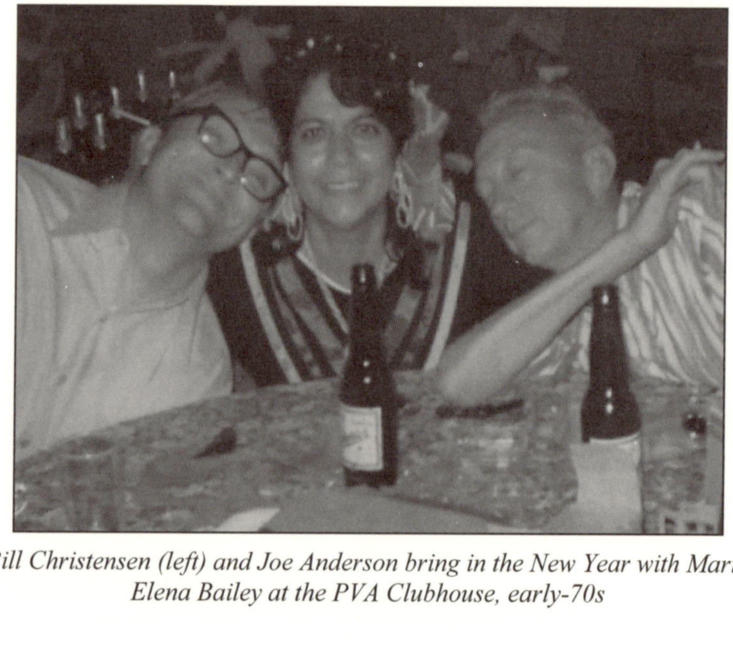

Bill Christensen (left) and Joe Anderson bring in the New Year with Maria Elena Bailey at the PVA Clubhouse, early-70s

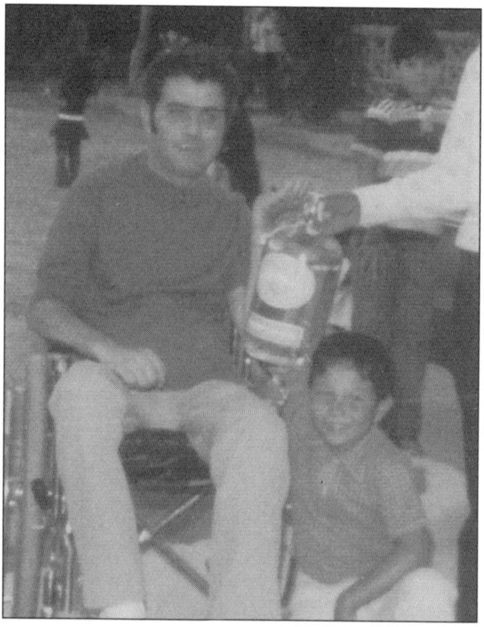

Frank Villani and stepson Marcos, early-70s
(Villani was murdered by one of his attendants a decade later)

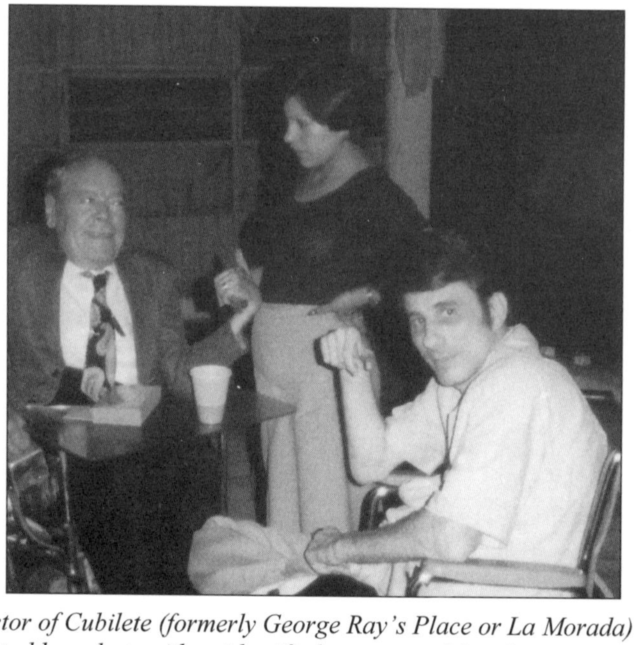

Proprietor of Cubilete (formerly George Ray's Place or La Morada) Kenny Ginsterblum chats with unidentified woman and Joe Cicero, early-70s

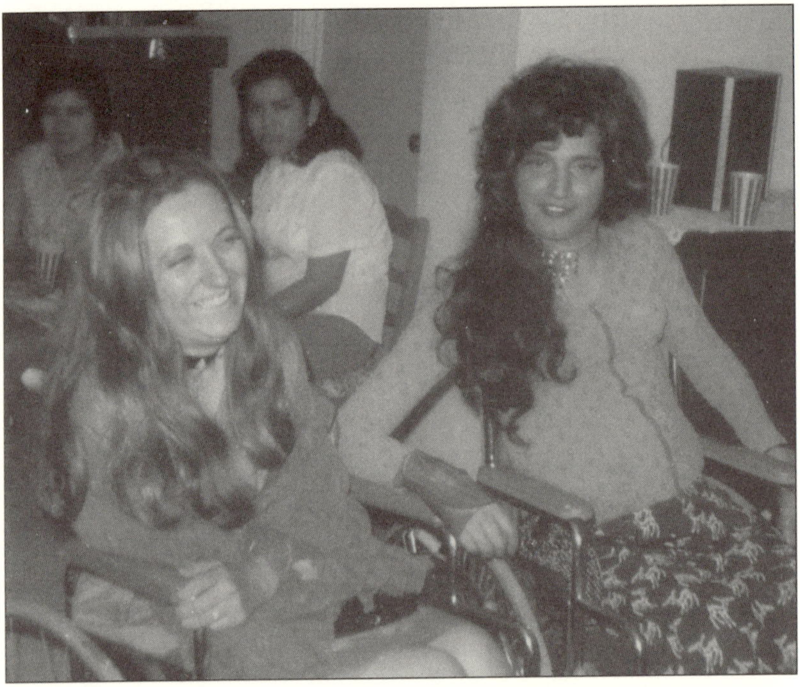

Paula Veilleux and Pete ("Don't I look great in orange?") Mirche are all smiles before costume party in February 1972. "No one at the party knew!" according to Mirche, who donned a wig and dressed as Paula's gal pal

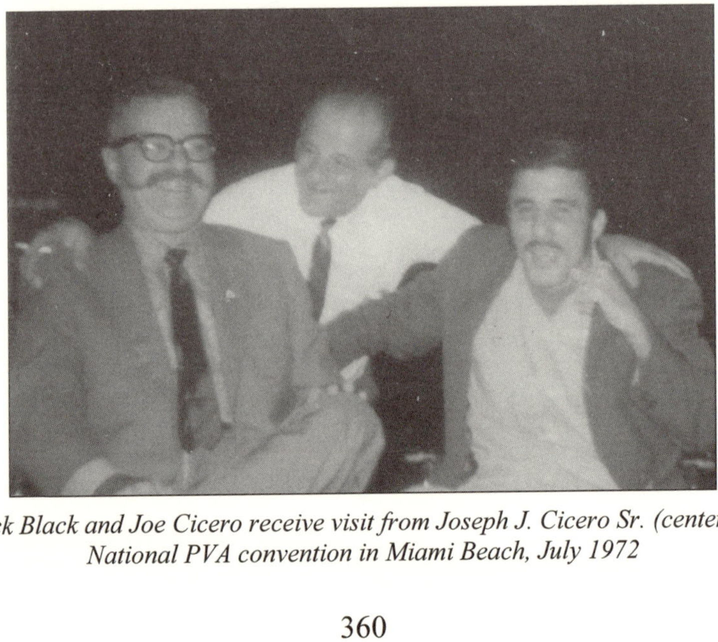

Jack Black and Joe Cicero receive visit from Joseph J. Cicero Sr. (center) at National PVA convention in Miami Beach, July 1972

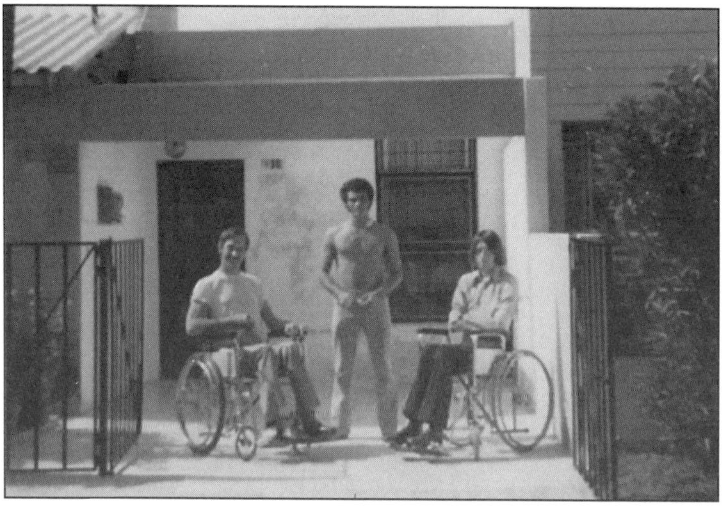

Vinnie Nash, Salvador, and Jack in front of their "new home" in November 1972
Three bedrooms with a phone for a whopping $40 per month!

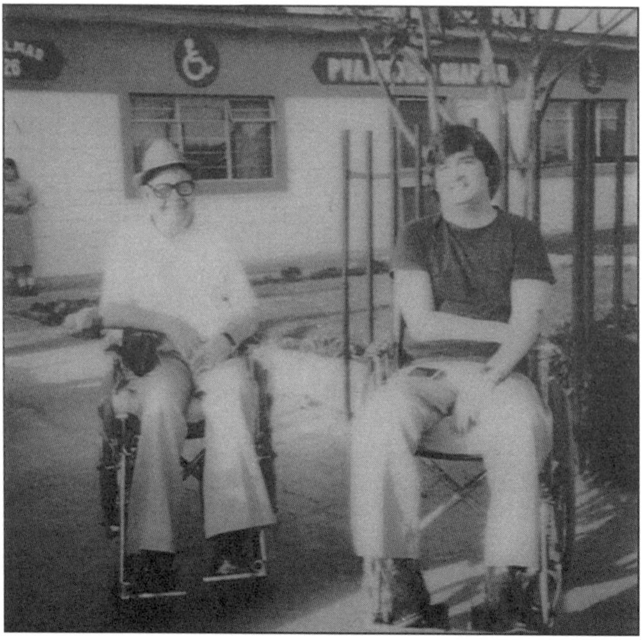

Charlie Gilliam and Jim Lietz in front of Mexico PVA Clubhouse

The tandem served the chapter as president and vice-president in fiscal '74 (June 1973 to June 1974)

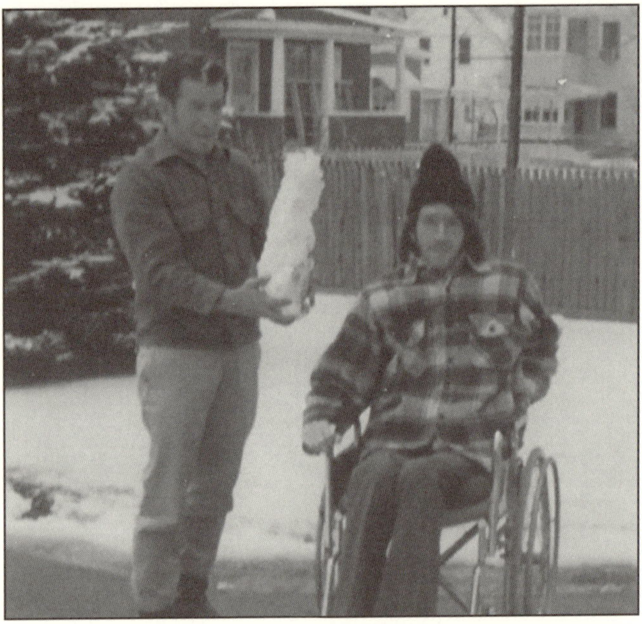

Alberto Navarro and Jack, Christmas 1975 visit with family in Rhode Island

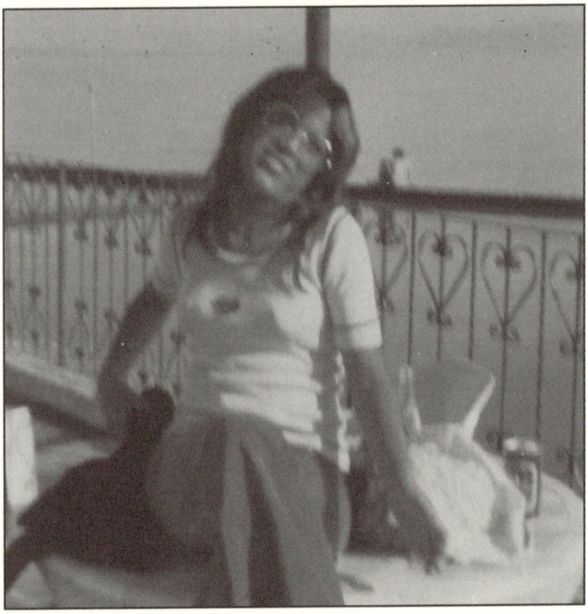

Bill and Maria Elena's niece, Teresa Cruz, on a mid-70s sunny day at San Juan Cosala with Lake Chapala in the background

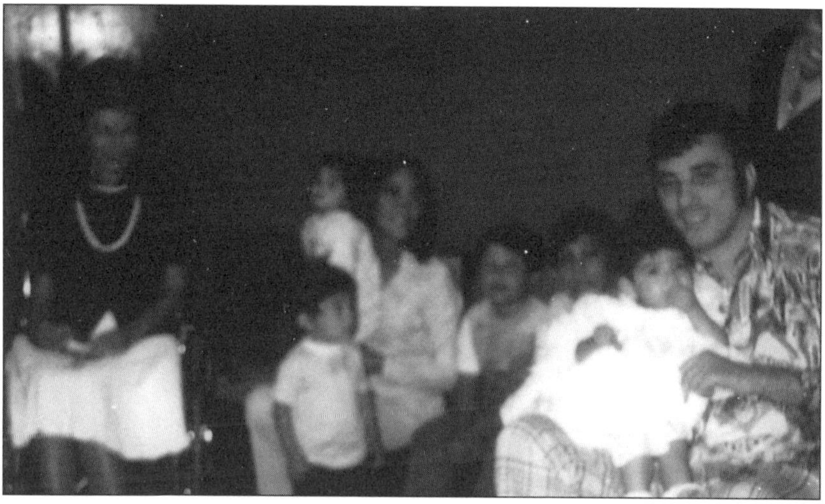

Proud Papa Joe Cicero holds daughter JoAnn as Eileen Van Albert (left) and other guests look on, mid-70s

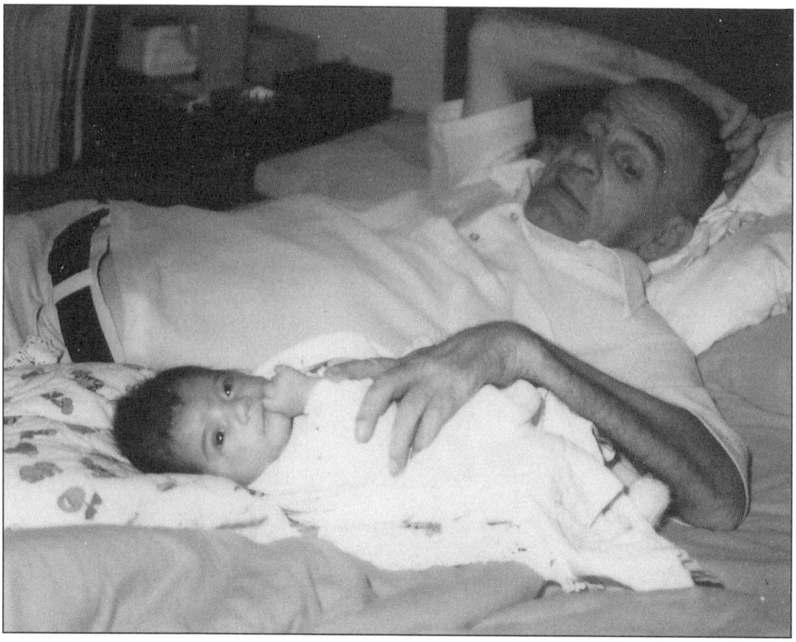

Cicero's brother-in-law Cliff Gulick is joined by niece JoAnn Cicero at siesta time, mid-70s

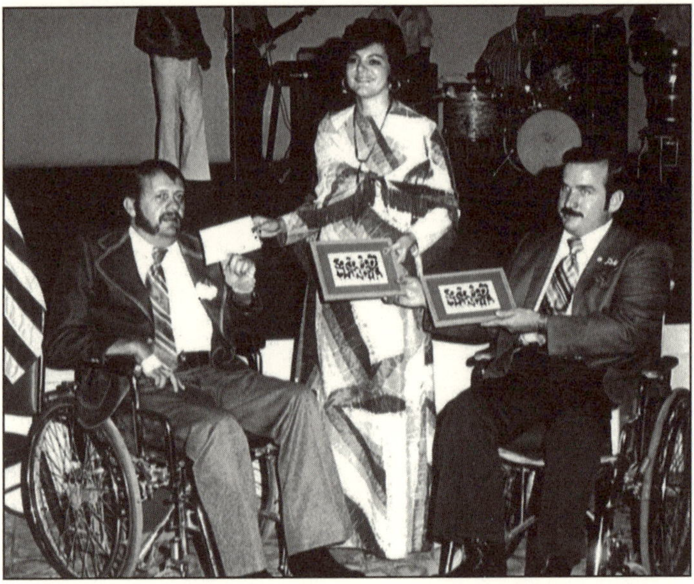

Keith Ziegler and Ray Clifford make donation and receive awards at a mid-70s Mexico PVA Annual Awards and Installation Banquet

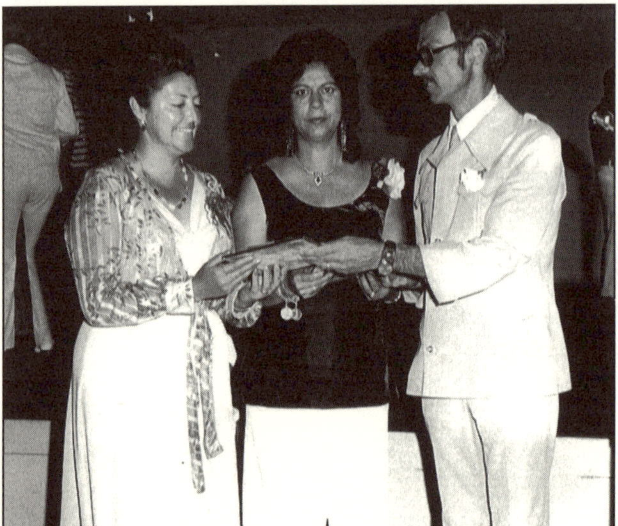

Josefina Ziegler and Maria Elena Bailey, two of the Mexico PVA's first ladies representing the women behind the men who kept chapter functions running smoothly, receive awards from an unidentified United States Consulate official at a mid-70s awards banquet

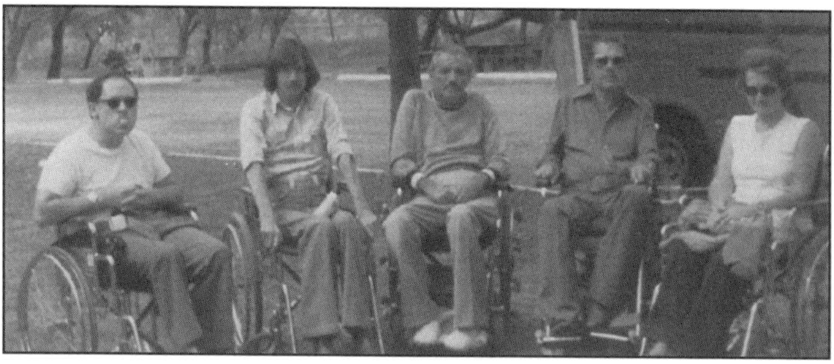

Buddy Pinsonnault, Jack, Tom Kirch, Bill Bailey, and JoAnn Kirch at Chimulco, a favorite park for Quadalajara residents about 20 miles from Quadalajara, with picnic areas, swimming pools, and plenty of fresh country air and sunshine, 1978

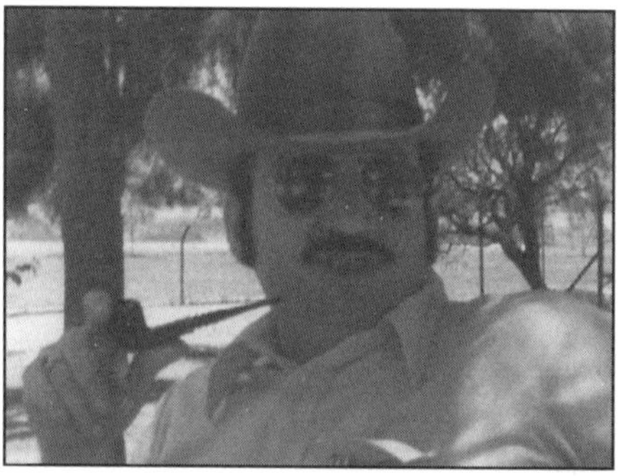

Ray Clifford, one of Mexico PVA's most dedicated workers enjoys a "Dia de Campo," a day in the countryside, at popular getaway Chimulco, 1978

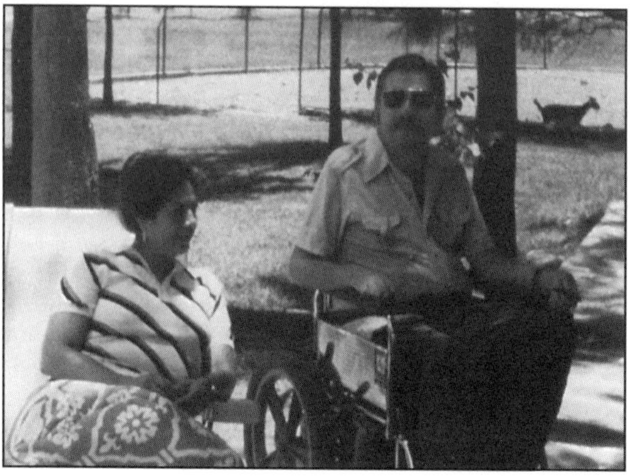

Maria Elena and Bill Bailey enjoy an afternoon at Chimulco, twenty years after their October 1958 wedding

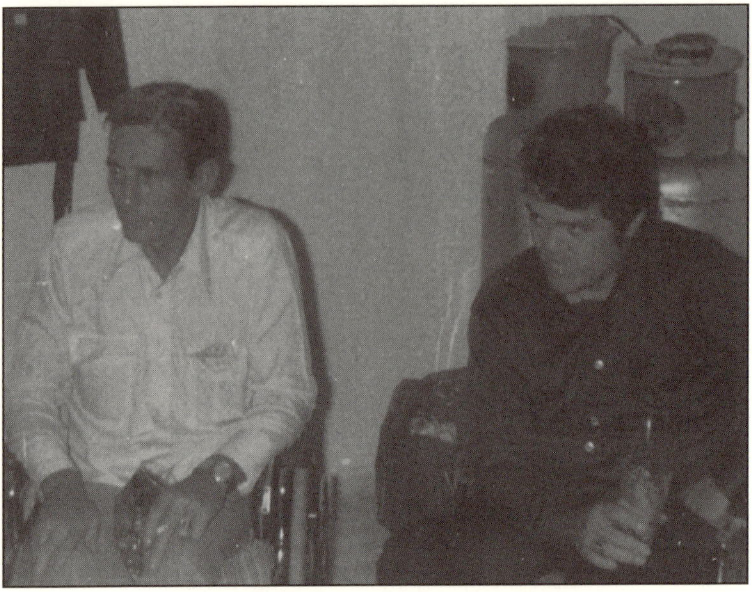

Mark Woods and Bob Flowers, 1978
"The Cowboy and the Marine," married cousins

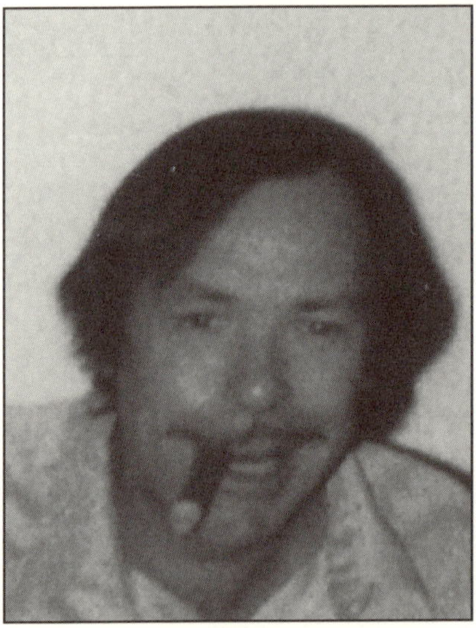

Jerry Andrews

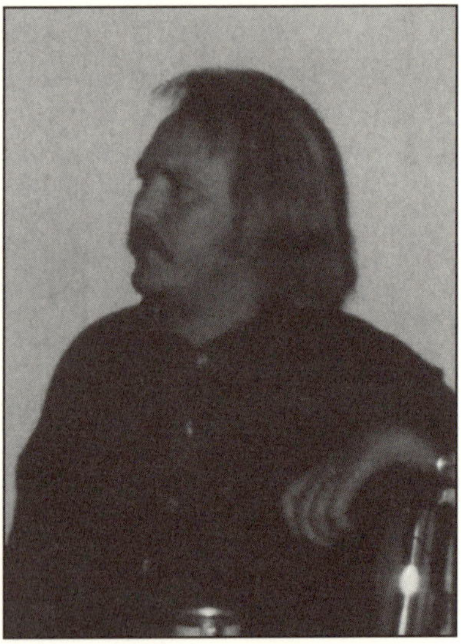

Darrell Roberson

Richmond VA Hospital alumni Flowers, Andrews, and Roberson were reunited in Quadalajara during the late-70s

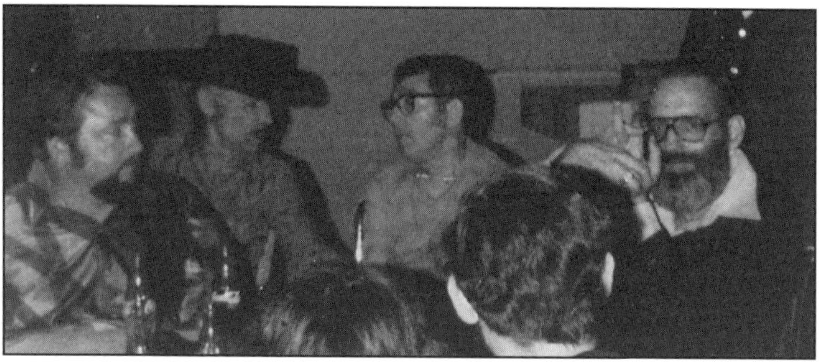

Joe Darichuk, Bill Baker, Bob Brassfield, John Rogers
Clubhouse social gatherings had a way of bringing people of diverse backgrounds and interests together

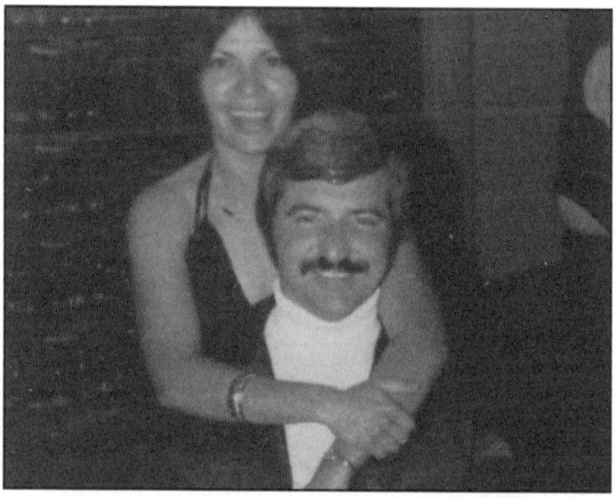

Steve and Guillermina Woosley at Mexico PVA Clubhouse

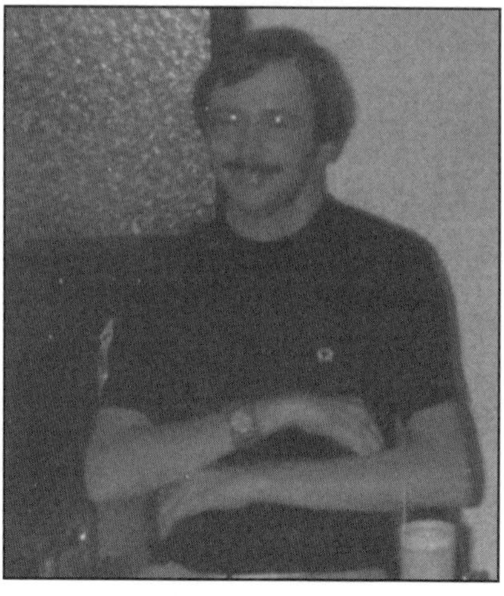

Richard Jaros

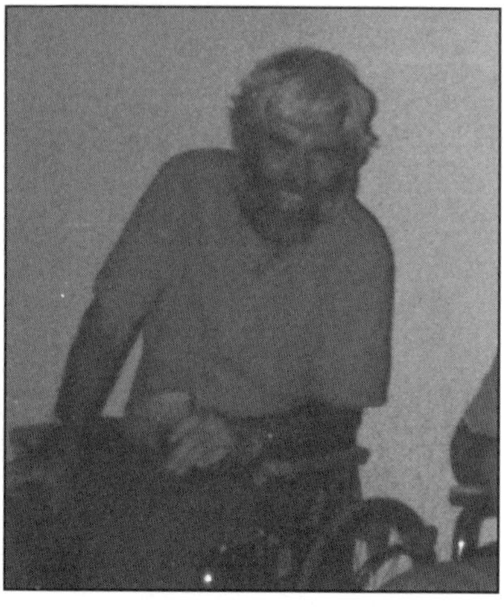

Dick "Wolfman" Wacholz 1978

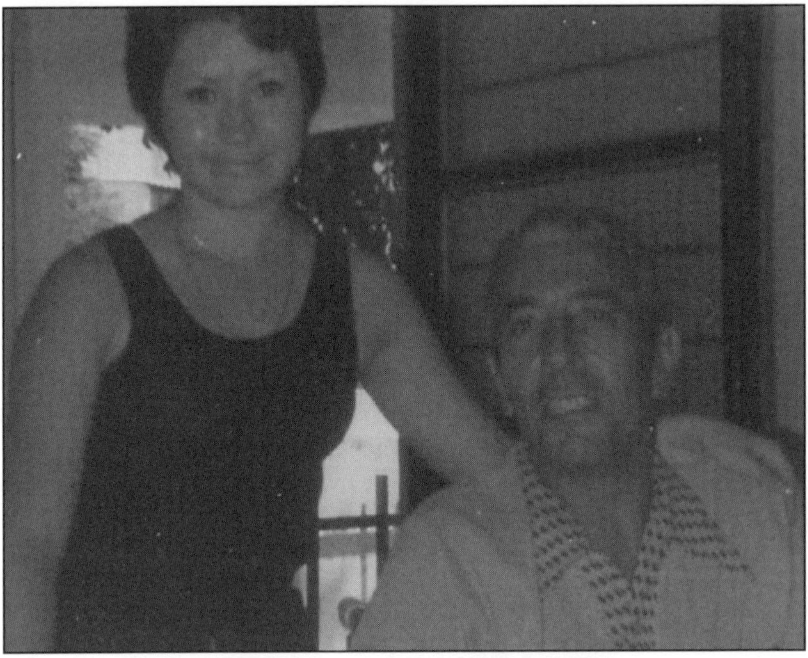

Pete Tanno and girlfriend Noemi, 1978

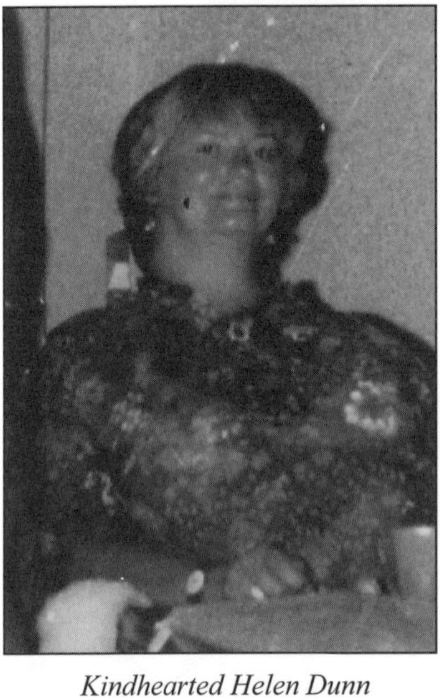

Kindhearted Helen Dunn

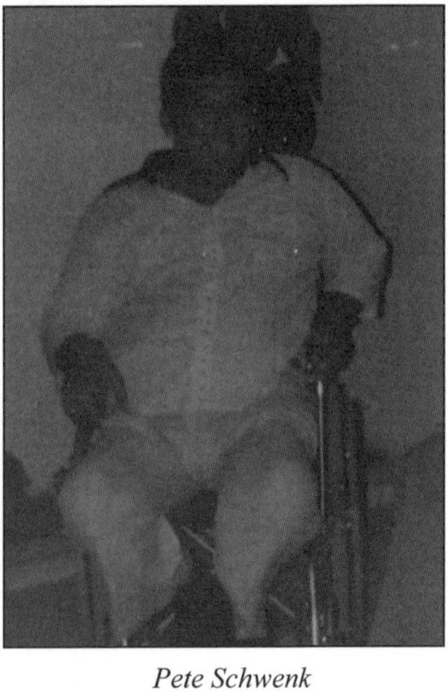

Pete Schwenk

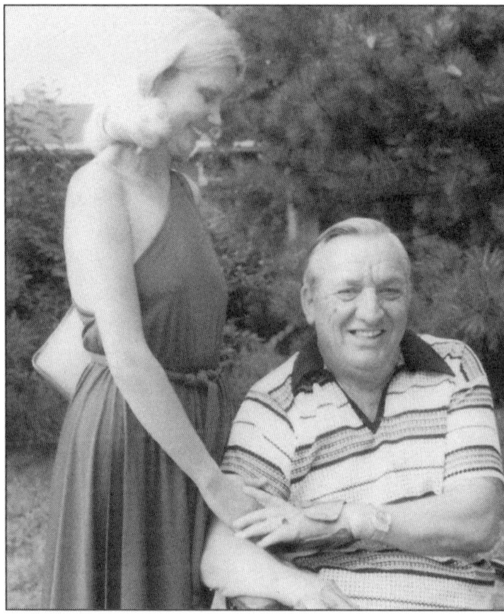

Founding member of Mexico PVA Stanley Pruncal visits his daughter in Pennsylvania, late-70s

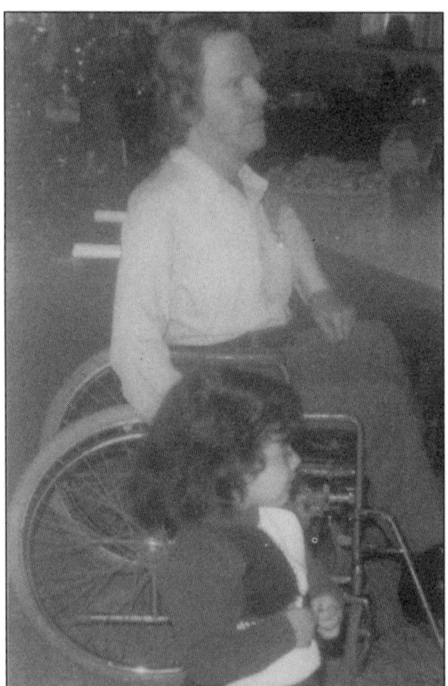

Herb Miller receives warm welcome from little JoAnn Cicero during late-70s visit

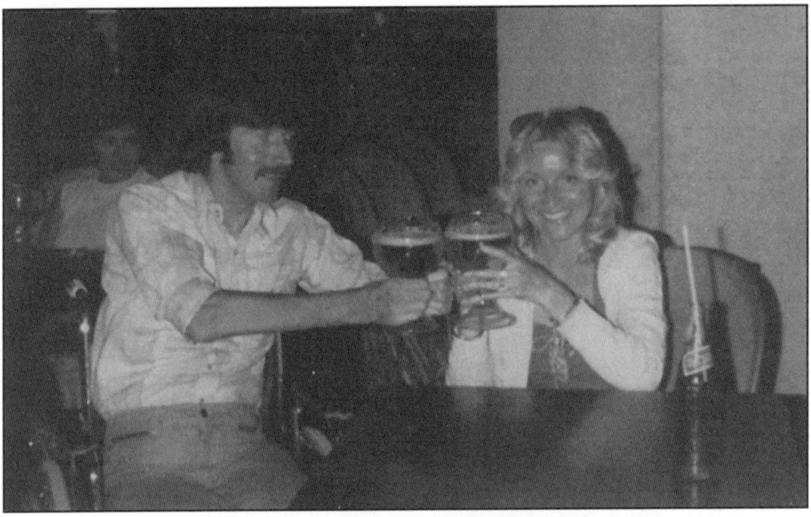

Jack and Sister Kathy toast her February 1979 visit to Quadalajara at Tlaquepaque's famous Mariachi Plaza, "El Parian"

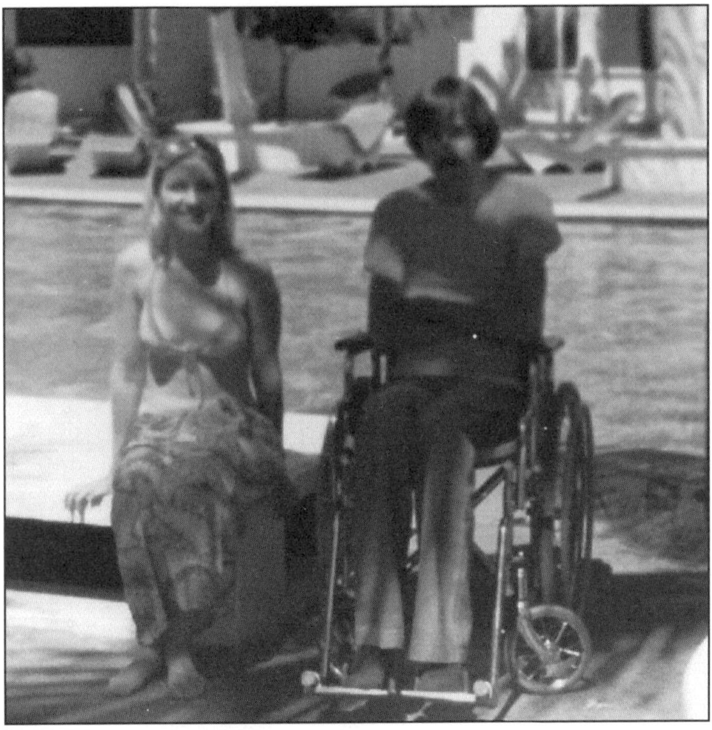

Kathy and Jack visit Manzanillo's Rancho Luna February 1979

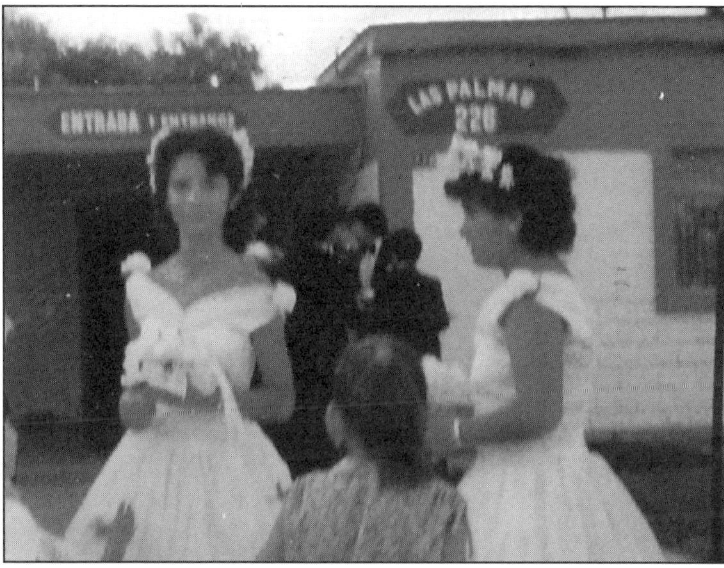

(left to right) Maria de la Paz Maldonado Cruz and Cousin Lucia Bailey Cruz (white dresses) outside of Mexico PVA Clubhouse prior to their double Quinceañera, traditional coming-of-age ceremony, including Catholic mass, for 15-year-old señoritas

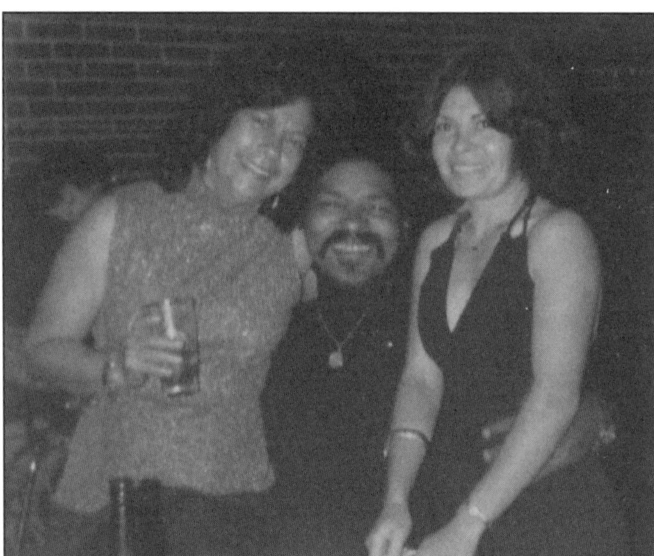

"Ladies Man" Harry "Chico" Wilson is flanked by Maria Elena Bailey and Guillermina Woosley at a PVA Clubhouse gathering

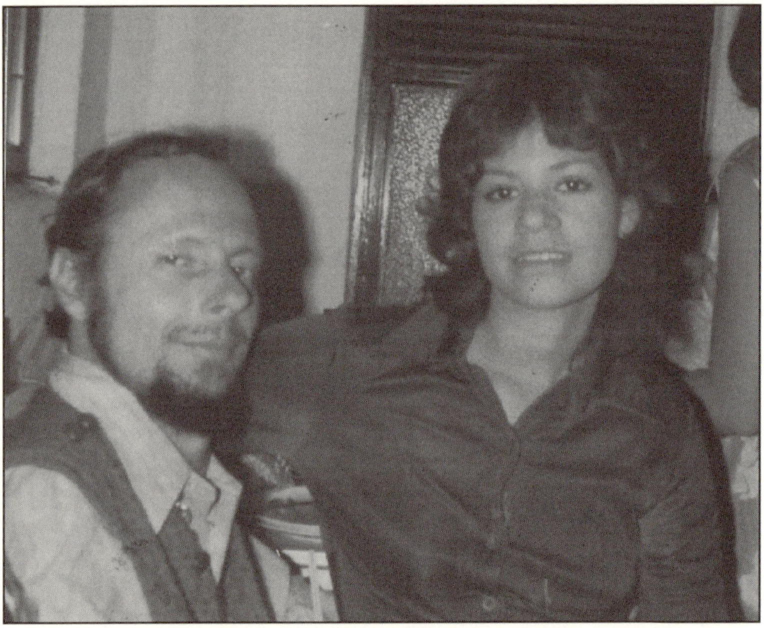

Don Bush and gal pal Adriana

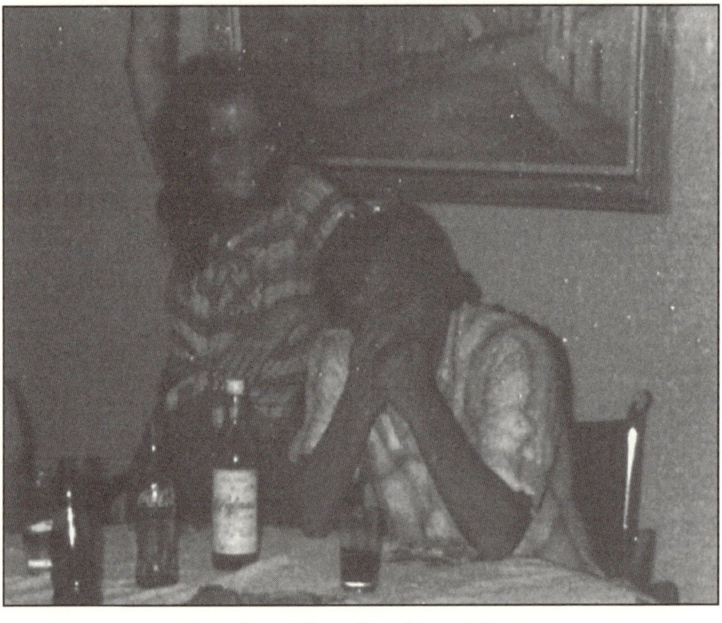

Greg Benisch and girlfriend Karen

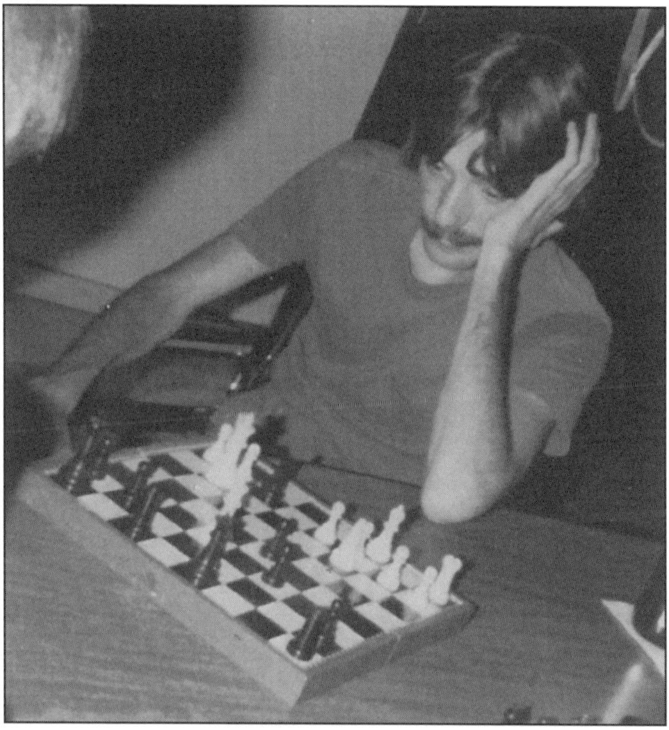

Chuck Hawkins ponders next move in seven-hour marathon chess match against friend and landlord Jack

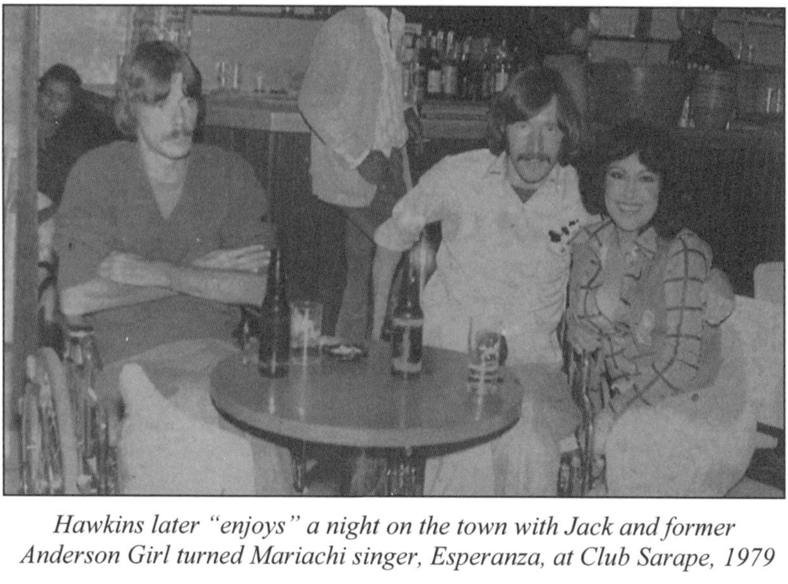

Hawkins later "enjoys" a night on the town with Jack and former Anderson Girl turned Mariachi singer, Esperanza, at Club Sarape, 1979

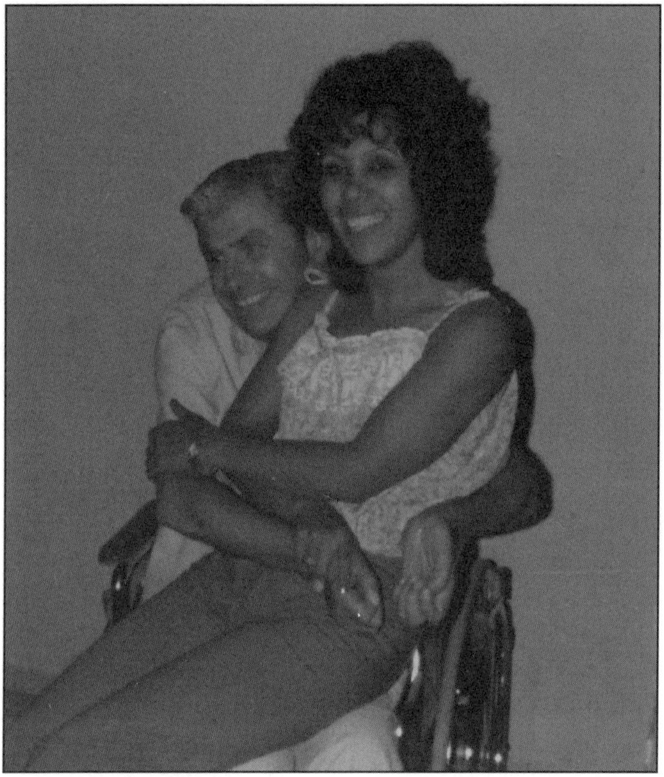

Eddie Lucier clowns around with the future Mrs. Jimmy Lietz, Sofia Peralta, at Mexico PVA Clubhouse

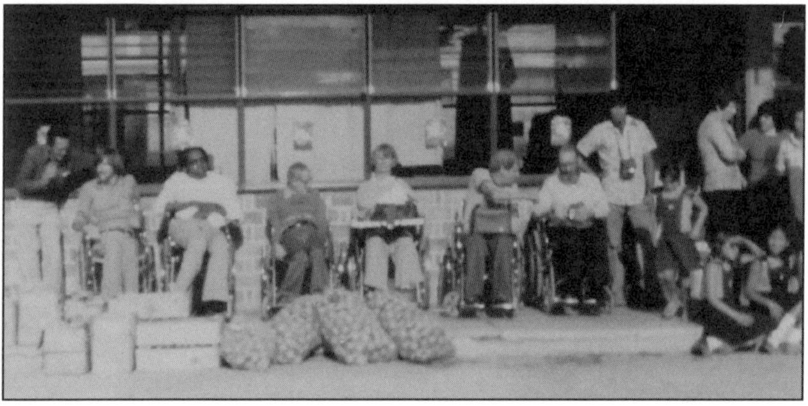

(left to right) Ciudad Granja official Enrique Gonzalez, Jack, Sandy Welborn, Norman Wilson, Helen Dunn, Eddie Lucier, John Rogers, Ruben Gomez (Lucier's attendant), faculty and students at 1979 Christmas Posada

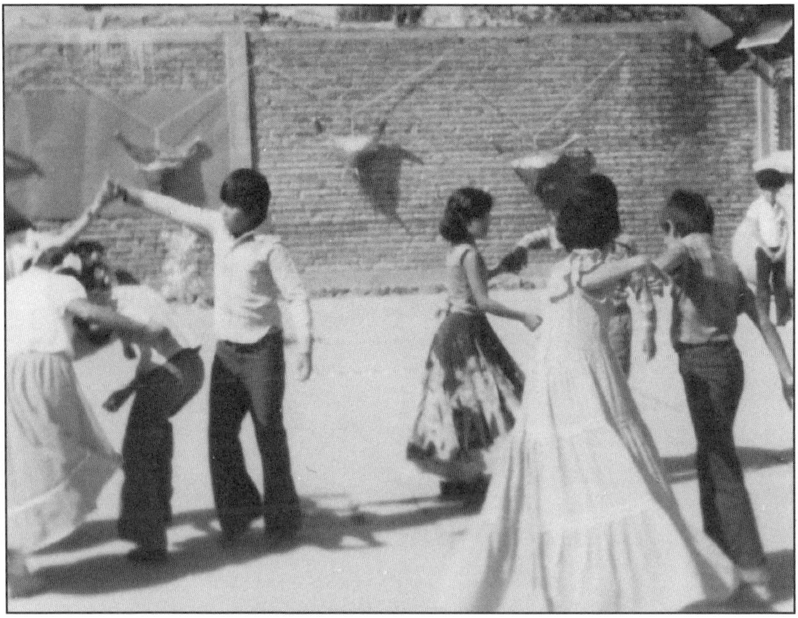

Dancing students entertain Mexico PVA members and friends
before breaking the hanging piñatas
1979 Christmas posada

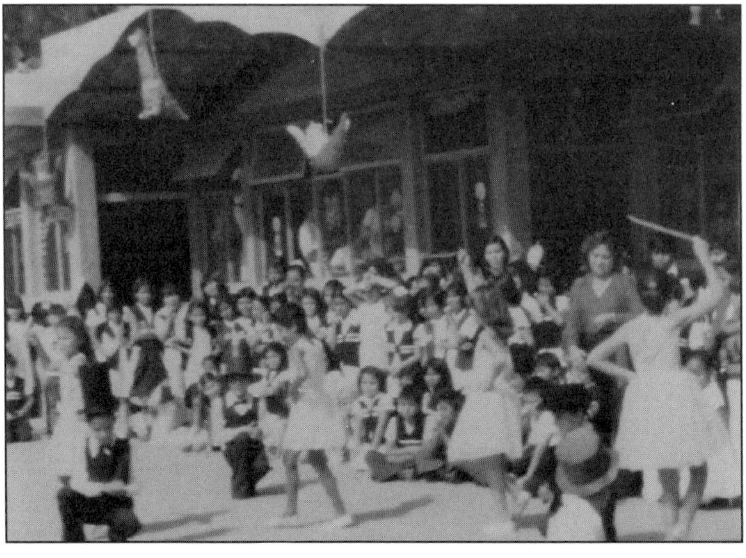

School children anticipate breaking the piñatas
1979 Christmas posada sponsored by Mexico PVA

'80s End of an Era

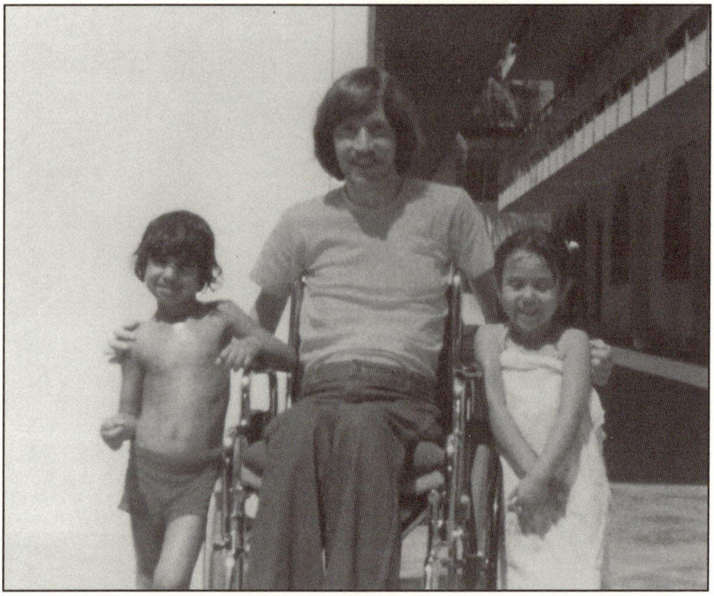

Paco, Jack, and Karina, Rincón de Guayabitos, 1980
Paco is Marta's nephew and Karina is the daughter of a former neighbor

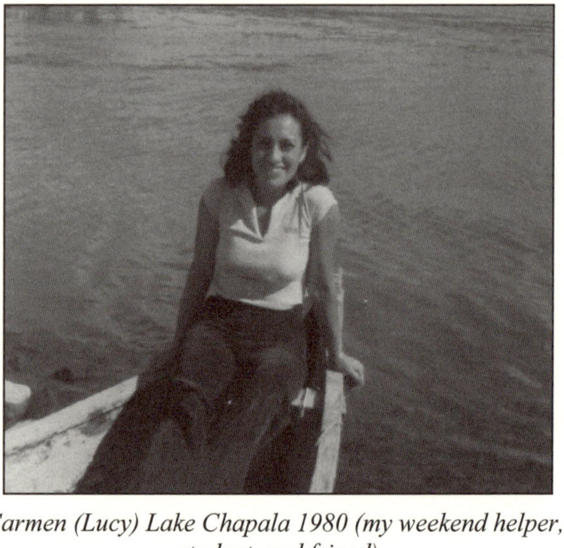

Luz del Carmen (Lucy) Lake Chapala 1980 (my weekend helper, medical student, and friend)

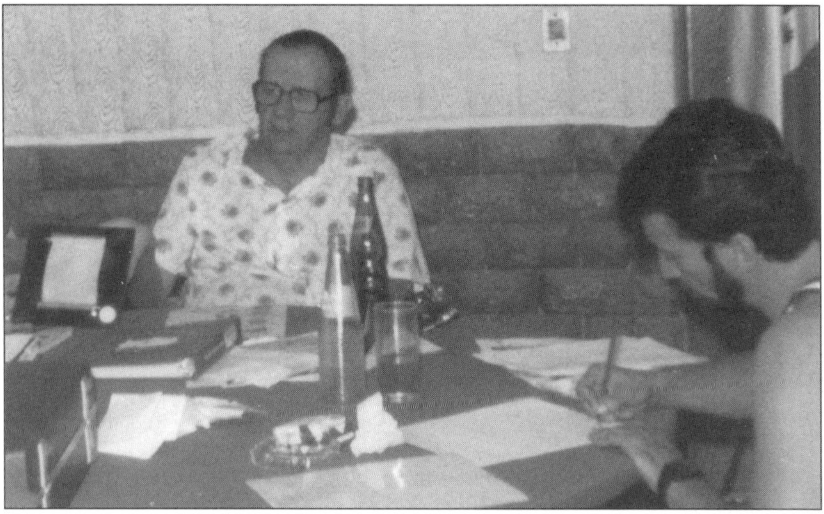

Mexico PVA President Keith Ziegler shows plaque of chapter's annual George E. Ray Award as Secretary Frank Stoppiello keeps minutes of membership meeting, early-80s

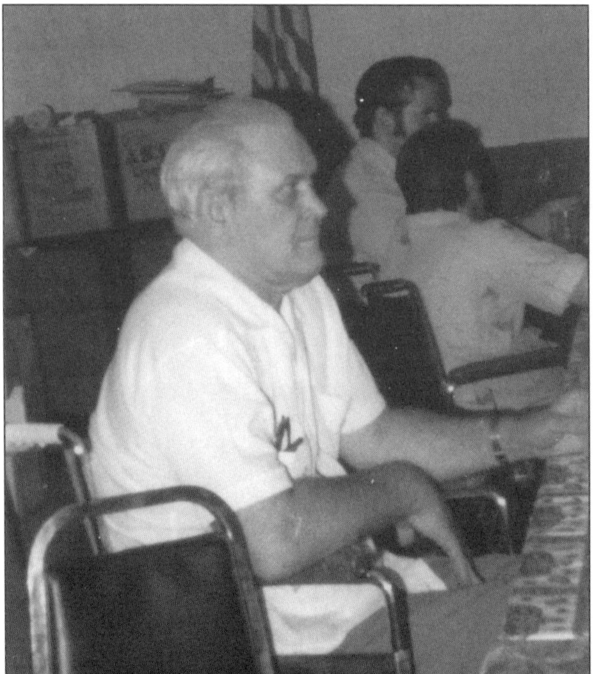

World War II veteran and Mexico PVA member Doyle Holt listens intently during an early-80s Clubhouse meeting

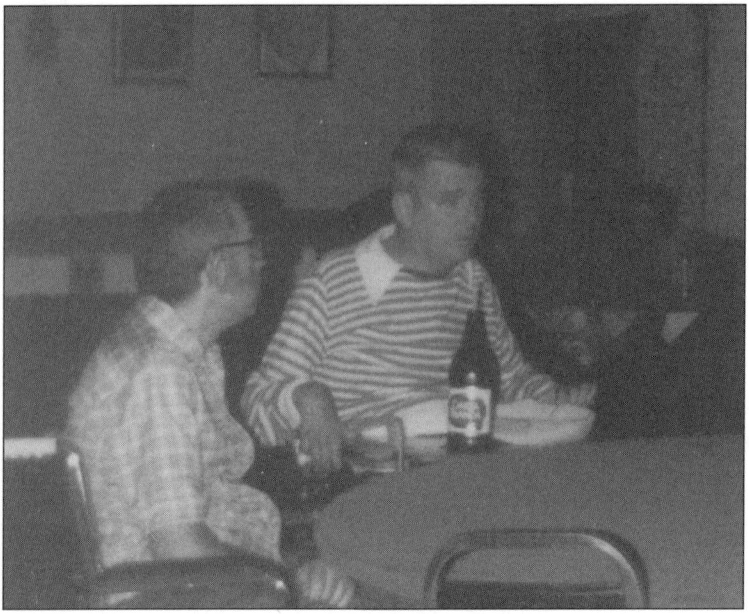

Bob Brassfield chats with a very thirsty Charlie Erickson (with beer in front of him) after an early-80s Mexico PVA meeting

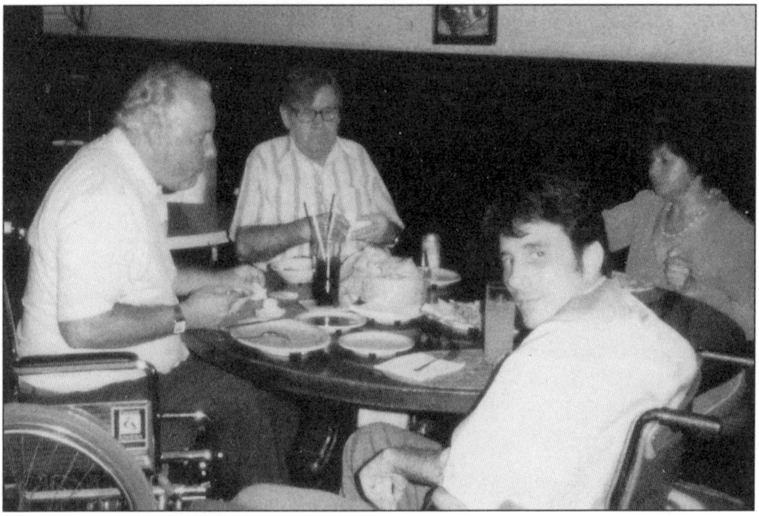

Roland Schellenberg, former proprietor of La Morada (after George Ray's death), visits with Paul Saine and Teresa and Joe Cicero at El Rodeo de Josepe restaurant, which Cicero purchased in the early-80s

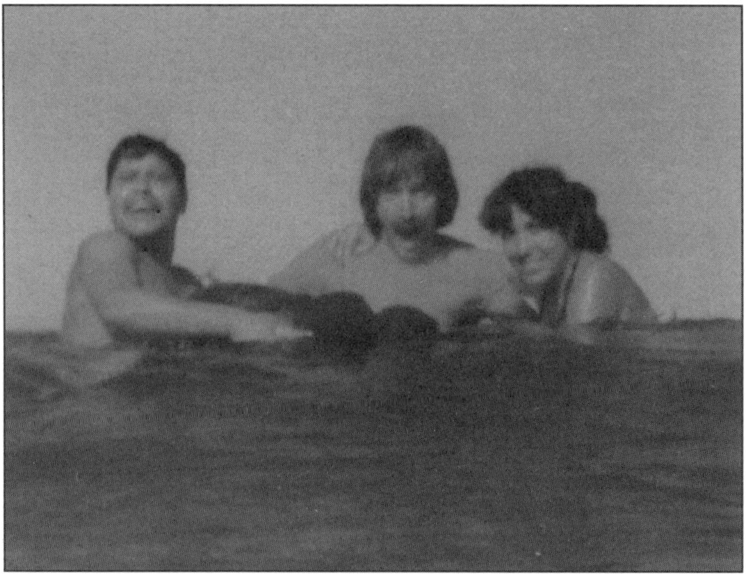

Juan Moreno, Jack, and Marta (the future Mrs. Dick Wacholz) ride out a wave at Rincón de Guayabitos, about 20 miles south of Puerto Vallarta, in chest-high waters some 50 yards from shore

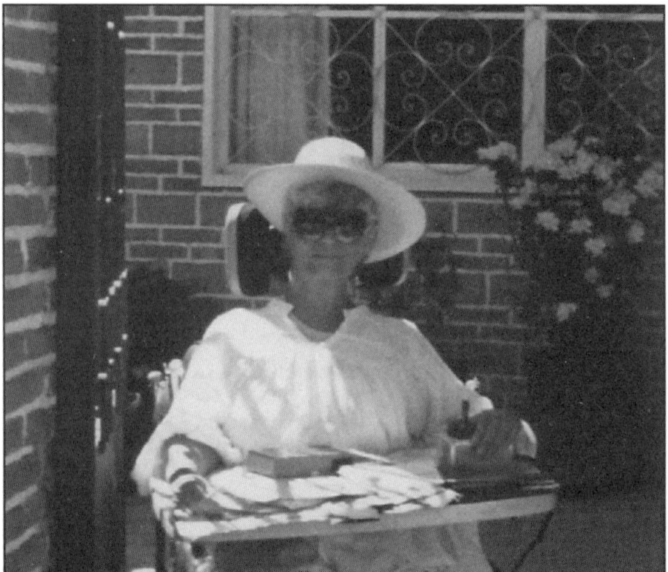

Helen Dunn at her post-Quadalajara home in Ajijic 1986

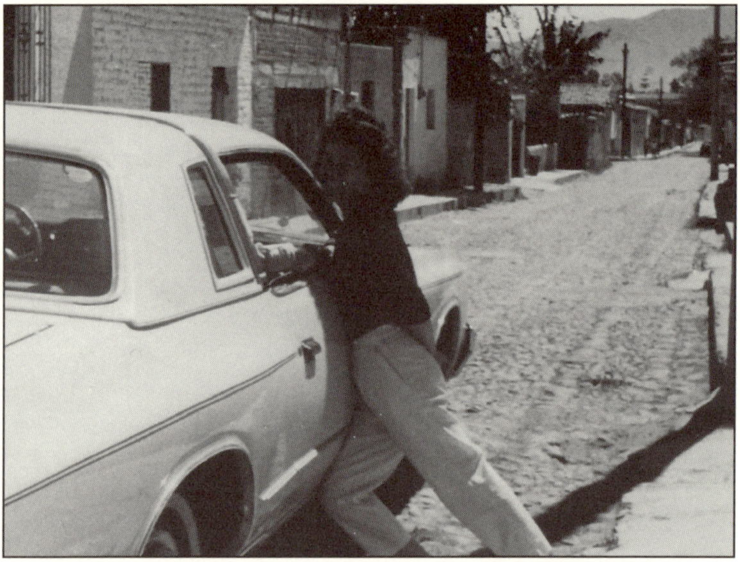

A surprised Cuca chats with her ex-fiancé at the Lakeside community of San Antonio 1986 (the narrow cobblestone street leads past the home of Barney and Alicia Vigil and to Lake Chapala)

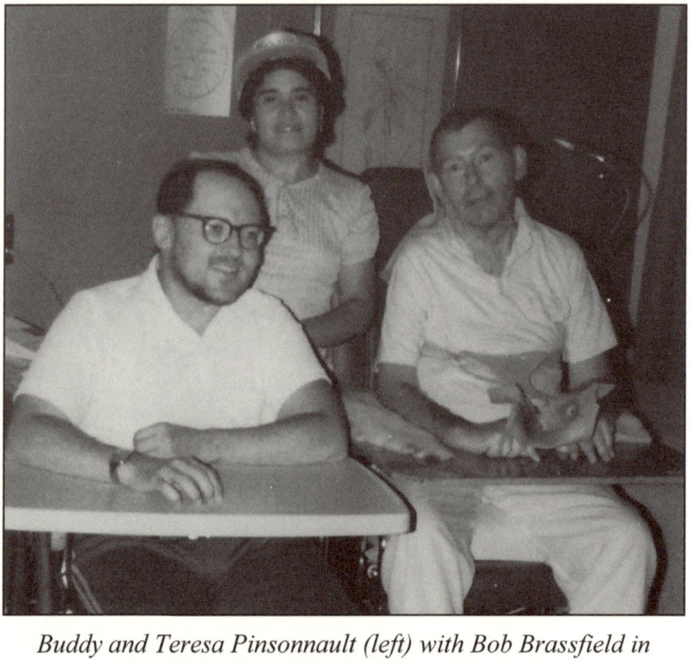

Buddy and Teresa Pinsonnault (left) with Bob Brassfield in San Diego late-80s, post-Quadalajara visit

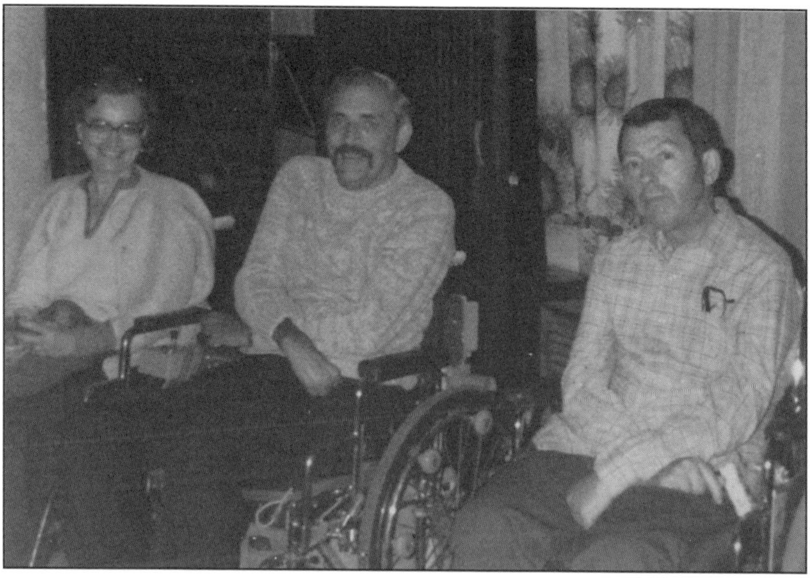

JoAnn Kirch, Tom Kirch, and Bob Brassfield

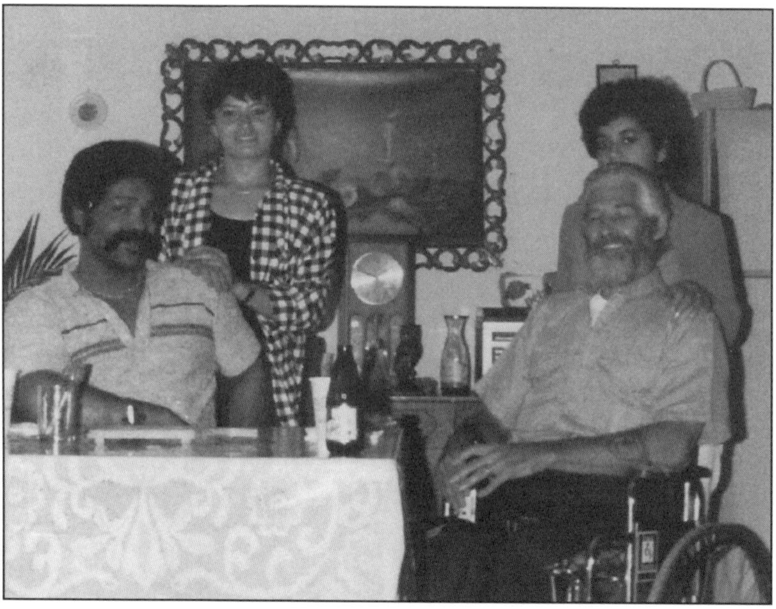

Chico Wilson (left) receives a post-Quadalajara late-80s visit from friend and former helper Paty Lopez, and Jerry and Martha Maurer in his Chapala area home

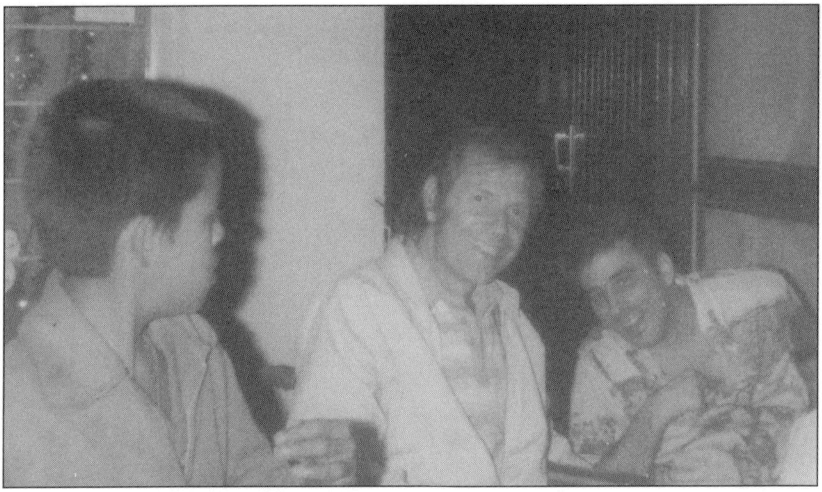

Jim Beletti and Joe Cicero post-Quadalajara (Beletti was later murdered outside of the city)

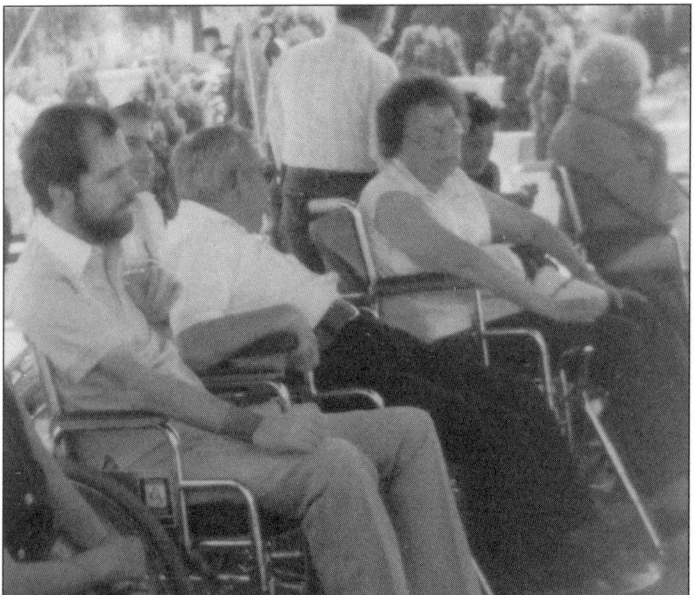

Las Fuentes wheelers Pat Kenny, unidentified man, and Rose and Sylvia Horowitz attend 1980s American Legion funeral

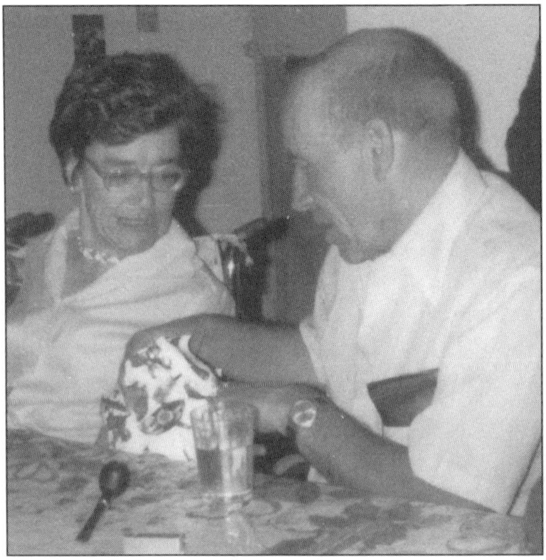

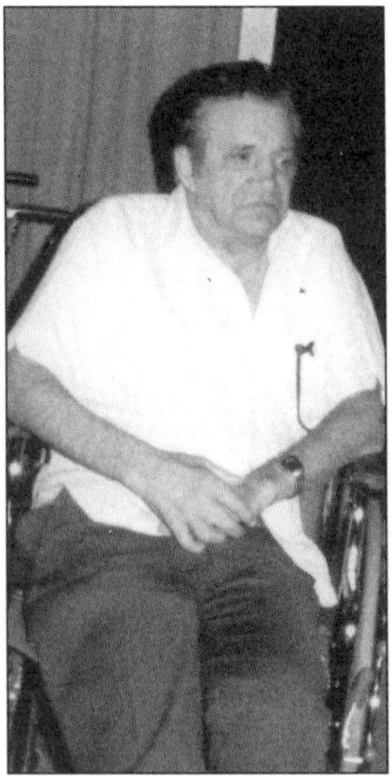

Mary Lou and Joe Fox prior to their 1980s move to Texas

Philadelphia's Joe Cella was a long-time snowbird and resident of Quadalajara's Motel Chapalita, 1980s

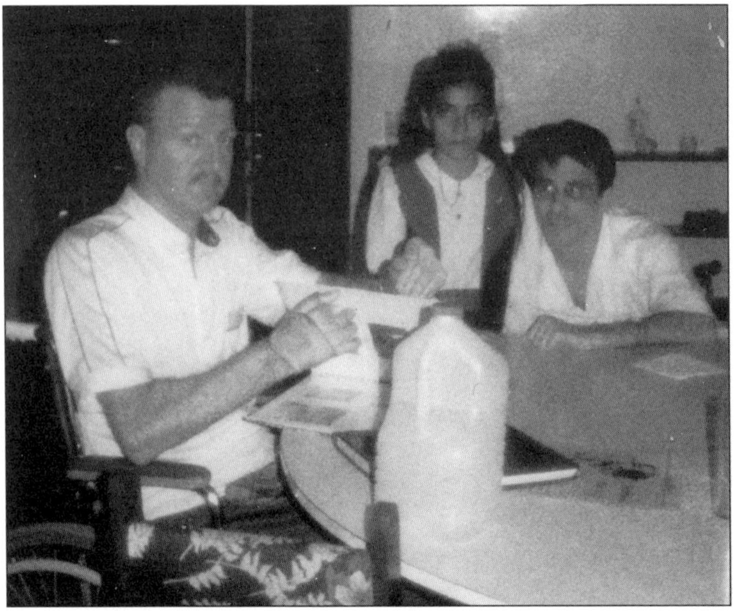

Dale "Nick" Nixon, JoAnn and Joe Cicero in '80s visit

Places of Quadalajara

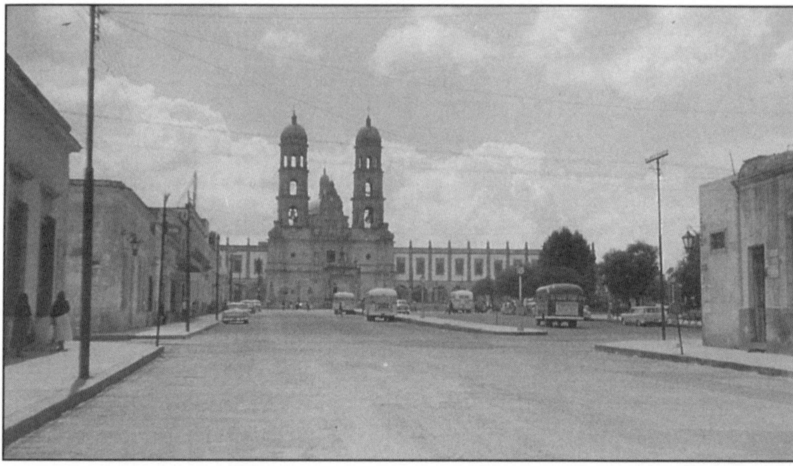

Basílica de Zapopan around 1960, was actually built in 1690

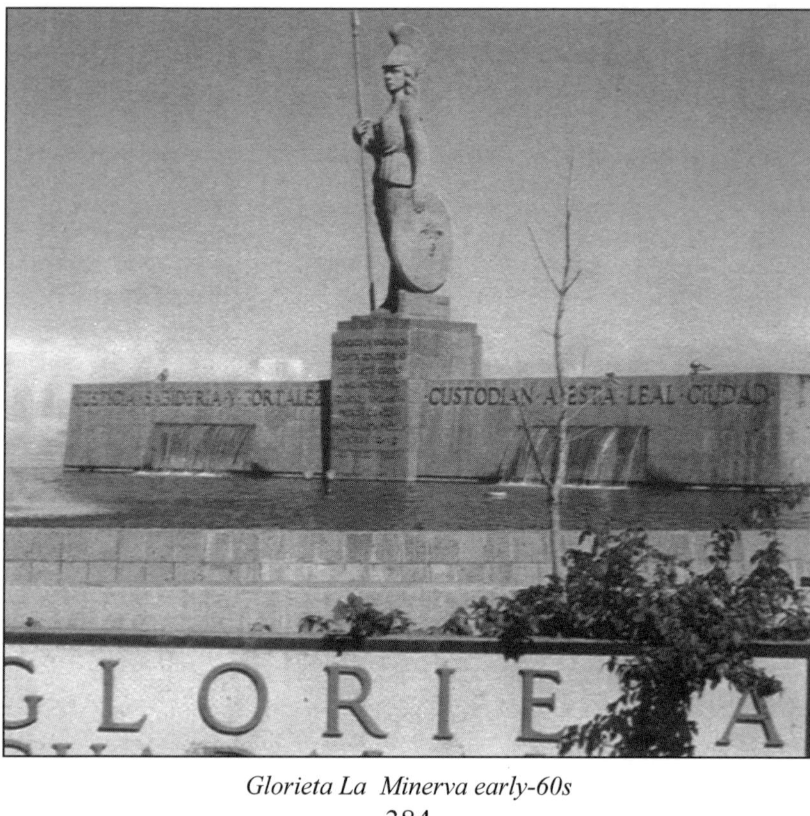

Glorieta La Minerva early-60s

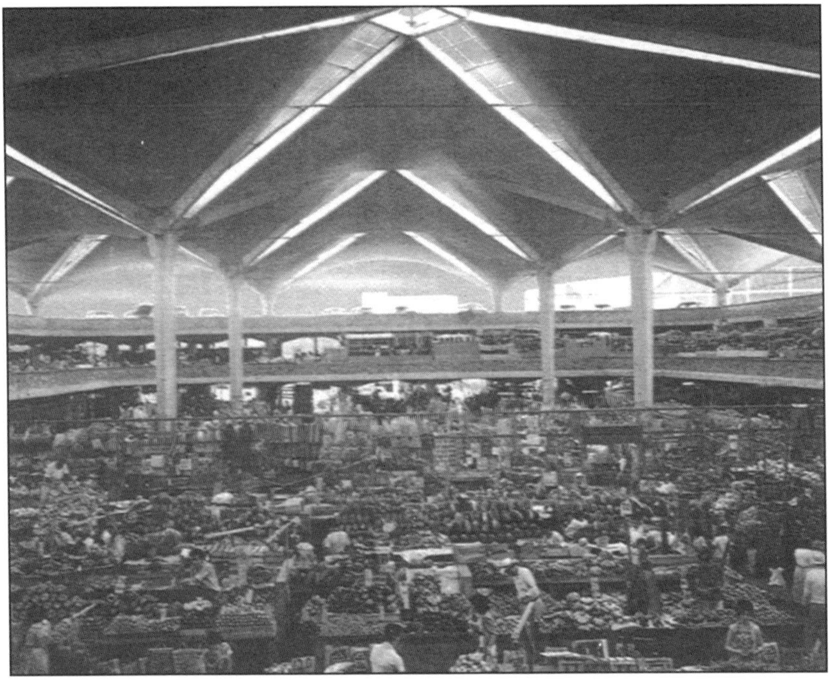

Mercado Libertad early-60s

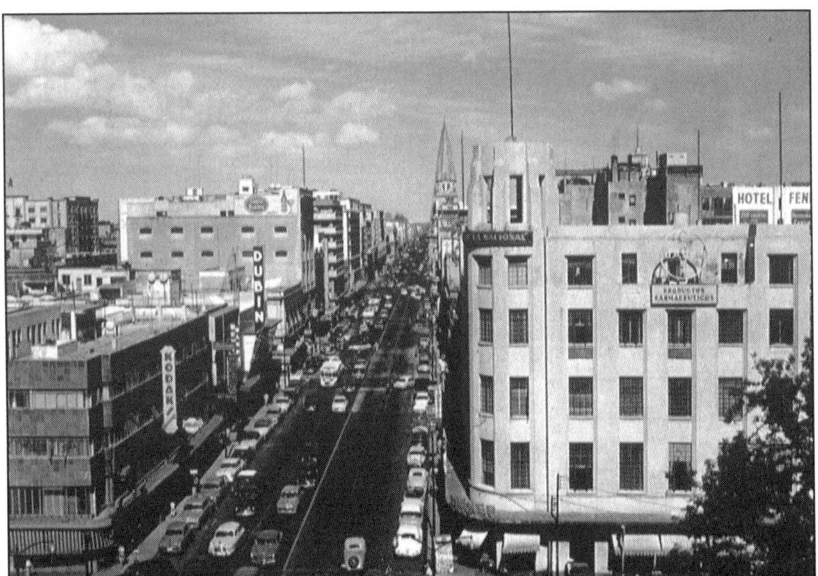

Avenida 16 de Septiembre, one of the city's more important avenues and commercial centers, early-60s

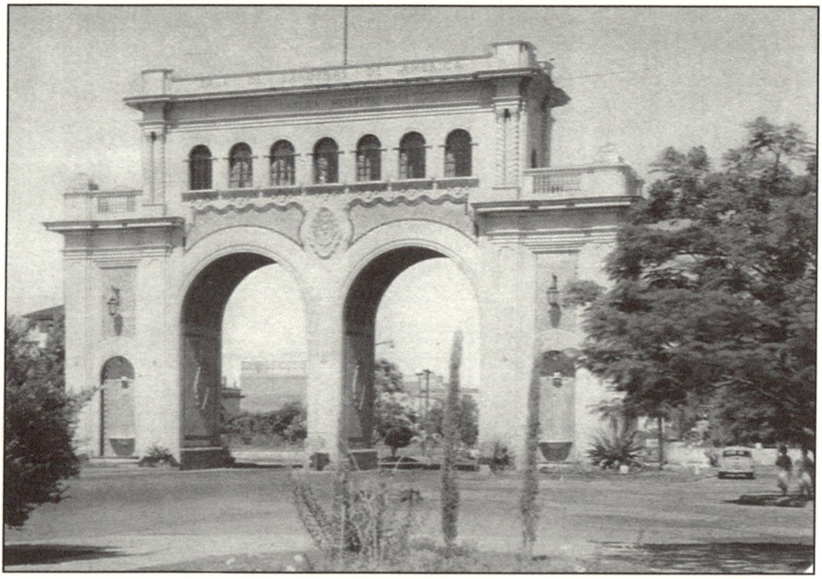

Quadalajara's Hospitality Arch "Los Arcos" (early-60s) was the originl entrance to the city

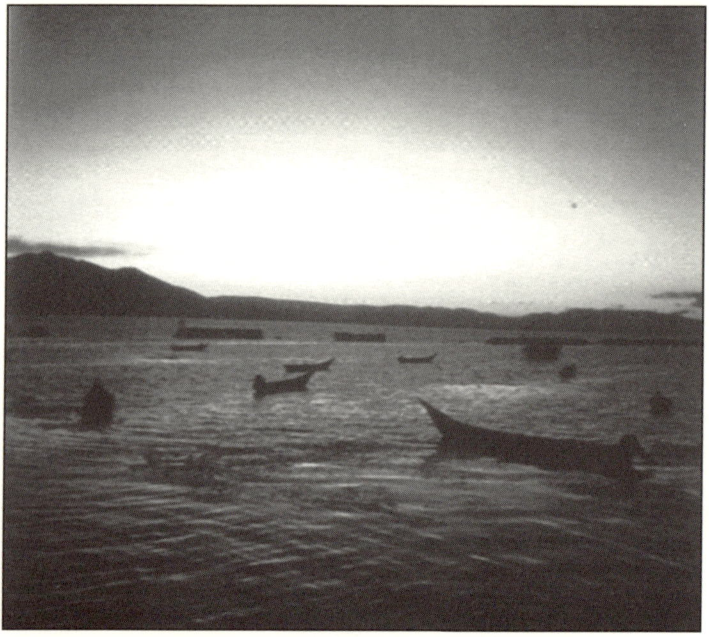

Lake Chapala at sunset 1964

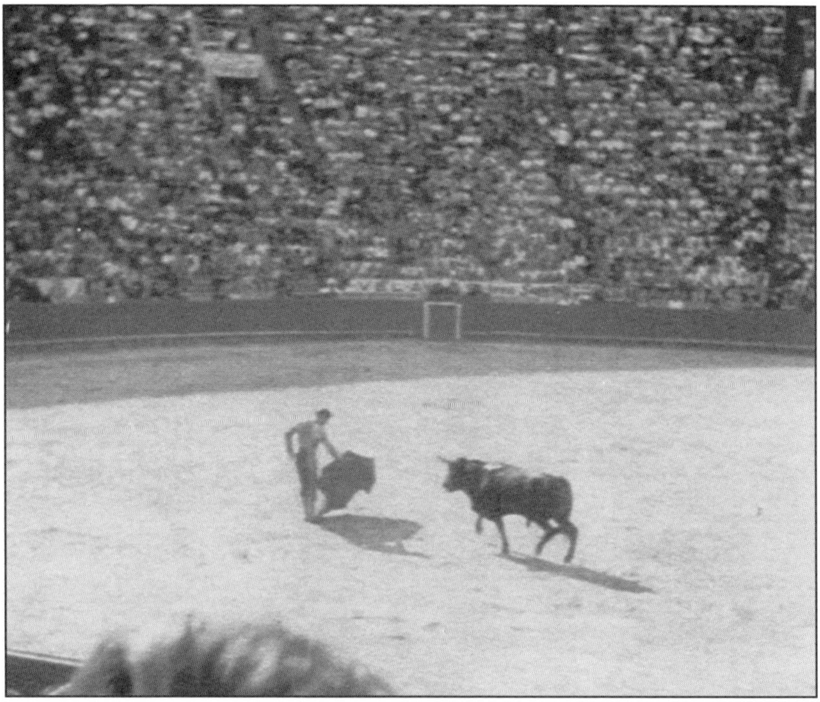

Bull Fight 1964

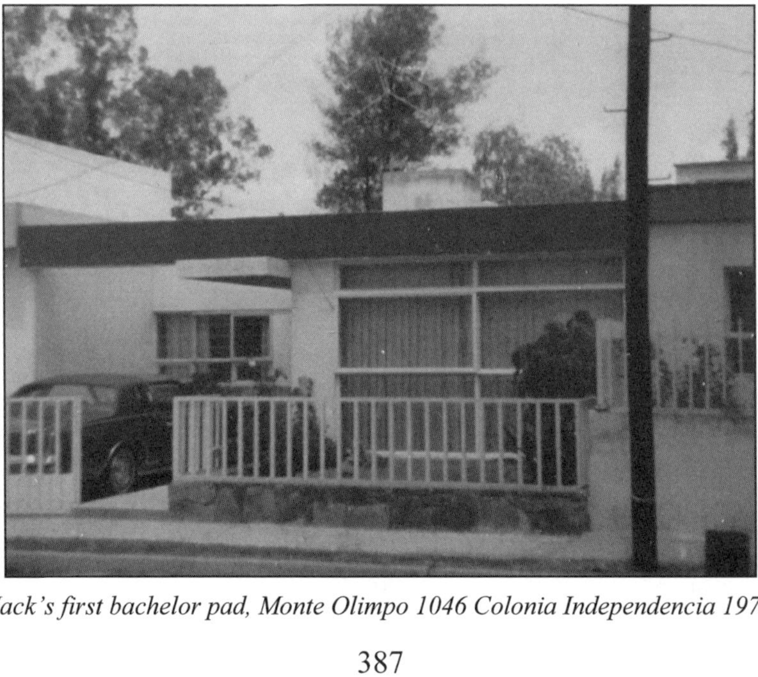

Jack's first bachelor pad, Monte Olimpo 1046 Colonia Independencia 1975

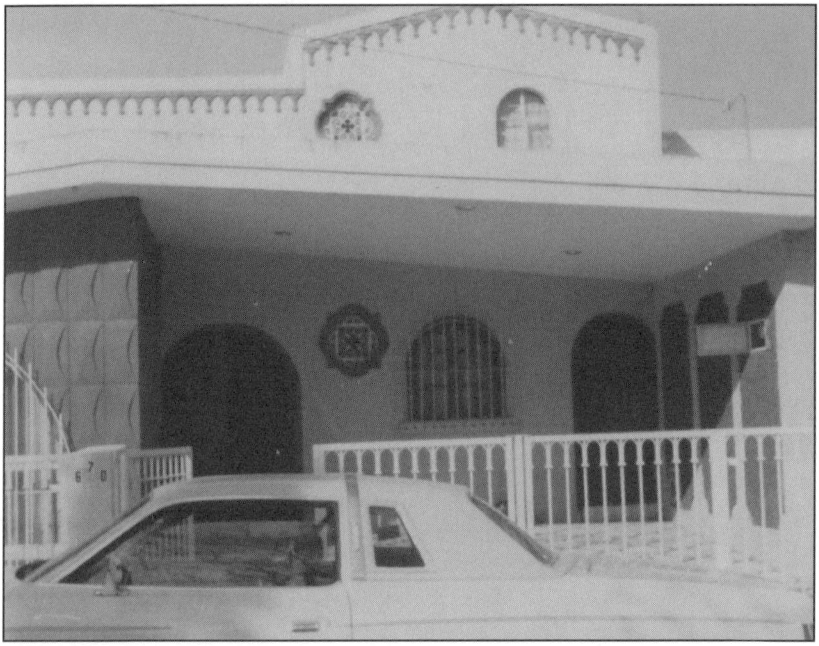

Jack's hacienda, Manuel Davalos Jardines Alcalde 1979

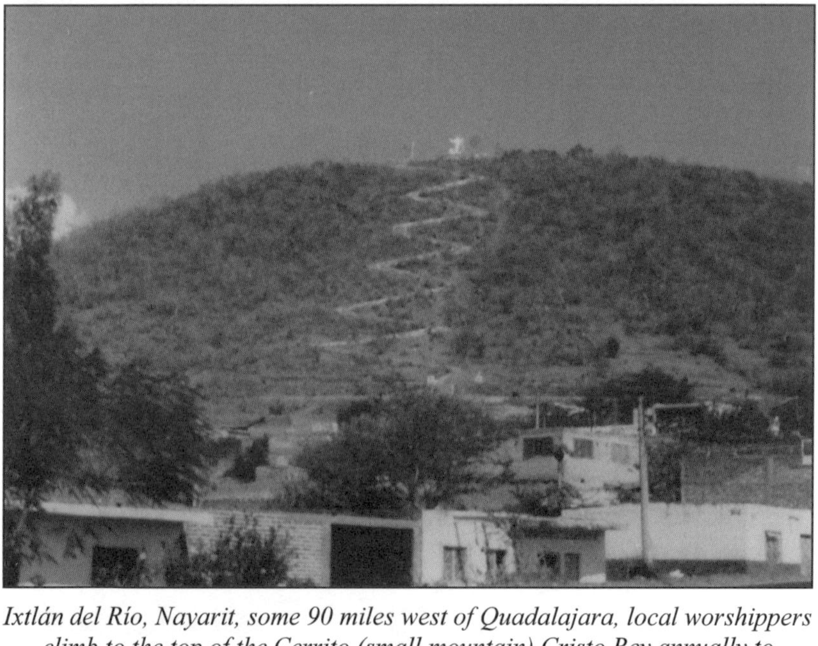

Ixtlán del Río, Nayarit, some 90 miles west of Quadalajara, local worshippers climb to the top of the Cerrito (small mountain) Cristo Rey annually to celebrate mass

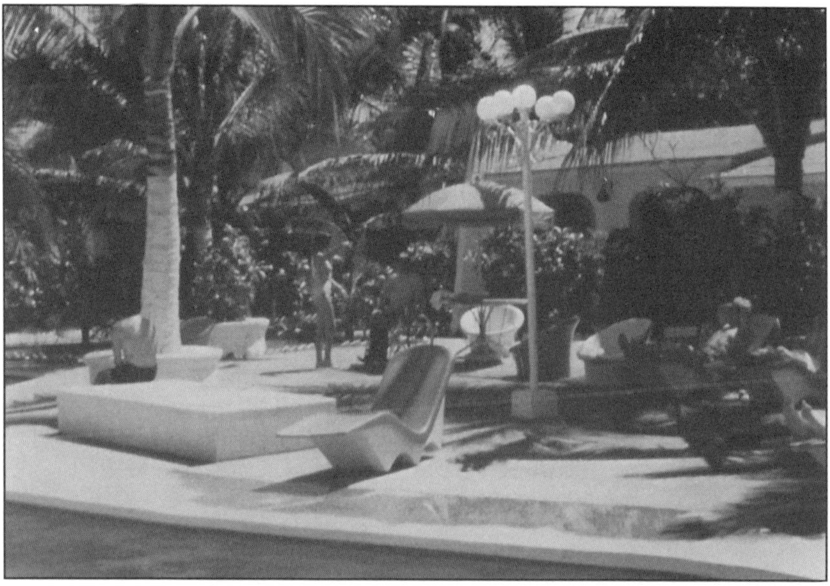

Rancho Luna, one of a number of places where one could rent a bungalow for a day, week, or longer—became a favorite spot in Manzanillo in the late-70s

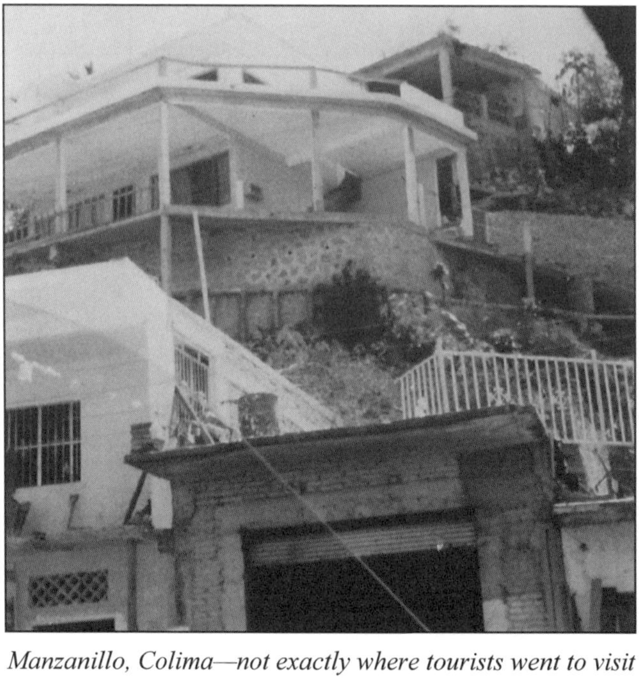

Manzanillo, Colima—not exactly where tourists went to visit

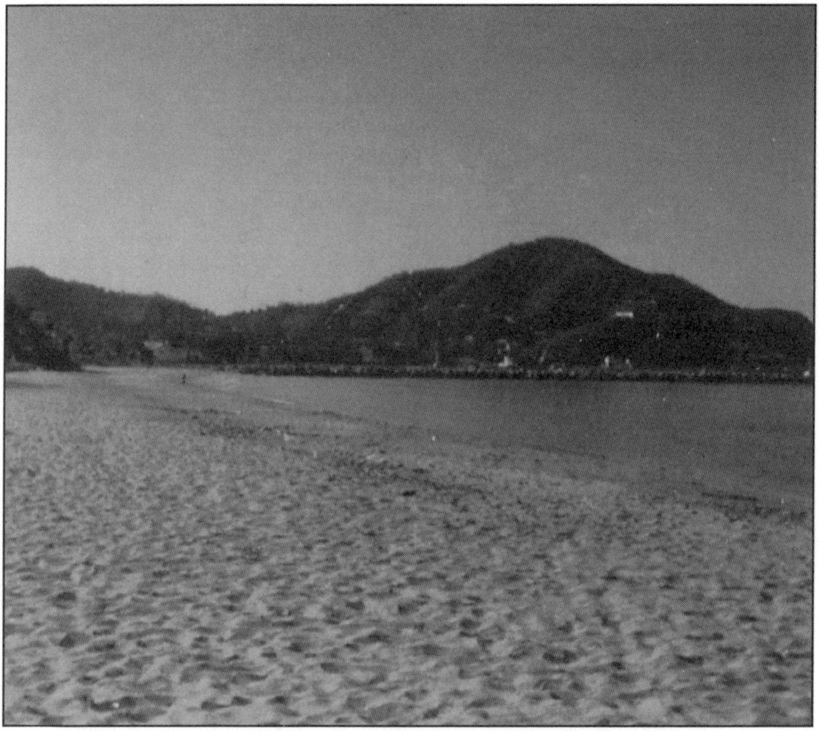

A quite afternoon along the Manzanillo shoreline

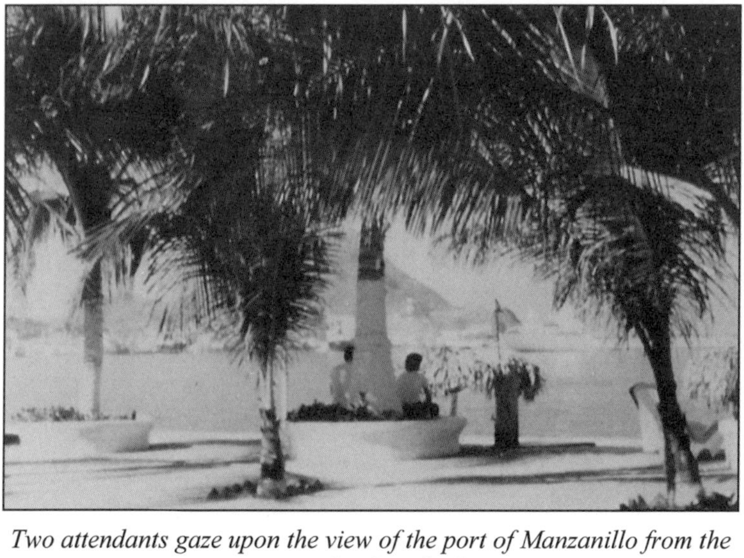

Two attendants gaze upon the view of the port of Manzanillo from the courtyard at Rancho Luna

Family Photos

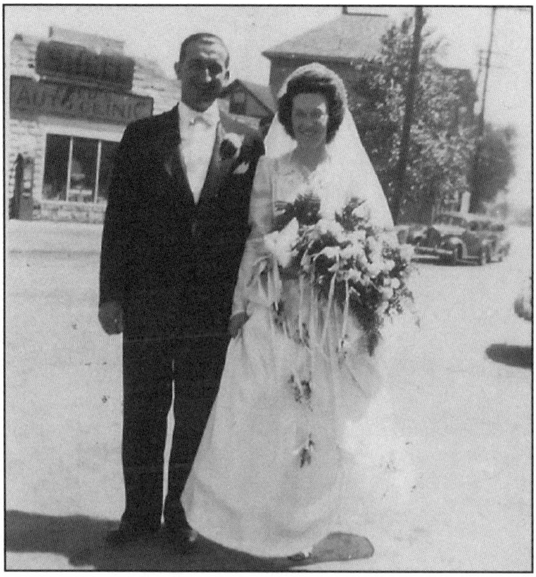

June 3, 1946 Wedding Day

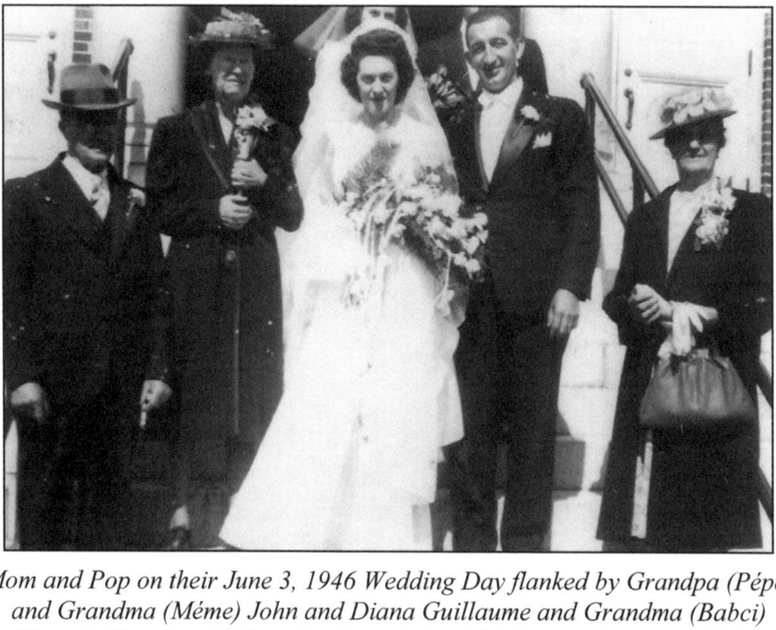

Mom and Pop on their June 3, 1946 Wedding Day flanked by Grandpa (Pépe) and Grandma (Méme) John and Diana Guillaume and Grandma (Babci) Victoria Tumidajski (Grandpa Joseph Tumidajski passed away in 1943)

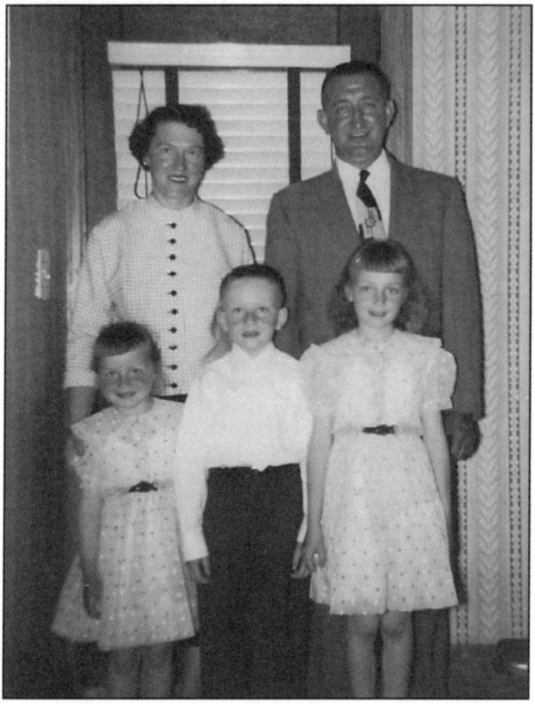

Mom and Pop with their first three "Baby Boomers" (left to right) Kathy, Jack, and Diane in our "Little House on Lauder," (early-50s)

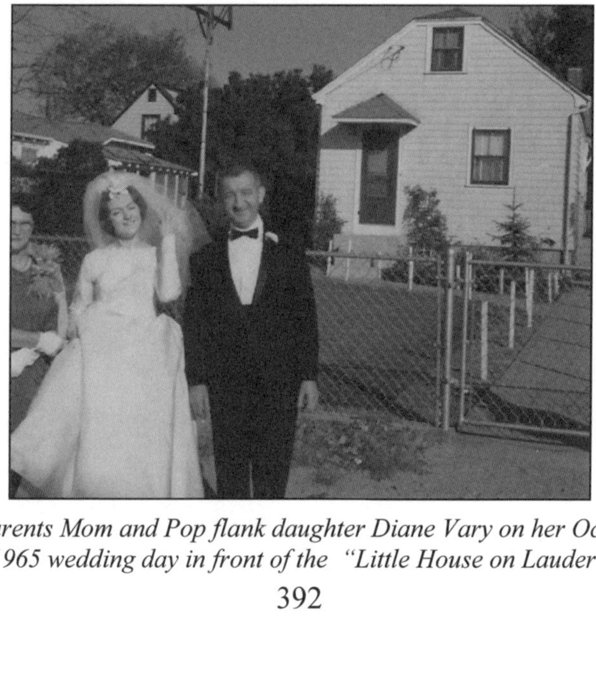

Proud parents Mom and Pop flank daughter Diane Vary on her October 30, 1965 wedding day in front of the "Little House on Lauder"

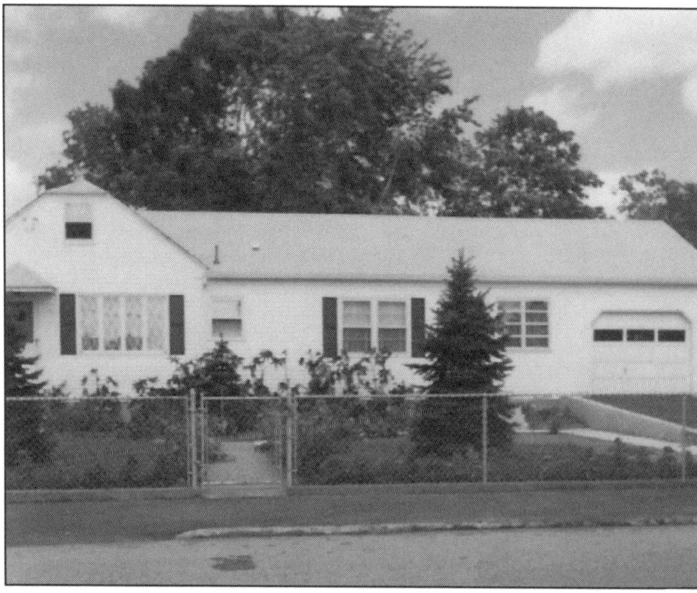

The 1970-71 extension to the former Aztec gold "Little House on Lauder" cost Pop his prized vegetable garden, but allowed Jack to leave the West Roxbury VA on March 26, 1971

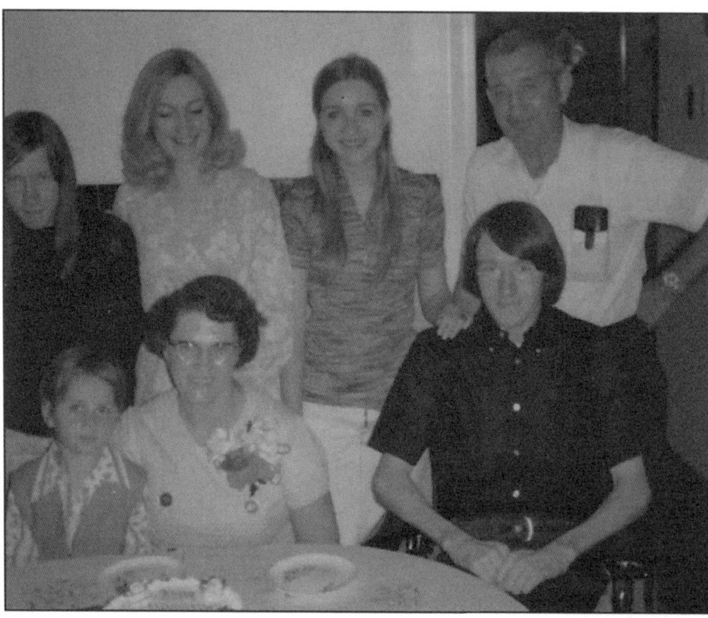

(Clockwise) Debbie, Diane, Kathy, Pop, Jack, Mom, and nephew David. Mom and Pop's 25th anniversary June 3, 1971(barely two months after going home)

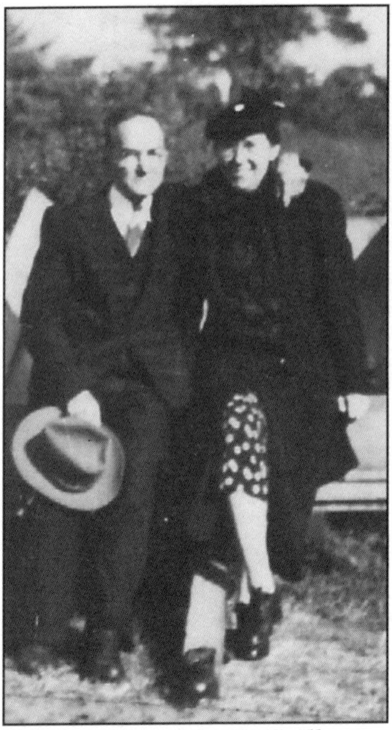

Mr. and Mrs. John B. Guillaume (Mom's father and mother)

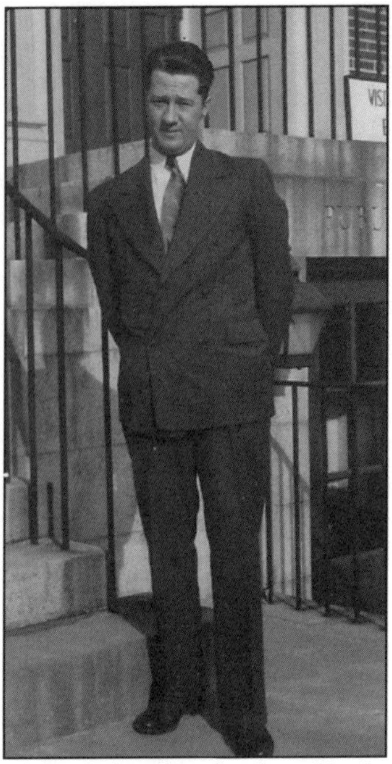

Mom's brother (and my Uncle "Buddy" passed away March 31, 1949 on the eve of my first birthday)

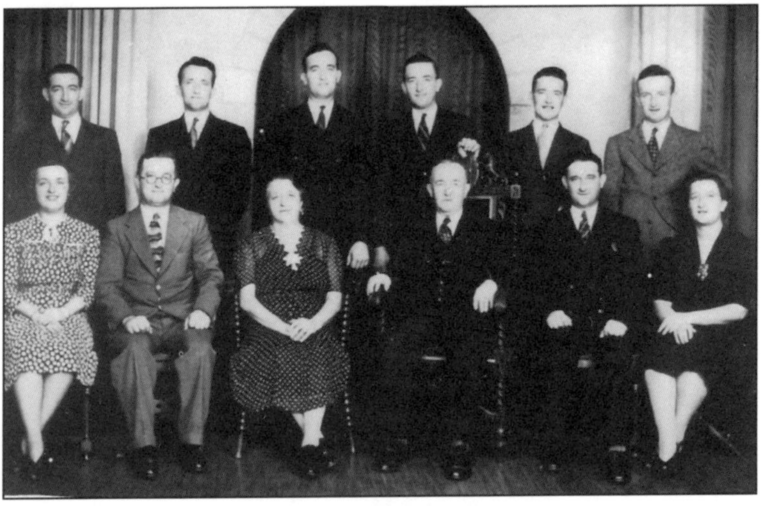

Tumidajski family front row (left to right) Catherine, Walter, (Mother) Victoria, (Father) Joseph, Ted, Tillie back row (left to right) future World War II Veterans John, Stanley, Joe, Adam, Matt, and Charlie (circa 1940)